Applied Nutrition for Young Pigs

To my wonderful wife, Efi,
for her unwavering support on this long-term project

Applied Nutrition for Young Pigs

Ioannis Mavromichalis, PhD

www.cabi.org

CABI is a trading name of CAB International

CABI Head Office
Nosworthy Way
Wallingford
Oxfordshire OX10 8DE
UK

Tel: +44 (0)1491 832111
Fax: +44 (0)1491 833508
E-mail: cabi@cabi.org
Website: www.cabi.org

CABI North American Office
875 Massachusetts Avenue
7th Floor
Cambridge, MA 02139
USA

Tel: +1 617 395 4056
Fax: +1 617 354 6875
E-mail: cabi-nao@cabi.org

A catalogue record for this book is available from the British Library, London, UK.

A catalogue record for this book is available from the Library of Congress, Washington DC.

ISBN-10: 1 84593 067 3
ISBN-13: 978 1 84593 067 7

Produced and typeset by Columns Design Ltd, Reading
Printed and bound in the UK by Cromwell Press, Trowbridge

Contents

About the Author

Dr Ioannis Mavromichalis holds graduate degrees on swine nutrition from Kansas State University (MSc) and University of Illinois (PhD), where his research and studies focused on the nutrition of the young pig, including work on sugars, amino acids, vitamins, minerals, sow's milk, feed processing and feeding management. He is the author of over 400 publications including journal papers, book chapters, reviews, articles, newsletters and columns in several technical magazines. He is the Director of Nutrition in a major international feed company, and his field work includes practical experiences from the USA and Europe.

Introduction

The nutrition of the piglet remains one of the most active scientific fields of swine nutrition throughout the world. As we continue to face problems associated with early weaning, we still fail to reap the full benefits of the tremendous potential for efficient early growth in young pigs. Despite its remarkable significance, the topic of young pig nutrition is barely covered in most swine nutrition textbooks and reference volumes, and even then only some aspects are presented.

This is a book about applied nutrition for young pigs with practical suggestions on how to achieve maximal performance at minimal cost under most commercial conditions. For this book, research reports, experience, current practices throughout the world, and financial considerations were taken into account to derive recommendations on how to best feed piglets under intensive commercial conditions.

To properly nourish the young pig, we need to understand its nutritional idiosyncrasies, its physiology and nutrient requirements, and how it responds to feedstuff and additive combinations. We must also realize that feeding goes beyond diet formulation, because diets must be properly processed, transported, stored, and finally presented for consumption before their potential is realized. Equally important is the development of a feeding program that includes the proper number of dietary changes and amount of each diet for each group of pigs to prevent under- or overfeeding. The ultimate goal is to economically produce a grower pig by exploring its potential with available means.

And a word of caution! Because the subject of piglet nutrition is such an active scientific field and full of debate, it is only logical to assume that there is more than one opinion on how to 'best' feed piglets. This book, therefore, can only offer but one such opinion. It has been said there is no wrong or right way to feed pigs, if certain nutritional principles are followed and profitability is ensured. But, what may be profitable to follow in one part of the world, may be illegal to implement in another. So, professional help from qualified nutritionists should be eagerly sought before implementing any of the contents of this book under your own circumstances.

Ioannis Mavromichalis, PhD
January 2006
Madrid,
Spain
ioannis@e-nutritionist.com
www.e-nutritionist.com

Acknowledgements

I would like to express my gratitude to my editors at CAB International, Rebecca Stubbs and Claire Parfitt, for their patience during the long time it took to complete this book. Many thanks also to the staff at CAB International for their work in transforming my manuscript into a publishable format. I would also like to thank all academic and commercial researchers and nutritionists who through their work have enriched the science and practice of piglet nutrition and, thus, enabled me to compile the present work.

Disclaimer

The contents of this book reflect the professional opinion of the author, without reference to his past or present employment and activities, based solely on information available in the public domain. The contents of this book do not necessarily reflect the philosophies or practices of any specific public or commercial institution, organization, company or person.

No representation or guarantee of performance or profitability is made here by the author or the publisher of this book. Neither the author nor the publisher make any warranty or accept any direct or indirect liability with respect to results from implementing the contents of this book. The author and the publisher strongly recommend seeking professional nutritional advice before using any of the information provided in this book.

1 Growth and Development

Introduction

Maximal growth is highly desirable in piglets. Not only is feed utilized more efficiently, but fast-growing piglets are also less susceptible to diseases, cope better with post-weaning trauma, adjust better to solid diets from sow's milk, and require less expensive diets to thrive. Maximal growth, however, is hardly ever realized in commercially raised piglets because insufficient quantities of milk limit neonatal growth, weaning at an early age depresses growth and appetite, gut capacity limits nutrient intake post-weaning, and many stress factors limit growth potential. Balanced nutrition is essential in achieving maximal growth in piglets under commercial conditions. Not only growth depends heavily on a constant supply of nutrients, but certain nutritional intervention strategies may also alleviate, at least partially, growth-depressing effects caused by modern husbandry practices.

Quantifying Growth

Growth may be defined as an increase in weight and size, associated with changes in shape, until pigs reach maturity. The most practical measurement of growth in young pigs is gain in body weight during a certain period of time, which is usually expressed as average weight gain per day (g/day). A less common way of expressing growth is weight gain as a percentage of initial body weight, which eliminates the effect of initial weight as heavier pigs tend to gain more weight than lighter pigs of the same age. With progressing age, weight gain rate (g/day) increases but percent weight gain rate (% of initial weight) decreases because growth rate develops slower than body weight. For example, a 6-kg pig that grows to 9 kg in 10 days has a growth rate of 300 g/day or 5% of its initial body weight. A 9-kg pig that grows to 12 kg in 8 days has a growth rate of 375 g/day, which is slightly above 4% of its initial body weight. Finally, it is always advisable to use distribution statistics, such as standard deviation, when describing growth to better assess variability in performance.

Weight gain rates are easily determined by weighing pigs at the initiation and end of a certain period. To monitor growth performance on a pen basis, at least 10% (but no less than 6%) of all pens randomly selected within each room should be weighed without excluding any pig. To monitor variation in growth, at least 10% of all pigs (but at least three pigs per pen) should be randomly selected, earmarked, scattered uniformly across all pens in each room and weighed at least twice. Weighing pigs at weekly intervals allows the determination of a uniform growth curve over time. This procedure should be performed in at least two different seasons each year.

There are three major ways to introduce errors in measuring weight gain in pigs: (i) human error in recording and calculations; (ii) unbalanced scales or use of scales that cannot counteract animal movement; and (iii) variability in the contents of the gastrointestinal tract (Lawrence and Fowler, 1997). Although it may be relatively easy to prevent or even correct human and mechanical problems, gastrointestinal fill is highly unpredictable and difficult to take into account in calculations. Gut fill is normally around 5% of body weight (Whittemore, 1998a). Equalizing gut fill among pigs is particularly important in trials when diets or management techniques may cause substantial differences in feed intake. To minimize variation in body weight due to gastrointestinal fill, the following have been suggested (Lawrence and Fowler, 1997):

1. Weigh pigs early in the morning.
2. Standardize weighing time in trials.
3. Withdraw feed for 6 to 12 h before weighing.
4. Weigh pigs on two consecutive days and average weights.

Modeling growth

It is now widely accepted that growth in pigs can be adequately described by mathematical models (Black, 1995; Whittemore, 1998a; Emmans and Kyriazakis, 1999), which predict potential growth under non-limiting conditions. Under most commercial conditions, however, actual growth patterns do not conform to ideal growth curves because several stress factors depress growth with variable effects. Nevertheless, this should not be considered as failure of mathematical models to adequately describe growth, but rather as an indication that pigs fail to grow to their potential due to restrictions imposed by husbandry practices. Indeed, when pigs are allowed to grow under non-limiting conditions they do exhibit patterns of growth that conform to theoretical assumptions (Emmans and Kyriazakis, 1997). Therefore, ideal growth curves can serve as guides in setting performance targets and in identifying factors that limit growth in pigs.

The Gompertz equation (Gompertz, 1825) provides the most widely recognized pattern of potential growth in pigs (Emmans and Kyriazakis, 1999), although other models are also equally applicable (Moughan and Verstegen, 1988; Black, 1995; van der Peet-Schwering *et al.*, 1999). The Gompertz equation:

$$\text{Weight gain (kg/day)} = \text{BW} \times B \times \log_e(\text{BW}/\text{BW}_m), \tag{1.1}$$

is based on the assumption that pigs will grow at maximal rates to reach maturity if nutrient supply or environmental conditions do not impose limits to this process. It describes growth as a function of mature body weight (BW_m) and a coefficient of growth (B) that determines maximal growth rates. The development of body weight (BW) over time as described by this model follows a sigmoid pattern (i.e. S-shaped) that is asymmetrical around its inflection point (Fig. 1.1a) and has three phases: (i) an accelerating phase that starts at conception; (ii) a linear portion; and (iii) a decelerating phase that overlaps with the late-finishing phase (80 to 120 kg) and reaches a plateau at maturity. The Gompertz curve for growth rate over time (Fig. 1.1b) is characterized by an accelerating and a decelerating phase, with its peak calculated by:

$$\text{Maximal weight gain (kg/day)} = (\text{BW}_m \times B)/e. \tag{1.2}$$

The exact values for parameters BW_m and B of the Gompertz equation depend on the genetic make-up of each specific line. For example, unimproved lines may be described by 220 kg (BW_m) and 0.009 (B), whereas modern lines may be described by 330 kg (BW_m) and 0.015 (B), as suggested by Whittemore (1998). The true growth potential of piglets, however, may not be accurately predicted by B values used for growing-finishing pigs because there have been incidents where B has been as high as 0.020 (Whittemore, 2001). Indeed, a B value of 0.015 would predict a growth rate of less than 600 g/day for fast-growing pigs (330 kg BW_m) between 3 and 30 kg body weight (Table 1.1).

In contrast, a B value of 0.020 would predict a growth rate of over 770 g/day for the same weight range, which is more realistic because it agrees well with actual maximal performance (Fig. 1.2) ever recorded in young pigs (Hodge, 1974; Harrell *et al.*, 1993). However, adoption of the same model for the entire grow-out period would predict a maximum growth rate of about 2400 g/day at 85 days of age, which is unrealistic.

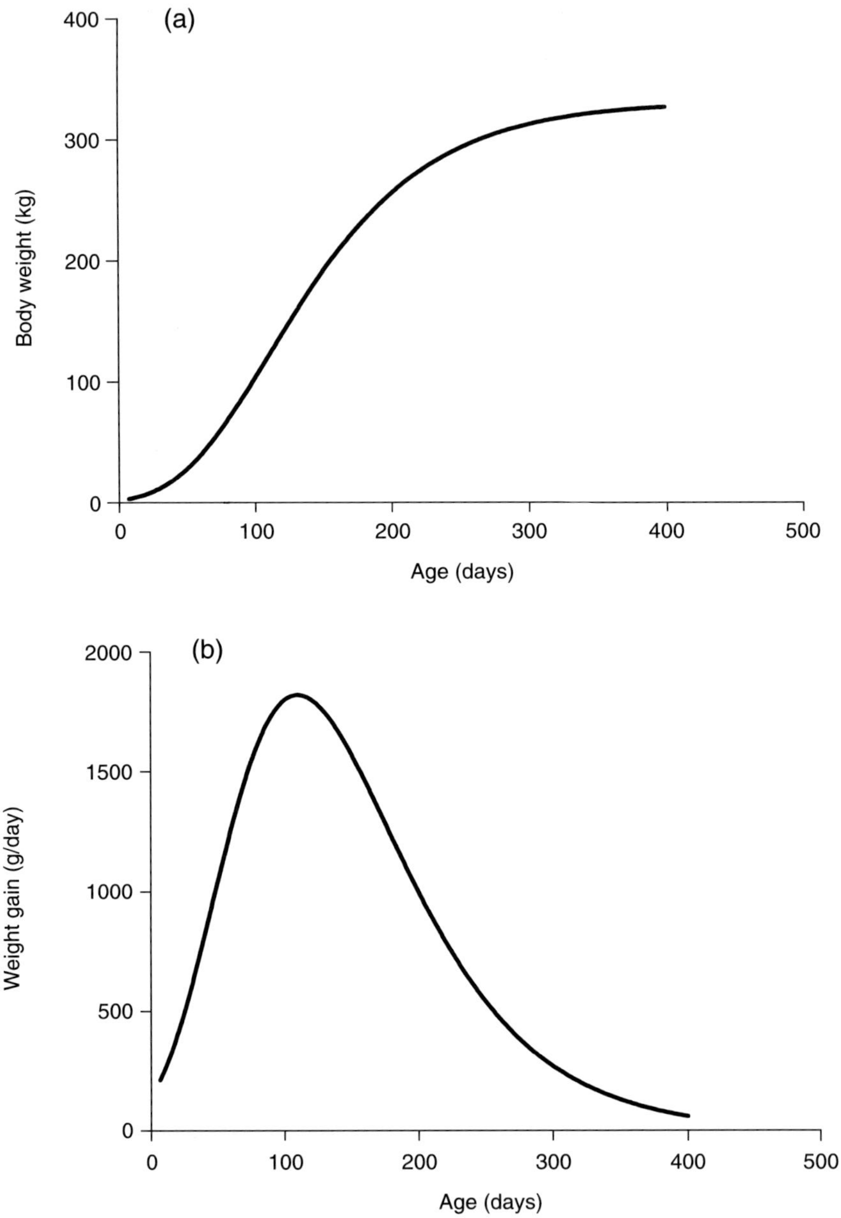

Fig. 1.1. Theoretical development of body weight (a) and weight gain rate (b) over time.

Table 1.1. Development of body weight (kg) in piglets as predicted by different Gompertz model parameters[a].

	Coefficient of growth (*B*)		
Age (days)	Currently (0.013)	Target (0.017)	Future (0.020)
14	4.5	5.0	5.4
21	6.5	7.9	9.2
28	9.0	12.0	14.5
35	12.3	17.2	21.7
42	16.3	23.9	30.8
49	21.1	32.0	41.8
56	26.8	41.4	54.6
63	33.3	52.0	69.0
70	46.2	73.2	96.2

[a] Calculations are based on Equations 1.1 and 1.2. It is assumed that mature body weight (BW_m) is equal to 330 kg and initial body weight at 7 days of age is equal to 3 kg.

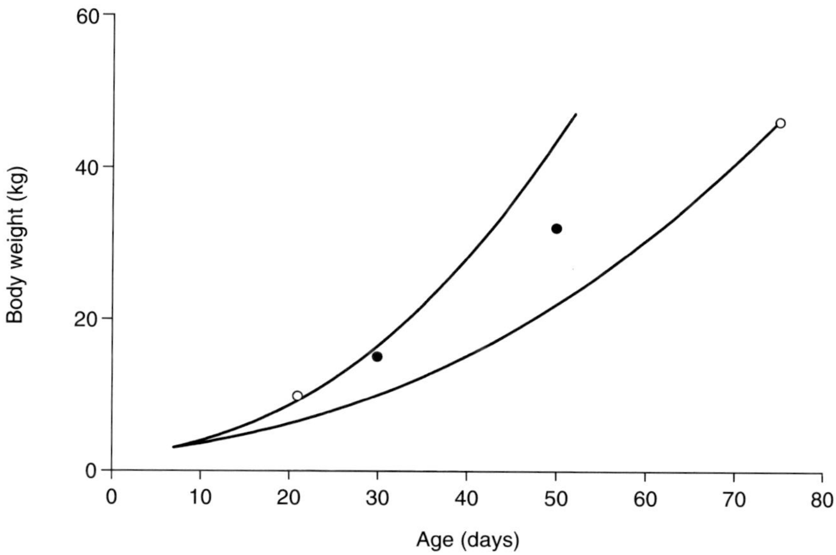

Fig. 1.2. Observed (●, Hodge, 1974; ○, Harrell *et al*., 1993) and theoretical estimates (——, Whittemore, 2001) of maximal body weight for age.

Growth Potential

That the growth potential of young pigs is severely compromised under commercial conditions has been repeatedly demonstrated in undisputable studies. It appears that the greatest loss in potential occurs during the suckling period, but it is highly debatable whether this reflects an amino acid imbalance or a supply deficit of sow's milk (Williams, 1995; Pluske and Dong, 1998; Mavromichalis *et al.*, 2001). Nevertheless, the biological potential for growth in neonatal pigs may be as much as 75% greater than that currently observed in sow-reared piglets (Boyd *et al.*, 1995). Field evidence supports such suggestions.

The fastest growth rates in young pigs were recorded by Hodge (1974), who offered reconstituted cow's milk (20% dry matter (DM)) for *ad libitum* consumption by pigs from 10 to 50 days of age. At 30 days of age, these pigs reached 25 kg with a growth rate of almost 600 g/day. Most modern pigs would still struggle to adapt to post-weaning diets at this age and, thus, they would not be expected to weigh more than 9 to 10 kg at best. In the same study, at 50 days of age pigs reached 32 kg with an astonishing growth rate of over 700 g/day. Again, most modern pigs receiving dry diets would not weigh more than 22 kg at the same age.

More recently, Harrell *et al.* (1993) indicated that 3-week-old pigs could easily reach 10 kg body weight under non-limiting conditions; in most commercial operations, pigs rarely exceed 7 kg at this age. In this study, a group of pigs was weaned at birth and fed a liquid milk replacer until weaning at 3 weeks of age. Another contemporary group of pigs was nursed by sows until weaning at the same age and all pigs received common dry diets after weaning (Fig. 1.3). The heaviest pigs from sow-nursed litters reached 6.4 kg at weaning and 37 kg at 75 days of age, whereas artificially reared pigs averaged 9.8 kg at weaning (+53%) and 46 kg at 75 days of age (+24%). These results indicate not only the great potential for growth in young pigs, but also the impediment in growth imposed by rearing pigs under sows.

In recent studies (Williams *et al.*, 1997a,b), individually penned pigs with high health status grew at about 700 g/day from 7 to 27 kg body weight at 40 days of age with conventional dry diets. In most commercial situations, 400–500 g/day would be satisfactory for the same weight range. Also, in the same studies, high-health pigs reared under segregated early-weaning schemes had growth rates approaching 550, 800, and 950 g/day at 10, 17, and 25 kg body weight, respectively.

In conclusion, the difference between potential and actual performance in piglets appears to be at least 50% up to 15 kg body weight, dropping to about 25% as pigs grow heavier. Clearly, there is a tremendous potential for growth that remains largely unexploited, especially during the suckling and post-weaning period.

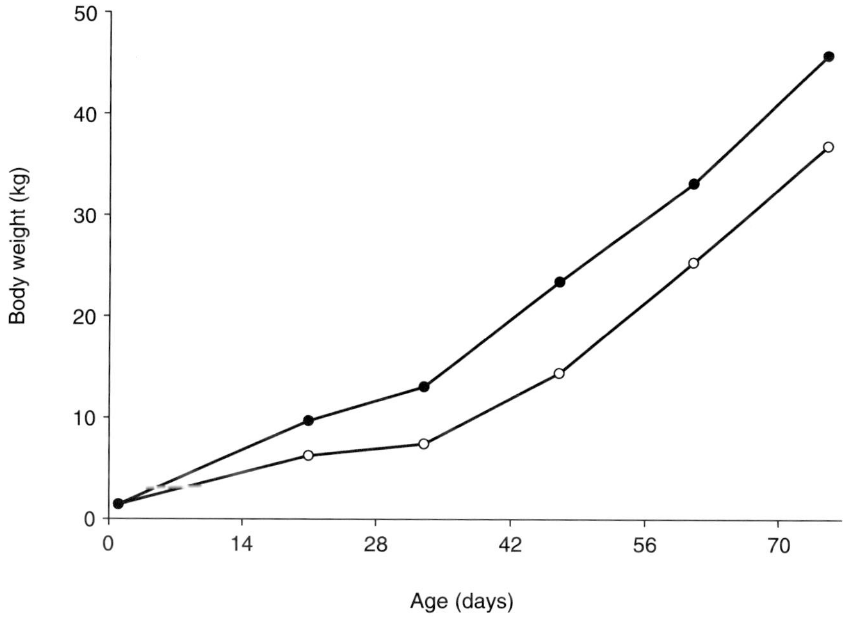

Fig. 1.3. Growth development in sow-reared (—○—) and artificially fed (with milk replacer, —●—) piglets. (From Harrell *et al.*, 1993.)

Factors Limiting Growth

Having established that young pigs fail to realize their full potential for growth, it is important to understand the factors that limit potential under commercial situations so that overall performance and profitability may be improved.

Nutrition

The major drive for growth in pigs is believed to be protein deposition to reach maturity, because fat deposition persists beyond maturity. Hence, protein growth over time can be described adequately by the Gompertz model (Emmans and Kyriazakis, 1999). Daily protein deposition (Fig. 1.4) responds linearly to increasing intake of a balanced diet until it plateaus at genetic potential (Bikker *et al.*, 1996a,b).

In the linear phase of daily protein deposition, lipid accretion is limited to amounts that are essential for normal tissue development. Lipid accretion accelerates rapidly, however, when nutrient supply exceeds requirements for maximal protein growth. In young pigs, protein deposition and growth respond linearly to feed intake (Fig. 1.5), because gut capacity almost invariably limits voluntary feed intake (Campbell *et al.*, 1975). Hence, nutrient-dense diets are usually beneficial for enhancing growth in young pigs.

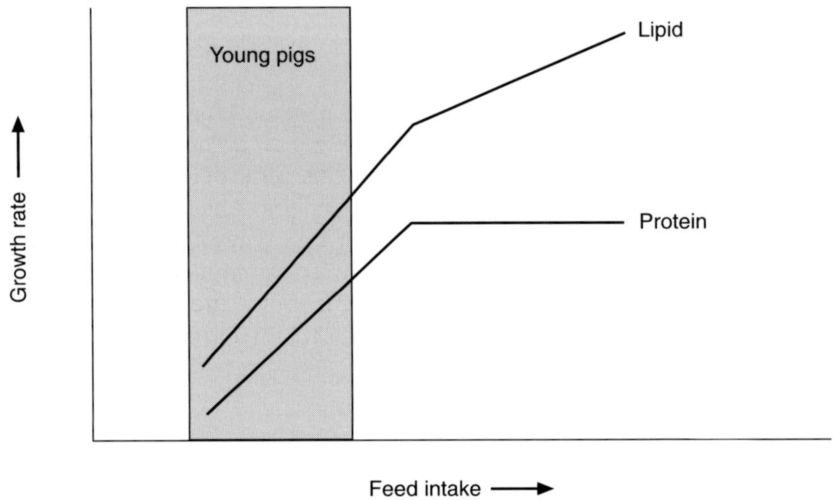

Fig. 1.4. Theoretical aspects of lipid and protein deposition in relation to feed intake and growth rate.

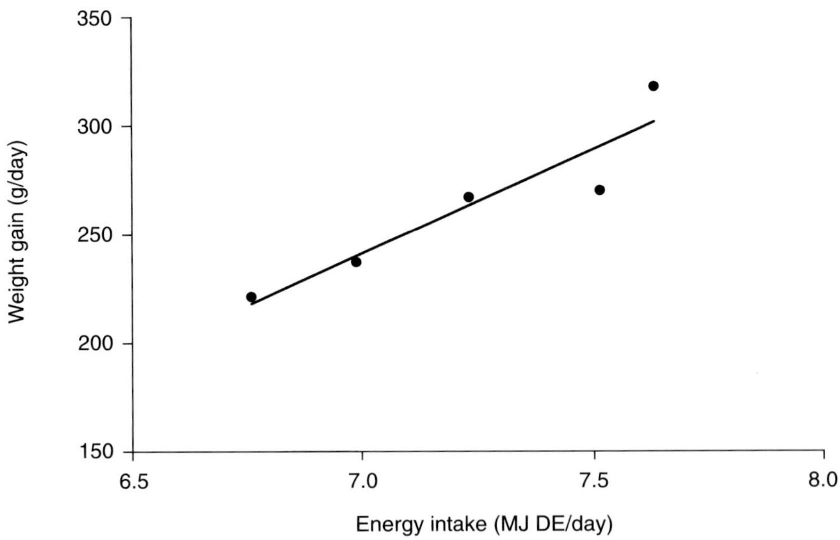

Fig. 1.5. Weight gain responds linearly to feed (digestible energy, DE) intake in piglets. (From Campbell *et al.*, 1975.)

Genetics

Genotype affects growth because it defines maximal potential for protein deposition rate under non-limiting conditions (Fig. 1.6). In general, young pigs with low potential for lean growth (i.e. older genotypes) eat more and are less efficient than modern pigs characterized by high potential for lean growth (Stahly *et al.*, 1994).

Among modern genotypes, the differences in early growth are small and difficult to detect under commercial conditions. This was demonstrated in a study by the National Pork Producers Council in the USA, in which several commercial pig genotypes were evaluated under comparable conditions (NPPC, 1995). Although there was a 15% difference between two extreme genotypes, all others exhibited comparable performance from 5 to 20 kg body weight (Fig. 1.7). This indicates that genetics plays a diminished role in defining growth in modern young pigs reared under limiting conditions and, therefore, genetic-specific dietary recommendations are not practical for commercial operations without actual growth and feed intake records.

Gender

Gender clearly affects protein deposition and feed intake (Campbell and Taverner, 1988). Boars are characterized by the highest protein deposition

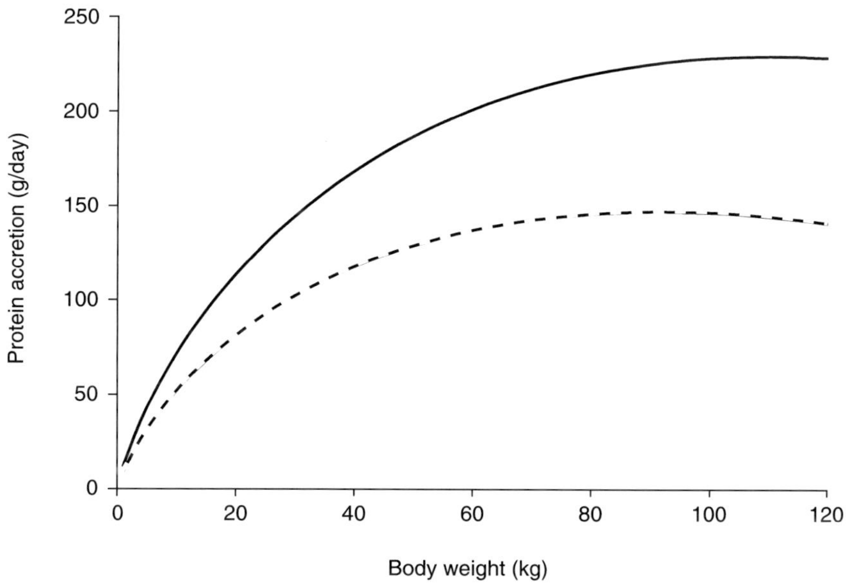

Fig. 1.6. Genotype greatly affects protein deposition rate (——, nucleus genotype; – – –, commercial medium-lean genotype).

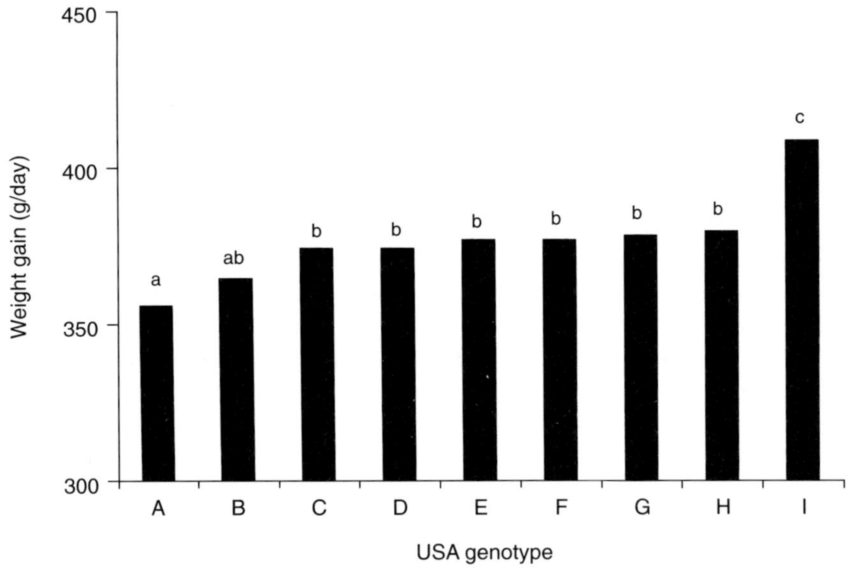

Fig. 1.7. Genotype has only a minimal effect on piglet performance (US test involving nine different genotypes; [a,b,c] bars with unlike superscript letters are different at $P < 0.05$). (From NPPC, 1995.)

rates and lowest feed intakes. Castrated males are the opposite, with gilts being intermediate. Although gender affects both the rate and composition of growth, this effect is more prevalent in pigs over 25 kg (Campbell *et al.*, 1988; Bikker *et al.*, 1996a,b). Below this threshold, modern pigs do not usually exhibit gender-associated growth patterns because their protein deposition rates do not usually reach genetic potential due to insufficient feed intake. Therefore, current dietary specifications and feeding programs for young pigs are not gender-specific, even though pigs may be kept occasionally in the nursery up to 35 kg body weight.

Immunological stress

Pigs are continuously exposed to a myriad of pathogenic and non-pathogenic microorganisms through their interaction with the environment and other animals. Even though disease may not always prevail, chronic exposure to antigens constantly triggers the immune system and causes subclinical disease symptoms that are difficult to identify and quantify (Johnson *et al.*, 2001). Antigenic stimuli activate the immune system and cause the release of pro-inflammatory cytokines that modulate the immune response and alter intermediate metabolism (Klasing, 1988). The most important cytokines are interleukin-1 (IL-1), interleukin 6 (IL-6), and tumor necrosis factor α (TNF-α) that are produced in massive amounts during immunological stress (Johnson, 1997). These cytokines, which are considered essential for the defense of the host, also reduce appetite, increase muscle protein degradation, reduce muscle protein synthesis, and divert nutrients to the synthesis of components of the immune system such as acute-phase proteins (Spurlock, 1997; Mitchell *et al.*, 2001). Thus, overall metabolism is switched from anabolism and growth in the healthy pig to catabolism and muscle loss in the challenged pig. The negative effects of chronic activation of the immune system (i.e. subclinical disease) in pigs reared under immunological stress are illustrated in Table 1.2.

From this study (Williams *et al.*, 1997a), it is apparent that pigs of high health status consume more feed, grow faster, and are more efficient than similar pigs under constant immunological stress. Healthy pigs also deposit more protein and proportionally less fat than challenged pigs. Increasing dietary lysine to counteract the negative effects of reduced feed intake in challenged pigs does not increase growth or protein deposition rates.

Management stress

In modern production systems, pigs are invariably exposed to several stress conditions caused by inappropriate management practices. Ambient temperature, humidity, and air velocity that define the micro-environment pigs experience daily seriously affect growth and feed intake in young pigs

Table 1.2. Health status affects performance and nutrient requirements in piglets[a]. (Adapted from Williams *et al.*, 1997a.)

Criterion	Health status	Dietary lysine concentration (%) 0.6	0.9	1.2	1.5	SEM	Effect
Weight gain (g/day)	High[c]	400	556	644	663	19	Lysine × health ($P < 0.01$)
	Low[d]	357	495	510	504		
Feed intake (g/day)	High	896	1025	1052	1002	36	Health ($P < 0.10$)
	Low	889	954	889	911		
Protein deposition (g/day)	High	48	78	101	111	3	Lysine × health ($P < 0.01$)
	Low	40	67	80	79		
Carcass lipid (%)[b]	High	22	16	12	11	1	Lysine ($P < 0.01$)
	Low	23	16	12	12		

SEM, standard error of the mean.
[a] Individually penned pigs (n = 5–6 pigs per treatment) from 6 to 27 kg body weight.
[b] Measured at 27 kg body weight.
[c] High, segregated early weaning accompanied with high levels of hygiene, medications, and vaccinations.
[d] Low, conventional weaning in a dirty continuous-flow nursery without medications and vaccinations.

(Noblet *et al.*, 2001). Inappropriate group size, stocking density, and pen design may increase stress and reduce growth or access to feed (Wolter *et al.*, 2000; Brumm and Gonyou, 2001). Frequent handling and mixing also increase stress and may depress performance in young pigs. In a recent study (Hyun *et al.*, 1998), pigs were exposed to multiple management stress factors that included high temperature, frequent mixing, and increased pen density. As expected, each stress factor applied alone depressed growth performance. However, stacking stress factors had an additive effect with each additional factor further depressing growth by about 10%.

The Trauma of Weaning

Wild boar piglets are weaned gradually between 8 and 20 weeks of age (Jensen and Recen, 1989). During this time, the contribution of nutrients from milk diminishes whilst that from solid feed increases, as foraging behavior develops via interaction and exploration. Interestingly, solid feed is first consumed, in small quantities, around 10 days of age. Therefore, weaning trauma as experienced by commercially reared piglets is not a natural event in the life of pigs and, hence, they are not prepared adequately to cope with it (Brooks and Tsourgiannis, 2003).

Under commercial conditions, weaning is an abrupt process that occurs between 2 and 5 weeks of age and involves separation from the sow, mixing with unfamiliar piglets, transferring to new facilities, and offering of dry diets in feeders and water via automatic drinkers. Therefore, a multiple number of concurrent stress factors disrupt the psychological, social, immunological, and nutritional status of early-weaned pigs. In response, piglets often fail to eat or drink and start losing weight for a period that may extent from a few hours to several days (Pluske *et al.*, 1995). It is now known that early-weaned pigs do not eat because of radical changes in feeding behavior, and diet composition and form. Before weaning, the sow was responsible for feeding the litter at frequent intervals and, thus, communal liquid feeding was the norm. After weaning, piglets are faced not only with a strange diet with different form and composition, but also with the decision of when and how much to eat. Moreover, weaned pigs are also required to distinguish thirst from hunger and to realize that these needs must be satisfied via separate media, as water is no longer provided in conjunction with solid matter as in sow's milk. In addition, passive immunity offered via colostrum and milk antibodies declines rapidly at about 3 weeks of age, whereas only then does active immunity start to slowly develop.

Depressed feed intake post-weaning is also associated with atrophy of the gastrointestinal tract and increased vulnerability to inflammation (Pluske *et al.*, 1996a,b). Allergenic reactions to antigens from legumes that may lead to nutritional diarrhea are also more prevalent in pigs with reduced appetites (McCracken *et al.*, 1995, 1999). Moreover, malnourished pigs usually take longer to recover from pathogenic diarrhea (Zijlstra *et al.*, 1997). A sudden increase in feed intake, usually observed between the second and fifth day post-weaning, occurs when piglets associate dry diets with nourishment. However, a sudden overload of the digestive tract is invariably followed by diarrhea because most of the feed passes undigested to the large intestine, where it serves as substrate for microbial proliferation.

Weaning trauma is more likely to affect pigs weaned at less than 3 weeks of age, because older pigs usually consume some creep feed and, thus, they have a more mature digestive system at weaning. Growth depression in early-weaned pigs was more common and pronounced until the early 1990s, after which time advances in feeding, housing, and managing greatly diminished but did not eliminate this problem. The recent abandonment of several growth-promoting agents (e.g. animal plasma, antimicrobial agents, zinc oxide, copper sulfate) in several parts of the world has intensified this problem and caused a surge of new research to address it.

Composition of Growth

Pigs are born with characteristically low body fat depots of less than 2%, compared to a physiological minimum of about 5% (Mitchell *et al.*, 2001). Yet, consumption of sow's milk increases lipid reserves rapidly to more than 15% at 3 to 4 weeks of age (de Lange *et al.*, 2001). It appears that lipid deposition is more important compared to protein growth for neonatal pigs as a mechanism of increasing their chances of survival in the wild. Therefore, the lipid to protein deposition ratio is equal to or even larger than one. Later in life, this ratio ranges between 0.5 and 1.0, depending on sex and genotype (Whittemore, 1998a), but for commercially reared piglets a ratio of 1:1 is deemed satisfactory for the nursery period (weaning to about 25 kg body weight).

The chemical composition of body weight (empty) in piglets is presented in Table 1.3. At about 3 to 4 weeks of age (most common weaning time), protein and lipid concentration are about the same at around 15%. Post-weaning growth depression, however, often draws from body lipid reserves to sustain life and to promote a minimum amount of protein growth. This depends on feed intake, protein (amino acid) concentration and digestibility in feed, and, of course, environmental temperature (Le Dividich and Seve, 2001).

It has been suggested that during post-weaning stasis, piglets actually deposit water in exchange for lipids catabolized to sustain life (Whittemore *et al.*, 1978). Indeed, Whittemore *et al.* (1981) demonstrated that, at weaning, pigs exhibiting zero weight gain rate actually mobilized 56 g lipids and gained 53 g water per day. Lipid deposition became positive only when weight gain exceeded 193 g/day.

Table 1.3. Chemical composition (%) of empty body weight in piglets. (Adapted from de Lange *et al.*, 2001.)

Component	Birth	7 kg	25 kg
Water	77	66	69
Protein	18	16	16
Lipid	2	15	12
Ash	3	3	3

Carryover Effects of Early Growth

High growth rate during early life assures survival and wellbeing, in that well-fed pigs are less susceptible to disease and cope better with environmental challenges. However, there is further merit in early growth, because pigs that grow fast in early life have accelerating growth rates throughout finishing.

Birth weight greatly affects growth rate and survivability. Weaning weight is positively related ($r = 0.56$) to birth weight; it increases by about 0.7 kg for every 0.1 kg increase in birth weight (Le Dividich, 1999). Heavier piglets initiate and sustain greater milk flow throughout the lactation period, and therefore they consume more milk than their lighter littermates (van der Steen and de Groot, 1992). Provision of creep in late-weaning schemes (over 21 days of age) diminishes the effect of birth weight on weaning weight ($r = 0.37$), as indicated by Sprent *et al.* (2001a). Caugant and Gueblez (1993) reported that among light piglets (less than 1 kg at birth) more than 50% died before weaning, and that heavy piglets (above 1.9 kg) grew about 4% faster, with 8% better feed efficiency, until market age compared to lighter littermates (below 1.2 kg).

Weaning weight, also, has a tremendous effect on post-weaning performance, although this effect diminishes with increasing age (Slade and Miller, 1999). Research at Ohio State University (Mahan and Lepine, 1991; Mahan, 1993; Mahan *et al.*, 1998) clearly demonstrated (Table 1.4) that heavy weaned pigs grow faster than lighter pigs of the same age, not only during the nursery phase (about +10%) but also during the growing-finishing phase (about +5%). This improvement in growth rate is derived mainly from increased feed intake throughout the grow-out period and partially from improved efficiency of feed utilization during the growing-finishing stage. Although prolonged provision of higher-quality diets to lighter pigs may reduce variation in weight gain within a group, heavy weaned pigs still reach market weight sooner than their lighter littermates. It is estimated that for every 1 kg extra weight at weaning, pigs reach market weight 3–5 days sooner. These experimental observations have recently been verified under commercial conditions (Sprent *et al.*, 2001b). That heavy pigs cope better with post-weaning trauma is attributed to increased

Table 1.4. The effects of weaning weight on subsequent growth performance. (Adapted from Mahan *et al.*, 1998.)

Item	Light pigs	Heavy pigs	Significance[a]
Weaning weight (kg)	5.5	7.5	
Weaning age (days)	23	24	
Nursery (5 weeks)			
Weight gain (g/day)	400	445	S
Feed intake (g/day)	686	774	S
Feed efficiency (g/kg)	583	575	S
Overall (weaning to market)			
Weight gain (g/day)	699	734	S
Feed intake (g/day)	2079	2133	S
Feed efficiency (g/kg)	336	345	S
Market weight (kg)	106	107	NS
Days to 105 kg	165	157	S

[a] S, means within a row are significantly different ($P < 0.05$); NS, means within a row are not different.

body fat reserves (Sloat *et al.*, 1985) and a more mature digestive system (Cranwell *et al.*, 1997).

Performance during the first week post-weaning is highly variable, yet independent of weaning weight (Pluske and Williams, 1991; Miller *et al.*, 1999). Weight gain during this period, however, is highly associated with subsequent performance during the entire nursery and even growing-finishing period. Research conducted at Kansas State University (Tokach *et al.*, 1992) demonstrated that pigs growing at least 230 g/day during the first week post-weaning reached market weight (105 kg) 10 days sooner than pigs barely maintaining their weaning weight (Fig. 1.8a). Put another way, fast-growing piglets were about 5 kg heavier at 56 days post-weaning and 8 kg heavier at market age (156 days) than littermates that did not gain weight during the first week post-weaning (Fig. 1.8b). These observations were later confirmed by other researchers (Dunshea *et al.*, 1999; Miller *et al.*, 1999). Pigs that do not grow during the first week post-weaning usually suffer from digestive upsets caused by abnormal feed intake patterns and, thus, take longer to recover and finish than pigs that grow normally during the same period.

Compensatory Growth

It is now well understood that pigs receiving inadequate amounts of feed (energy deprivation) or imbalanced diets (nutrient deprivation) grow slower than well-fed pigs. Malnourishment also affects composition of weight gain; energy deprivation decreases lipid deposition, whereas protein deprivation

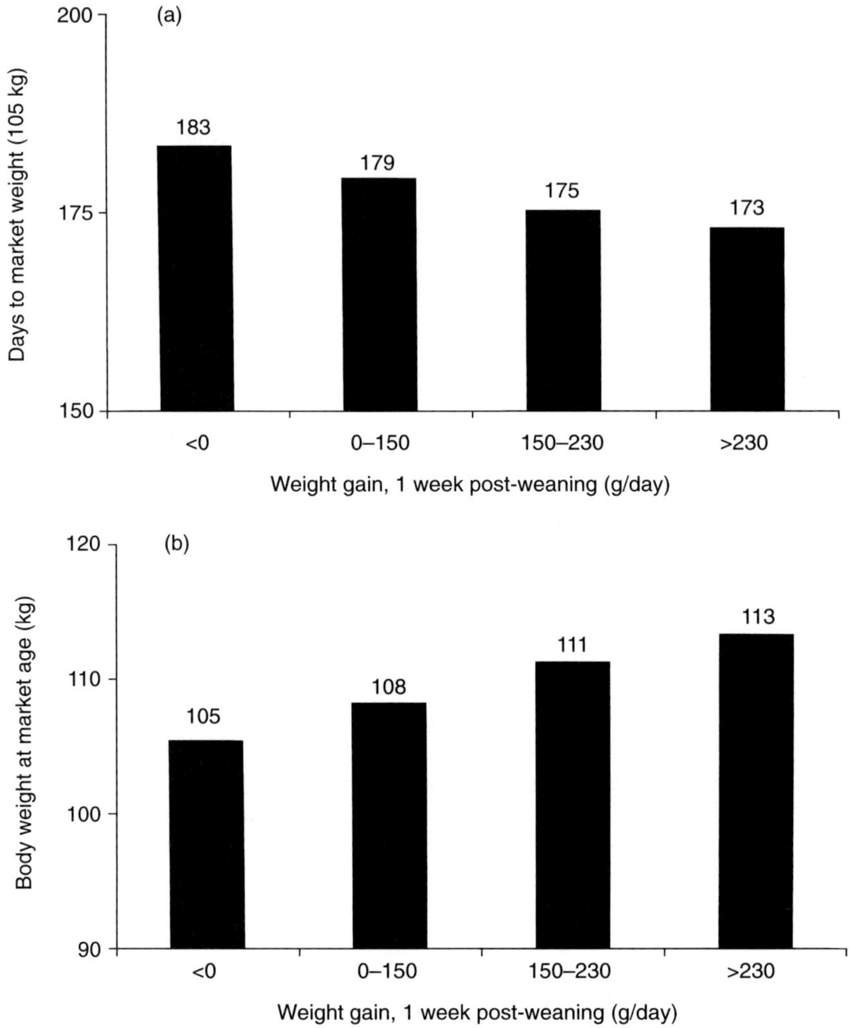

Fig. 1.8. The significance of early growth post-weaning on overall performance in pigs.

decreases protein deposition. Prolonged malnourishment causes severe deviations from normal body composition. Thus, energy- or feed-deprived pigs will become leaner, albeit lighter, than pigs fed *ad libitum*. In contrast, protein-deprived pigs will be fatter, and perhaps heavier if fed *ad libitum*, than normal pigs (Whittemore, 1998a). Given enough time, stunned pigs may attain mature weight and body composition after rehabilitation.

Because pigs grow to attain certain body weight and composition, any deviations from this target must be corrected. Thus, rate and composition of gain during rehabilitation depend on the magnitude of malnourishment and its effects on body composition. Energy malnourishment, therefore, increases fat deposition, whereas protein malnourishment increases protein deposition, during rehabilitation. This is compensatory growth, a phenomenon documented in many species. Although there is no doubt today that compensatory growth occurs in severely malnourished pigs, considerable debate still exists regarding its practical importance during the limited lifespan of commercial pigs and its effects on lean-tissue growth.

Young pigs invariably experience malnourishment during the post-weaning period via reduced feed intake or provision of low-quality diets. Reduced feed intake may be a voluntary reaction to weaning stress, or imposed as a measure against diarrhea. Low-quality diets limit nutrient intake and (or) absorption because they may have anti-nutritional factors and toxins, severe nutritional imbalances, or reduced ingredient complexity and, thus, nutrient digestibility. Diets of reduced ingredient complexity may be less digestible than complex diets, but they appeal to least-cost production schemes because they are relatively inexpensive. The question, therefore, is whether pigs that receive suboptimal nutrition during the post-weaning period can exhibit sufficient compensatory growth to reach the weight and body composition of well-fed pigs of similar age.

The answer to this dilemma came from research at the Scottish Agricultural College, Edinburgh (Stamataris *et al*., 1991), in which pigs were given either *ad libitum* access to feed or were restricted to 55% *ad libitum* intake from 6 to 12 kg body weight. As expected (Table 1.5), restricted-fed pigs grew slower (–60%) and were less efficient (–29%) than *ad libitum*-fed pigs. Thus, they took longer (+158%) and consumed more feed (+38%) to reach 12 kg body weight, at which stage they had less gut fill, increased body protein to lipid ratio, and lighter digestive tract. During the rehabilitation period (12 to 24 kg body weight), when all pigs had *ad libitum* access to feed, malnourished pigs grew faster (+29%) and were more efficient (+13%) than control pigs, but without fully recovering body composition. Malnourished pigs also had more gut fill, but comparable internal organ weights, at 24 kg. Interestingly, compensatory growth was evident only during the first week of the rehabilitation period. Even then, it was directed toward body fat and organs. There was no protein compensatory growth.

Protein deprivation is less common in young pigs reared under commercial conditions. However, husbandry practices that dilute complete diets with barley or oats to prevent or control diarrhea induce a period of artificial protein malnourishment. Prolonged protein malnutrition reduces weight gain, feed efficiency, protein deposition, and increases time to reach market weight. Lipid deposition rate and relative body lipid content, however, both increase with protein deprivation. During rehabilitation, pigs correct their body protein and lipid concentrations by adjusting protein and lipid deposition rates. Thus, growth rate and feed efficiency are improved during the initial phase of rehabilitation. The magnitude of compensatory growth is analogous to the state of the pig at the end of the malnourishment period and the protein concentration of the rehabilitation feed (Kyriazakis *et al*., 1991).

Table 1.5. Feed deprivation and compensatory growth in weaned pigs. (Adapted from Stamataris *et al.*, 1991.)

Item	*Ad libitum*-fed pigs	Restricted-fed pigs	Significance[a]
Restriction period (6–12 kg)			
Days taken	13	32	S
Weight gain (g/day)	480	190	S
Feed intake (g/day)	543	300	S
Feed efficiency (g/kg)	888	633	S
Gut fill (kg)	1.19	0.56	S
Gastrointestinal tract (kg)	0.95	0.73	S
Liver (kg)	0.51	0.35	S
Body lipid (%)	9.30	5.92	S
Body protein (%)	15.04	16.61	S
Rehabilitation period (12–24 kg)			
Days taken	18	13	S
Weight gain (g/day)	686	972	S
Feed intake (g/day)	964	1178	S
Feed efficiency (g/kg)	712	825	S
Gut fill (kg)	1.74	2.15	S
Gastrointestinal tract (kg)	1.44	1.43	NS
Liver (kg)	1.02	1.07	NS
Lipid deposition (g/day)	92	139	S
Protein deposition (g/day)	116	126	NS
Internal organ deposition (g/day)	75	148	S
Skin deposition (g/day)	117	164	S
Body lipid (%)	11.87	10.96	NS
Body protein (%)	16.43	15.82	S

[a] S, means within a row are significantly different ($P < 0.05$); NS, means within a row are not different.

In conclusion, there is no doubt that compensatory growth is a natural process that aims to correct body composition after a period of malnourishment. However, compensatory growth is directed toward organs and fat tissues unless a severe depletion of muscle protein is experienced by protein malnutrition, and this applies even to growing-finishing pigs (Crister *et al.*, 1995; Bikker *et al.*, 1996a,b). Under commercial conditions, young pigs are most likely to be more energy- than protein-deficient.

Runt Piglets

Piglets that weigh less than half of their littermates are frequently classified as runts (Mitchell *et al.*, 2001). There are two causes that produce runt piglets:

(i) insufficient prenatal development due to decreased nutrient supply to the fetus (Warshaw, 1990); and (ii) insufficient postnatal nutrition due to inadequate ingestion of nutrients from sow's milk or solid feed. Runt piglets are more common in sows that receive a protein-deficient diet throughout gestation (Schoknecht *et al.*, 1993). In addition, a large number of piglets (2 to 5%) that are otherwise normal may fail to thrive after weaning at an early age and be classified as runts or fallbacks. Mortality among runt piglets is extremely high (up to 75%) and, thus, special management and nutrition practices are required for these pigs to survive and grow.

Piglets born weighing less than one-third of their littermates are characterized by relatively smaller organ size compared to well-developed littermates. For example (Widdowson, 1971), in newborn runt piglets (625 g) the relative weight of quadriceps muscles (31%), small intestine (25%), liver (27%), and stomach (46%) was significantly lower than that in large littermate piglets (1606 g). Thus, runt piglets contain relatively less protein and DNA, lower protein to DNA ratio, and smaller and fewer muscle fibers compared to normal piglets (Mitchell *et al.*, 2001). Runt piglets that survive grow more slowly (–10%) and take longer to reach market weight with a carcass that eventually is as lean (Hegarty and Allen, 1978) or sometimes even fatter (Powell and Aberle, 1980) than that from normal piglets. During the first two postnatal weeks, runt pigs exhibit compensatory growth, in terms of improved feed efficiency, but they still fail to achieve average weaning weight (Ritacco *et al.*, 1997).

Management of runt piglets is crucial for their survival (England, 1974). Runt piglets that are fostered together to good-milking sows have increased chances of survival and wellbeing compared to runt piglets left to compete with well-developed littermates. Enhanced nutritional management (e.g. oral supplements, liquid milk replacers, milk-based creep diets, prolonged lactation period) may further increase the chances of recovery. Alternatively, some large operations may set a minimum birth weight below which piglets are euthanized. Piglets that become runts after weaning usually recover faster than piglets stunted at birth. Weaning weight and age cannot predict the chances of a normal piglet to develop runting. Weaned runt piglets are characterized by sunken abdomens, dehydration, lethargy, and severe weight loss because they suffer the most from post-weaning trauma. Penning all runt piglets together and offering them a liquid milk replacer diet is the most practical way to manage runt piglets after weaning (Fig. 1.9). An increased allowance of the first solid diet post-weaning, gruel feeding and (or) mat-feeding are also recommended for increased nutrient uptake and faster recovery. Medication treatments may also be required to prevent onset of farm-specific diseases in the entire population due to the high susceptibility of runt pigs to endemic diseases. Again, some larger operations that are short on labor prefer not to handle piglets that fail to thrive after a specific period post-weaning.

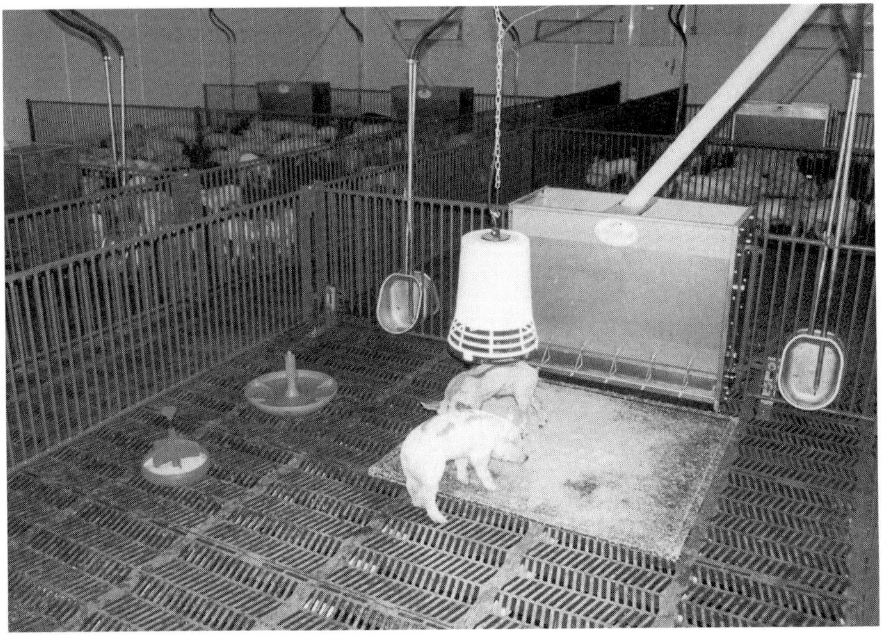

Fig. 1.9. Piglets too small for their age are best cared for in a special 'hospital' pen.

Variation in Body Weight

Variability in weight is part of the natural selection process, and some degree of variability should be acceptable even under commercial conditions. Variability is usually measured by the standard deviation (SD) or the coefficient of variation (CV), which is calculated as standard deviation divided by the mean. The standard deviation increases with age because the absolute difference between light and heavy pigs increases as pigs grow. The coefficient of variation, however, is more stable because it is independent of pig weight, and, thus, it is a more reliable measure of variability throughout the production cycle. A reasonable target for coefficient of variation of body weight would be about 15% for all phases of production (de Grau *et al.*, 2001).

Excess variability in pig weight is undesirable at every phase of production because it intensifies management inputs and compromises pig flow (Fig. 1.10). Variability increases pig sorting and mixing, and time to reach market weight, whereas pigs light for their age may be sold with a discount at slaughter. Because variation increases the number of pigs with nutrient requirements different from those of the average pig, feeding programs with increased nutrient density are required to properly nourish the majority of the population (Edwards, 1999).

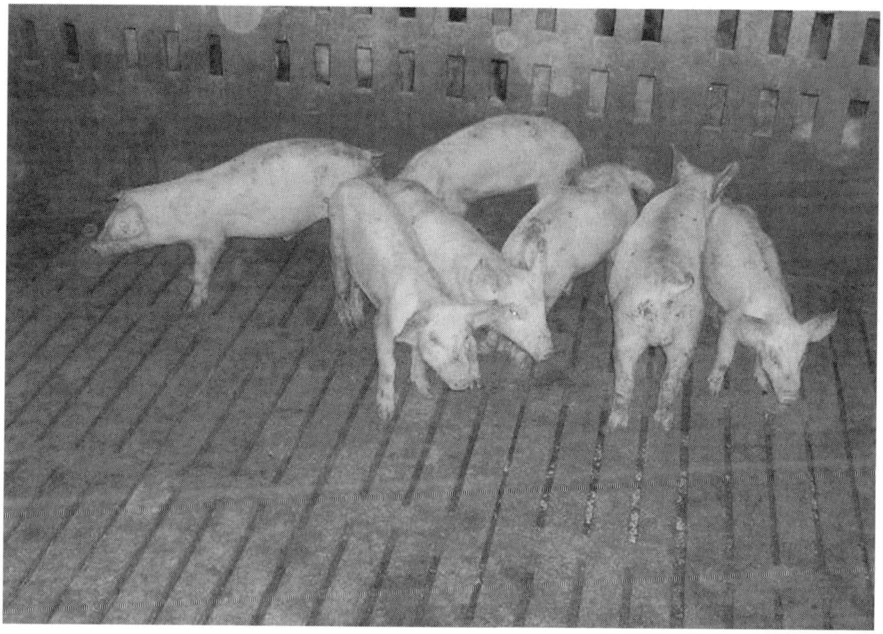

Fig. 1.10. Nutritional, management, facility, and health factors all may contribute to uneven growth within a group.

Variability is affected by genotype, nutrition, disease status, use of in-feed antimicrobial agents, age spread within groups, management, facilities, environmental conditions, weight at entry, and season (Payne *et al.*, 1999). Measures that increase growth rate usually reduce variability also. Variability in nursery pigs is further increased when pigs fail to thrive immediately after weaning. A Canadian study, which involved nine commercial farms, indicated that the difference in body weight between the lightest 25% and heaviest 25% of pigs was about 2, 6, and 26 kg at weaning (14 to 28 days of age), 7, and 20 weeks of age, respectively (de Grau *et al.*, 2001). These authors also indicated that under commercial conditions weight variation was affected mostly by the presence of endemic diseases. For example, farms with all-in all-out pig flow had 12% CV at weaning and 19% CV at 7 weeks of age, whereas farms with continuous pig flow had 26% CV from weaning to 7 weeks of age.

Body weight distribution at weaning follows the pattern of normal distribution (Toplis *et al.*, 2001) as indicated in Fig. 1.11. Increased variability flattens and spreads the bell-shaped curve, whereas reduced variability raises and narrows the curve around the average. Variability at weaning is usually taken into account in designing feeding programs with the goal of reducing the difference between heavy and light pigs. Although weaning weight is very variable, field evidence indicates that standard deviation is less variable and about 1 kg for pigs weaned between 2 and 4 weeks of age. The average weaning weight and its standard deviation are used to calculate the number of pigs expected to be in different weight groups. For example, with an average weaning weight of 6 kg and SD of 1 kg, 68% of the pigs are expected to be between 5 and 6 kg (BW±1SD), 16% less than 5 kg, and 16% above 7 kg (BW±2SD). This information is used to estimate feed allowances for each group to avoid overfeeding of expensive diets to heavy pigs and allow light pigs to catch up (see Chapter 4 for more details).

Commercial Growth Targets

Despite growth's variable nature, it is necessary to establish targets to monitor performance and evaluate nutrition and management practices. Adopting targets within reach is the first step to success. Although performance in some operations already exceeds targets commonly used in the industry, such as these described here, there is always room for improvement as the full genetic potential of the young pig is still untapped.

Birth weight

Average birth weight is reduced as litter size increases. Energy and protein intake during pregnancy may affect birth weight, but only in severely

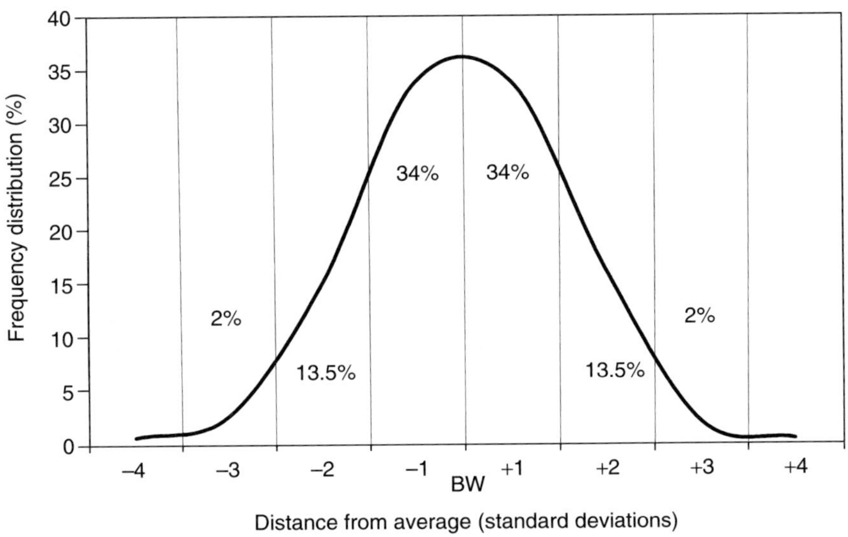

Fig. 1.11. Normal distribution pattern of body weight (BW) at weaning with a standard deviation of 1 kg.

depleted sows (Pluske *et al.*, 1995). Gilts are more sensitive than sows to malnutrition during pregnancy, and, thus, they tend to produce lighter pigs. Addition of fat (up to 10%) or increasing feed allowance (up to 2 kg extra) during late pregnancy may improve birth weight and reduce mortality of light piglets in farms with below-average performance (Pettigrew, 1981; Aherne and Kirkwood, 1985; Whittemore, 1998b).

Commercial records indicate that average birth weight is about 1.4 kg with SD of about 0.15 kg. Indeed, 12,000 farms under a commercial record-management system in the USA reported 1.45 kg average birth weight with ten piglets per litter. Likewise, a British record-keeping system reported an average birth weight of 1.35 kg with 12 pigs per litter. Pigs weighing below 1 kg at birth usually fail to thrive, whereas those below 0.8 kg frequently die within the first few days after birth, and these pigs should be candidates for artificial rearing (English, 1974) or be euthanized upon birth.

Pre-weaning growth

Typical growth rates of suckling pigs range from 200 g/day for conventional genotypes to 300 g/day for modern genotypes, with two patterns of growth usually observed during a 4-week lactation period (King *et al.*, 1999). The early period, which is associated with accelerating but highly variable growth rate (Thompson and Fraser, 1988), corresponds roughly with the first week of life. During this period, growth rates increase gradually from about 50 g/day up to 200 g/day, depending on litter size, sow performance, and environmental conditions. The rest of the lactation period is characterized by a plateau in piglet growth rate at 200–300 g/day, indicating the inadequacy of milk supply to cover the increasing needs of piglets (King *et al.*, 1999).

Pre-weaning growth rates are closely associated with milk consumption, especially with weaning ages around 3 to 4 weeks (Williams, 1995). Piglets require on average 4 kg of milk per kg of growth, based on the fact that sow's milk contains 5.5 MJ metabolizable energy (ME)/kg and litter growth requires 22 MJ ME/kg (Whittemore, 1998a). Milking ability of the sow, on the other hand, is affected mainly by her voluntary feed intake and dietary composition, when environmental and health conditions are satisfactory. For sow energy intakes between 20 and 70 MJ ME/day, average litter growth is expected to increase about 9 g/MJ, which is equivalent to 36 g of extra milk per day (Williams, 1995). Milk production is also related positively to litter size, although individual milk intake is reduced with each additional piglet (Aldquist *et al.*, 1994):

$$\text{Milk yield (kg)} = 5.98 + 0.689 \times \text{litter size } (r^2 = 0.95). \tag{1.3}$$

Based on Equation 1.3 it can be predicted that the average daily milk yield for a litter of six piglets would be about 10.1 kg or 1.7 kg per piglet. If the same litter had 14 piglets, average daily milk yield would be increased to

15.6 kg, but milk intake would now be only 1.1 kg per piglet. Sow milk yield is also associated with milking intensity, in that heavier piglets initiate and sustain a greater milk flow during suckling and as a consequence they consume more milk than their lighter littermates (van der Steen and de Groot, 1992).

The benefits of creep feeding are marginal at best when the lactation period is around 2–3 weeks. Intake of creep feed before this age is minimal, highly variable, and accounts for less than 5% of daily energy intake (Aherne *et al.*, 1982; Pajor *et al.*, 1991; Pluske *et al.*, 1995). Creep feeding, however, becomes an important source of nutrients for growth and development when pigs are weaned closer to 4–5 weeks of age (Appleby *et al.*, 1992), as creep feed can contribute up to 17% of total energy intake (Pluske *et al.*, 1995). Based on the amount of feed wastage usually observed with creep feeding, such diets would be better reserved for management schemes that practice late weaning.

Offering liquid milk replacers or skim milk before weaning can also enhance growth rates pre-weaning (King *et al.*, 1998). But, this is more likely to happen during the summer, when intake of the milk replacer can be four times greater than in the rest of the year (Azain *et al.*, 1996), or when sow milk yield is diminishing or litter size exceeds the milking capacity of the sow (Williams, 1995).

Weaning weight

Weaning weight is closely associated with weaning age. For pigs weaned below 3 weeks of age, for every extra day of lactation, weaning weight increases by about 0.25 kg per piglet. For later weaning ages, weaning weight is further increased by creep feeding and can easily exceed 0.5 kg/day in pigs weaned at 5 weeks of age.

In the USA, weaning weight is about 5.5 (± 1) kg at an average age of about 18 (± 6) days, although some farms wean as young as 10 days of age. In Europe, average weaning weight is 5–7 kg at an average age of 21–28 days, with a trend toward later weaning. In some parts of the world minimum weaning age is dictated by law. For example, it is 5 weeks in Sweden and 3 weeks in Canada. In the EU, the trend has been toward increasing weaning age to balance the absence of antimicrobial agents in post-weaning diets and it is currently set by law at 4 weeks.

Nevertheless, it is clear now that weaning weight is limited by milk supply. Therefore, there is ample room for improvement via the provision of creep diets and liquid feeding, especially during the later stages of lactation. Targets for weaning weight according to age presented in Table 1.6 should be used only as guidelines to set up initial farm-specific performance targets.

Table 1.6. Targets for weaning weight according to age.

Age (days)	Body weight (kg)	Weekly growth rate (g/day)
Birth	1.5	
7	2.5	150
14	4.5	290
21	6.5	290
28	9.0[a]	350
35	12.0[a]	430

[a] Without creep feeding, weaning weight targets should be 8 and 10 kg for pigs weaned at 28 and 35 days, respectively.

Post-weaning growth

The success or failure of any commercial piglet nutrition program depends on the degree it reaches its targets in terms of growth performance, which often is used as an indicator of profitability under intensive production conditions. An example of a commercial set of performance targets is presented in Table 1.7. There are three levels of projected performance targets, but due to natural variability and different levels of management many farms certainly fall in between these levels.

- *Level 1*. Farms with severe health and management problems belong to this group. Also, farms following older nutritional guidelines but using modern genetics and facilities often experience unrealized growth potential (and profit) and, thus, they are often grouped in this category.
- *Level 2*. This is the group that incorporates the majority of commercial farms that follow most nutrition, health, and management guidelines. What is keeping these operations from achieving greater performance is often a more aggressive nutritional program in terms of nutrient density and ingredient complexity, which of course is more expensive in cost per unit weight of feed.
- *Level 3*. The most progressive farms usually attain the highest levels of performance. In these farms, management realizes that cost per kilo of feed is not as important as cost per kilo of live weight gain. A high-density, high-quality feeding program that appears to be the most expensive option often yields the lowest cost per kilo weight gain.

Another way of looking at performance targets, often practiced in the USA, is by exit weight. Many farms know the exit weight and age of a certain batch of pigs and, in conjunction with feed delivery records, estimate actual growth rate, feed intake, and feed to gain ratio. Actual performance may be gauged against performance targets in Table 1.8, suitable for above-average farms.

Table 1.7. Example of commercial European weekly performance targets.

	Level 1			Level 2			Level 3		
Age (days)	Weight (kg)	Gain (kg/week)	Feed (kg/week)	Weight (kg)	Gain (kg/week)	Feed (kg/week)	Weight (kg)	Gain (kg/week)	Feed (kg/week)
21	5.0			6.5			7.0		
28	6.0	1.0	1.0	8.0	1.5	1.5	9.0	2.0	2.0
35	7.5	1.5	2.0	10.0	2.0	2.5	11.5	2.5	3.0
42	9.5	2.0	3.0	12.5	2.5	3.5	14.5	3.0	4.0
49	12.0	2.5	4.0	15.5	3.0	4.5	18.0	3.5	5.0
56	15.0	3.0	5.0	19.0	3.5	5.5	22.0	4.0	6.0
63	18.5	3.5	6.0	23.0	4.0	6.5	26.5	4.5	7.0
70	22.5	4.0	7.0	27.5	4.5	7.5	32.0	5.0	8.0
Overall		17.5	28.0		21.0	31.5		24.5	35.0

Level 1, below-average farms in terms of health, management, nutrition, facilities; Level 2, average farms that achieve satisfactory results; Level 3, exceptional farms.

Table 1.8. Example of commercial US growth performance targets according to nursery exit weight[a].

Exit weight (kg)	Weight gain (kg/day)	Feed intake (kg/day)	Feed/gain	Gain/feed (g/kg)	Duration (days)	Age (days)
18	0.41	0.57	1.400	714	33	47
20	0.42	0.60	1.425	702	37	51
22	0.43	0.62	1.450	690	41	55
24	0.44	0.65	1.475	678	44	58
26	0.45	0.68	1.500	667	48	62
28	0.46	0.70	1.525	656	51	65
30	0.47	0.73	1.500	645	54	68
32	0.48	0.76	1.575	635	57	71

[a] Assuming initial body weight of 4.5 kg at 14–16 days of age.

References

Aherne FX, Danielson V, and Nielsen HE (1982) The effects of creep feeding on pre- and post-weaning pig performance. *Acta Agricultura Scandinavia Section A* 32:155–160.

Aherne FX and Kirkwood RN (1985) Nutrition and sow prolificacy. *Journal of Reproduction and Fertility* S33:169–183.

Aldquist DE, Morrish L, Thompson M, and King RH (1994) Response of sows to varying litter size. *Proceedings of the Nutrition Society of Australia* 18:175.

Appleby MC, Pajor EA, and Fraser D (1992) Individual variation in feeding and growth of piglets: effects of increased access to creep food. *Animal Production* 55:147–152.

Azain MJ, Tomkins T, Sowinski JS, Arentson RA, and Jewell DE (1996) Effect of supplemental pig milk replacer on litter performance: seasonal variation in response. *Journal of Animal Science* 74:2195–2202.

Bikker P, Verstegen MWA, Kemp B, and Bosch MW (1996a) Performance and body composition of finishing gilts (45 to 85 kilograms) as affected by energy intake and nutrition in earlier life: I. Growth of the body and body components. *Journal of Animal Science* 74:806–816.

Bikker P, Verstegen MWA, and Campbell RG (1996b) Performance and body composition of finishing gilts (45 to 85 kilograms) as affected by energy intake and nutrition in earlier life: II. Protein and lipid accretion in body components. *Journal of Animal Science* 74:817–826.

Black JL (1995) Modelling energy metabolism in the pig – critical evaluation of a simple reference model. In: *Modelling Growth in the Pig*, by Moughan PJ, Verstegen MWA, and Visser-Reyneveld MI (ed), 87–102. Wageningen Pers, Wageningen, The Netherlands.

Boyd RD, Kensinger RS, Harrell RJ, and Bauman DE (1995) Nutrient uptake and endocrine regulation of milk synthesis by mammary tissue of lactating sows. *Journal of Animal Science* 73(Supplement 2):36.

Brooks PH and Tsourgiannis CA (2003) Factors affecting the voluntary feed intake of the weaned pig. In: *Weaning the Pig – Concepts and Consequences*, by Pluske JR, Le Dividich J, and Verstegen MWA (ed), 81–116. Wageningen Academic Publishers, Wageningen, The Netherlands.

Brumm MC and Gonyou HW (2001) Effects of facility design on behavior and feed and water intake. In: *Swine Nutrition* (2nd edn), by Lewis AJ and Southern LL (ed), 499–518. CRC Press LLC, Boca Raton, FL.

Campbell RG, Taverner MR, and Mullaney PD (1975) The effect of dietary concentrations of digestible energy on the performance and carcass characteristics of early-weaned pigs. *Animal Production* 21:285–294.

Campbell RG and Taverner MR (1988) Genotype and sex effects on the relationship between energy intake and protein deposition in growing pigs. *Journal of Animal Science* 66:676–686.

Campbell RG, Taverner MR, and Curic DM (1988) The effects of sex and liveweight on the growing pig's response to dietary protein. *Animal Production* 46:123–130.

Caugant A and Gueblez R (1993) Influence of piglet weight at birth on subsequent production traits. *Journees de la Recherche Porcine en France* 25:123–128.

Cranwell PD, Pierzynowski SG, Rippe C, Pluske JR, Power GN, Campbell RG, Kerton DJ, King RH, and Dunshea FR (1997) Weight and age at weaning influence pancreatic size and enzymatic activity. In: *Manipulating Pig Production VI*, by Cranwell P (ed), 66. Australasian Pig Science Association, Werribee, Australia.

Critser DJ, Miller PS, and Lewis AJ (1995) The effects of dietary protein concentration on compensatory growth in barrows and gilts. *Journal of Animal Science* 73:3376–3383.

de Grau AF, Dewey CE, and Friendship RM (2001) Effect of pig management on weight variation in grower-finisher pigs. *32nd Annual Meeting of the American Association of Swine Veterinarians*, 521–526. American Association of Swine Veterinarians, Perry, IA.

de Lange CFM, Birkett SH, and Morel PCH (2001) Protein, fat, and bone tissue growth in swine. In: *Swine Nutrition* (2nd edn), by Lewis AJ and Southern LL (ed), 65–81. CRC Press LLC, Boca Raton, FL.

Dunshea FR, Kerton DJ, Eason PJ, and King RH (1999) Supplemental skim milk before and after weaning improves growth performance of pigs. *Australian Journal of Agricultural Research* 50:1165–1170.

Edwards AC (1999) Feed processing and feeding management to enhance nutrient utilization in commercial livestock production. *Recent Advances in Animal Nutrition in Australia* 12:137–144.

Emmans GC and Kyriazakis I (1997) Models of pig growth: problems and proposed solutions. *Livestock Production Science* 51:119–129.

Emmans GC and Kyriazakis I (1999) Growth and body composition. In: *A Quantitative Biology of the Pig*, by Kyriazakis I (ed), 181–197. CAB International, Wallingford, UK.

England DC (1974) Husbandry components in prenatal and perinatal development in swine. *Journal of Animal Science* 38:1045–1049.

Gompertz B (1825) On the nature of the function expressive of the law of human mortality and on a new method of determining the value of life contingencies. *Philosophical Transactions of the Royal Society* 55:155–166.

Harrell RJ, Thomas MJ, and Boyd RD (1993) Limitations of sow milk yield on baby pig growth. *Proceedings of the Cornell Nutrition Conference for Feed Manufacturers*, 156–164. Cornell University, Ithaca, NY.

Hegarty PVJ and Allen CE (1978) Effect of pre-natal runting on the post-natal development of skeletal muscles in swine and rats. *Journal of Animal Science* 46:1634–1640.

Hodge RW (1974) Efficiency of food conversion and body composition of the preruminant lamb and the young pig. *British Journal of Nutrition* 32:113–126.

Hyun Y, Ellis M, Riskowski G, and Johnson RW (1998) Growth performance of pigs subjected to multiple concurrent environmental stessors. *Journal of Animal Science* 76:721–727.

Jensen P and Recen B (1989) When to wean – observations from free-ranging domestic pigs. *Applied Animal Behaviour Science* 23:49–60.

Johnson RW (1997) Inhibition of growth by pro-inflammatory cytokines: an integrated view. *Journal of Animal Science* 75:1244–1255.

Johnson RW, Escobar J, and Webel DM (2001) Nutrition and immunology of swine. In: *Swine Nutrition* (2nd edn), by Lewis AJ and Southern LL (ed), 545–562. CRC Press LLC, Boca Raton, FL.

King RH, Boyce JM, and Dunshea FR (1998) Effect of supplemental nutrients on the growth performance of sucking pigs. *Australian Journal of Agricultural Research* 49:883–887.

King RH, Le Dividich J, and Dunshea FR (1999) Lactation and neonatal growth. In: *A Quantitative Biology of the Pig*, by Kyriazakis I (ed), 155–180. CAB International, Wallingford, UK.

Klasing KC (1988) Nutritional aspects of leukocytic cytokines. *Journal of Nutrition* 118:1436–1446.

Kyriazakis I, Stamataris C, Emmans GC, and Whittemore CT (1991) The effects of food protein content on the performance of pigs previously given foods with low or moderate protein contents. *Animal Production* 52:165–173.

Lawrence TLJ and Fowler VR (1997) *Growth of Farm Animals*. CAB International, Wallingford, UK.

Le Dividich J (1999) Neonatal and weaner pig: management to reduce variation. In: *Manipulating Pig Production VII*, by Cranwell P (ed), 135–155. Australasian Pig Science Association, Werribee, Australia.

Le Dividich J and Seve B (2001) Energy requirements of the young pig. In: *The Weaner Pig*, by Varley MA and Wiseman J (ed), 17–44. CAB International, Wallingford, UK.

Mahan DC and Lepine AJ (1991) Effect of pig weaning weight and associated nursery feeding programs on subsequent performance to 105 kilograms body weight. *Journal of Animal Science* 69:1370–1378.

Mahan DC (1993) Effect of weight, split-weaning, and nursery feeding programs on performance responses of pigs to 105 kilograms body weight and subsequent effects on sow rebreeding interval. *Journal of Animal Science* 71:1991–1995.

Mahan DC, Cromwell GL, Ewan RC, Hamilton CR, and Yen JT (1998) Evaluation of the feeding duration of a phase I nursery diet to three-week-old pigs of two weaning weights. *Journal of Animal Science* 76:578–583.

Mavromichalis I, Parr TM, Gabert VM, and Baker DH (2001) True ileal digestibility of amino acids in sow's milk for 17-day-old pigs. *Journal of Animal Science* 79:707–713.

McCracken BA, Gaskins HR, Ruwe-Kaiser PJ, Klasing KC, and Jewell DE (1995) Diet-dependent and diet-independent metabolic responses underlie growth stasis of pigs at weaning. *Journal of Nutrition* 125:2838–2845.

McCracken BA, Spurlock ME, Roos MA, Zuckermann FA, and Gaskins HR (1999) Weaning anorexia may contribute to local inflammation in the piglet small intestine. *Journal of Nutrition* 129:613–619.

Miller HM, Toplis P, and Slade RD (1999) Weaning weight and daily live weight gain in the week after weaning predict piglet performance. In: *Manipulating Pig Production VII*, by Cranwell P (ed), 130. Australasian Pig Science Association, Werribee, Australia.

Mitchell AD, Scholz AM, and Mersmann HJ (2001) Growth and body composition. In: *Biology of the Domestic Pig* (2nd edn), by Pond WG and Mersmann HJ (ed), 225–308. Cornell University Press, Ithaca, NY.

Moughan PJ and Verstegen MWA (1988) The modelling of growth in the pig. *Netherlands Journal of Agricultural Science* 36:145–166.

Noblet J, Le Dividich J, and Milgen JV (2001) Thermal environment and swine nutrition. In: *Swine Nutrition* (2nd edn), by Lewis AJ and Southern LL (ed), 519–544. CRC Press LLC, Boca Raton, FL.

NPPC (1995) *Genetic Evaluation: Terminal Line Program Results*. National Pork Producers Council, Des Moines, IA.
Pajor EA, Fraser D, and Kramer DL (1991) Consumption of solid food by suckling pigs: individual variation and relation to weight gain. *Applied Animal Behaviour Science* 32:139–155.
Payne HG, Mullan BP, Trezona M, and Frey B (1999) Variation in pig production and performance. In: *Manipulating Pig Production VII*, by Cranwell P (ed), 13–26. Australasian Pig Science Association, Werribee, Australia.
Pettigrew JE (1981) Supplemental dietary fat for peripartal sows: a review. *Journal of Animal Science* 53:107–117.
Pluske JR and Williams IH (1991) Which piglets perform the best after weaning? In: *Manipulating Pig Production III*, by Batterham ES (ed), 148. Australasian Pig Science Association, Werribee, Australia.
Pluske JR, Williams IH, and Aherne FX (1995) Nutrition of the neonatal pig. In: *The Neonatal Pig: Development and Survival*, by Varley MA (ed), 187–235. CAB International, Wallingford, UK.
Pluske JR, Williams BL, and Aherne FX (1996a) Maintenance of villous height and crypt depth in piglets by providing continuous nutrition after weaning. *Animal Science* 62:131–144.
Pluske JR, Williams IH, and Aherne FX (1996b) Villous height and crypt depth in piglets in response to increases in the intake of cows' milk after weaning. *Animal Science* 62:145–158.
Pluske JR and Dong GZ (1998) Factors influencing the utilization of colostrum and milk. In: *The Lactating Sow*, by Verstegen MWA, Moughan PJ, and Schrama JW (ed), 45–70. Wageningen Pers, Wageningen, The Netherlands.
Powell SE and Aberle ED (1980) Effect of birth weight on growth and carcass composition of swine. *Journal of Animal Science* 50:860–868.
Ritacco G, Radecki SV, and Schoknecht PA (1997) Compensatory growth in runt pigs is not mediated by insulin-like growth factor I. *Journal of Animal Science* 75:1237–1243.
Schoknecht PA, Pond WG, Mersmann HJ, and Maurer RR (1993) Protein restriction during pregnancy affects postnatal growth in swine progeny. *Journal of Nutrition* 123:1818–1825.
Slade RD and Miller HM (1999) Influence of litter origin and weaning weight on post-weaning piglet growth. In: *Manipulating Pig Production VII*, by Cranwell P (ed), 131. Australasian Pig Science Association, Werribee, Australia.
Sloat DS, Mahan DC, and Roehrig KL (1985) Effect of pig weaning weight on postweaning body composition and digestive enzyme development. *Nutrition Reports International* 31:627–634.
Sprent M, Varley MA, and Cole MA (2001a) The effect of birth weight on subsequent performance in piglets. *The Weaner Pig – Nutrition and Management*, 41. BSAS Occasional Meeting, University of Nottingham, Nottingham, UK.
Sprent M, Varley MA, and Cole MA (2001b) The effect of weaning weight on growth to slaughter for growing pigs. *The Weaner Pig – Nutrition and Management*, 40. BSAS Occasional Meeting, University of Nottingham, Nottingham, UK.
Spurlock ME (1997) Regulation of metabolism and growth during immune challenge: an overview of cytokine function. *Journal of Animal Science* 75:1773–1783.

Stahly TS, Williams NH, and Swenson S (1994) Impact of genotype and dietary amino acid regimen on growth of pigs from 8 to 25 kg. *Journal of Animal Science* 72(Supplement 1):165.

Stamataris C, Kyriazakis I, and Emmans GC (1991) The performance and body composition of young pigs following a period of growth retardation by food restriction. *Animal Production* 53:373–381.

Thompson BK and Fraser D (1988) Variation in piglet weight: weight gains in the first days after birth and their relationship with later performance. *Canadian Journal of Animal Science* 70:1864–1872.

Tokach MD, Goodband RD, Nelssen JL, and Kats LJ (1992) Influence of weaning weight and growth during the first week post-weaning on subsequent pig performance. *Agricultural Experiment Station Report No. 667*:15–17. Kansas State University, Manhattan, KS.

Toplis P, Miller HM, Redfern EJ, and Jacques M (2001) Knowledge of variation in piglet weaning weights as an aid to nutritional management. *The Weaner Pig – Nutrition and Management*, 43. BSAS Occasional Meeting, University of Nottingham, Nottingham, UK.

van der Peet-Schwering CMC, den Hartog LA, and Vos HJPM (1999) Application of growth models for pigs in practice. *Pig News and Information* 20(2):49N–54N.

van der Steen HAM and de Groot PN (1992) Direct and maternal effects on growth and milk intake in piglets: Meishan versus Dutch breeds. *Livestock Production Science* 30:361–373.

Warshaw JB (1990) Nutritional correlates of fetal growth. *Developmental Pharmacology and Therapeutics* 15:153–158.

Whittemore CT, Aumaitre A, and Williams IH (1978) Growth of body components in young weaned pigs. *Journal of Agricultural Science (Cambridge)* 91:681–692.

Whittemore CT, Taylor HM, Henderson R, Wood JD, and Brock DC (1981) Chemical and dissected composition changes in weaned piglets. *Animal Production* 32:203–210.

Whittemore CT (1998a) *The Science and Practice of Pig Production* (2nd edn). Blackwell Science Ltd, Oxford, UK.

Whittemore CT (1998b) Influence of pregnancy feeding on lactation performance. In: *The Lactating Sow*, by Verstegen MWA, Moughan PJ, and Schrama JW (ed), 183–200. Wageningen Pers, Wageningen, The Netherlands.

Whittemore CT (2001) Growth of the young weaned pig. In: *The Weaner Pig – Nutrition and Management*, by Varley MA and Wiseman J (ed), 1–15. CAB International, Wallingford, UK.

Widdowson EM (1971) Intra-uterine growth retardation in the pig. *Biology of the Neonate* 19:329–340.

Williams IH (1995) Sow milk as a major nutrient source before weaning. In: *Manipulating Pig Production V*, by Hennessy DP and Cranwell P (ed), 107–113. Australasian Pig Science Association, Werribee, Australia.

Williams NH, Stahly TS, and Zimmerman DR (1997a) Effect of level of chronic immune system activation on the growth and dietary lysine needs of pigs fed from 6 to 112 kg. *Journal of Animal Science* 75:2481–2496.

Williams NH, Stahly TS, and Zimmerman DR (1997b) Effect of chronic immune system activation on the rate, efficiency, and composition of growth and lysine needs of pigs fed from 6 to 27 kg. *Journal of Animal Science* 75:2463–2471.

Wolter BF, Ellis M, Curtis SE, Parr EN, and Webel DM (2000) Group size and floor-space allowance can affect weanling-pig performance. *Journal of Animal Science* 78:2062–2067.

Zijlstra RT, Donovan SM, Odle J, Gelberg HB, Petschow BW, and Gaskins HR (1997) Protein–energy malnutrition delays small-intestinal recovery in neonatal pigs infected with rotavirus. *Journal of Nutrition* 127:1118–1127.

2 Digestive Physiology

Introduction

The volume of published material on digestive physiology in pigs merits a separate book on its own. Indeed, there are excellent studies providing in-depth coverage both for young and mature pigs (Lindberg and Ogle, 2001; Blok *et al.*, 2002; Xu and Cranwell, 2003). However, it is worth repeating here the basic concepts of digestive physiology in piglets, especially those that create practical obstacles in the adaptation to solid diets post-weaning.

The central focus of this discussion is the abrupt change at weaning from sow's milk to a cereal-based diet with a different nutrient composition. In nature, where pigs are weaned gradually over a long(er) period of time, the digestive system matures gradually and, thus, digestive upsets are not as frequent as under modern husbandry practices. Digestive upsets in piglets are manifested through nutritional and (or) pathogenic diarrheas, with further implications on growth performance, overall health, and survival rate.

Gastric pH

Gastric pH in mature monogastric animals is controlled by secretion of hydrochloric acid from gastric mucosa (Kidder and Manners, 1978). Hydrochloric acid is required to initiate protein digestion by activating pepsinogen to pepsin, the major gastric protease. Mature animals have a relatively low gastric pH (2–3), which virtually eliminates pathogens entering the digestive system through feed and water (Clemens *et al.*, 1975).

Neonatal pigs have a rather high gastric pH (5–6) facilitated by the strong buffering capacity of colostrum (Smith and Jones, 1963). This allows passage of ingested environmental bacteria from the stomach to the small and large intestines for the establishment of a normal gastrointestinal microflora. Usually, the predominant bacteria in the stomach are lactobacteria and bifidobacteria, whereas in the intestines there is a mix of bacteria (Smith and Jones, 1963). After the first few hours of suckling, gastric pH drops to around 3.5–5 to remain there for the first four weeks post-weaning (Cranwell *et al.*, 1976). Afterwards, gastric pH drops gradually to mature levels (2–3) even without the provision of any solid feed (Schicketanz and Richter, 1967; cited by Kidder and Manners, 1978).

A gastric pH of 3.5–5 in suckling pigs is favorable for the activation of chymosin (rennin), the enzyme responsible for the clotting of milk in the stomach (Shen and Liechty, 2003). Without the action of chymosin, milk would pass quickly and largely undigested into the small intestine. Although pepsin can also clot milk, albeit at reduced efficacy than chymosin, the latter has weaker proteolytic activity, which protects milk immunoglobulins from digestion (Kidder and Manners, 1978). Having a gastric pH of 3.5–5 also benefits proliferation of lactobacteria while excluding other pathogenic organisms (Cranwell *et al.*, 1968). A healthy population of lactobacteria produces a copious quantity of lactic acid that stabilizes gastric pH and further depresses the production of hydrochloric acid. Thus, suckling piglets exhibit limited capacity for secretion of hydrochloric acid, which is not strongly stimulated by sow's milk (Cranwell *et al.*, 1976).

At weaning, gastric pH (3–4) remains relatively higher than what is needed for efficient digestion of plant- and animal-derived proteins (other than milk), as the activity of pepsin peaks at pH 2 and 3.5 (Kidder and Manners, 1978). Some proteins are digested only at the lower optimum pH, whereas no significant digestion of proteins occurs above pH 4. Provision of dairy products in post-weaning diets has been shown to reduce gastric pH in weaned pigs compared to suckled littermates (Polivoda *et al.*, 1973). Dietary protein concentration also affects gastric pH, with low-protein diets supporting lower gastric pH due to their lower buffering capacity (Manners, 1970).

Protein indigestion in the young pig not only reduces efficiency of feed utilization but also gives rise to intestinal microflora populations that thrive on protein, and especially to opportunistic pathogens such as *Escherichia coli* (Smith and Jones, 1963). This situation usually ends with the development of scours, and occasionally death, unless pigs are treated with antimicrobial agents (antibiotics, zinc oxide, copper sulfate, organic acids, and essential oils) that control intestinal pathogens.

To prevent protein indigestion in newly weaned pigs, several measures are proposed. First, low-protein diets composed of highly digestible protein sources are strongly recommended for the first few days post-weaning. Second, if *ad libitum* feeding overloads the immature digestive system with proteins, restricted feeding may be employed for a limited period of time (usually, 2 to 5 days post-weaning is enough). Finally, addition of lactic (Geary *et al.*, 1999) and other acids (Mroz, 2003; Koch, 2005) in post-weaning diets has been shown repeatedly to improve animal performance, mostly due to their antimicrobial properties and less due to any lowering of gastric pH.

Enzymes

The enzymatic apparatus of the suckling piglet is clearly geared toward digesting sow's milk (Lindemann *et al.*, 1986; Cranwell, 1995). Indeed, the specific activity of lactase (the major enzyme responsible for the digestion of lactose, the primary sugar in milk) is high throughout the early lactation period and starts to decline at about 3 weeks of age (Fig. 2.1). Likewise, the major gastric proteinase (chymosin) is predominant early on with pepsins becoming prevalent with increasing age (Kidder and Manners, 1978). Lipase activity in the stomach is rather high, justified by the abundance of lipids in sow's milk, but pancreatic lipase is not secreted in any significant quantities in suckling piglets (Shen and Liechty, 2003). Finally, enzymes responsible for the digestion of starch, such as α-amylase and maltase, are extremely low in the neonatal pig, but their activity increases with age (Lindemann *et al.*, 1986).

Creep feeding has the potential for inducing enzymatic maturation of the digestive system to handle nutrients different from those found in sow's milk (Friend *et al.*, 1970; Shields *et al.*, 1980; Hampson and Kidder, 1986). It has been also demonstrated that enzymatic secretion is influenced by

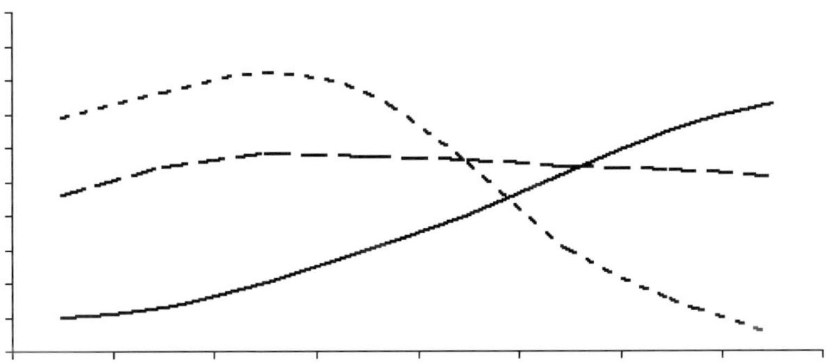

Fig. 2.1. Schematic representation of the development of the digestive enzymatic system (- - -, lactase; ——, amylase/proteases; – – –, lipase) in piglets. (From Lindemann *et al.*, 1986.)

substrate availability (Corring, 1980; Graham *et al.*, 1981; Hampson, 1986b). For example (Kidder and Manners, 1978), when pigs were offered a starch-free diet based on lipids, the concentration of gastric lipase increased dramatically compared to that of α-amylase. The opposite was found when pigs were offered a fat-free diet based on starch. It has been estimated that in growing pigs it takes about 3 to 5 days for the enzymatic system to adapt to changes in substrate (Corring and Saucier, 1972), during which time efficiency of nutrient utilization is, of course, limited. It should be logical to assume that when weaned pigs experience low feed intake and digestive upsets, this adaptation period may be even longer.

At weaning, piglets without prior exposure to creep feeding are faced with novel nutrients (mainly of vegetable origin) which are difficult to digest with the available milk-oriented enzymes. For this reason, it is advisable to offer piglets a post-weaning diet based on milk-derived products such as whey, skim milk, and lactose. This regimen provides nourishment while the appropriate enzymes are induced to handle the less digestible ingredients. Thus, as the digestive system matures, the complexity of diet can be decreased accordingly. Under practical conditions, this process usually takes from 2 to 5 weeks, during which time indigestion frequently leads to diarrheas.

The case for lipid digestibility

Although suckling pigs are well adapted to digest lipids in sow's milk, the ability of the young pig to utilize animal and vegetable fats has been strongly debated. Earlier studies (Eusebio *et al.*, 1965; Leibbrandt *et al.*, 1975) proposed that young pigs were unable to utilize dietary fat calories as efficiently as carbohydrate calories. When piglets were offered high-lipid diets, growth performance was reduced and energy required per unit of weight gain was increased. However, in these experiments lipids were replacing carbohydrates on a weight basis (i.e. instead of an isocaloric basis), thus creating an energy/nutrient imbalance, which of course confounded the results (Allee *et al.*, 1971). In contrast, when young pigs were offered lipid-based diets that were well balanced for other nutrients, they were able to utilize lipid calories as efficiently as carbohydrate calories (Cline *et al.*, 1977; Lawrence and Maxwell, 1983).

Work conducted at Ohio State University (Cera *et al.*, 1988b, 1989) indicated that weaned piglets utilize lipid sources with a varying degree of efficiency. Indeed, during the first 4 weeks post-weaning, fat digestibility depended largely on the degree of saturation and chain length in component fatty acids. Animal fats were the least digestible, followed by vegetable oils, and coconut fat being the most digestible. Although coconut fat (an oil that is solid at room temperature) is highly saturated, it is composed mainly of medium-chain fatty acids, which like those in sow's milk are readily absorbed and metabolized (Odle, 1998). From the same university work, it was also demonstrated that digestibility of all types of lipids increased gradually during the first 4 weeks post-weaning (Fig. 2.2). It was finally established that lipid digestibility affected efficiency of feed utilization, with animal fats supporting the worst feed/gain ratio (Fig. 2.3), apparently due to reduced energy availability.

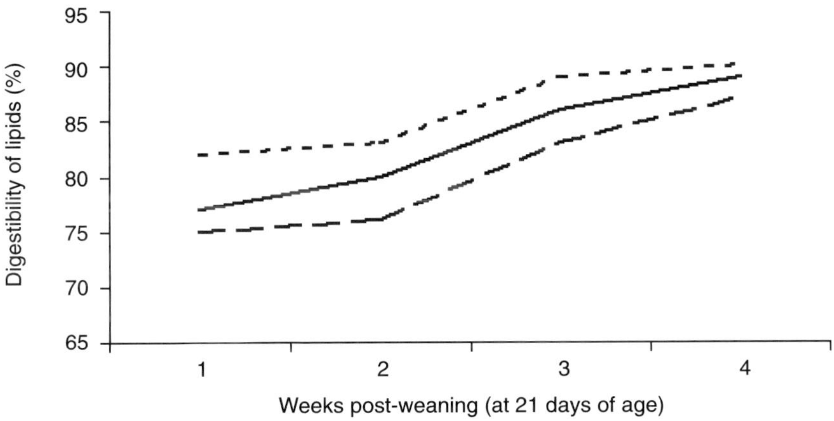

Fig. 2.2. Lipid digestibility is strongly affected by source (- - -, coconut; ——, vegetable; – – –, animal). (From Cera *et al.*, 1988b, 1989.)

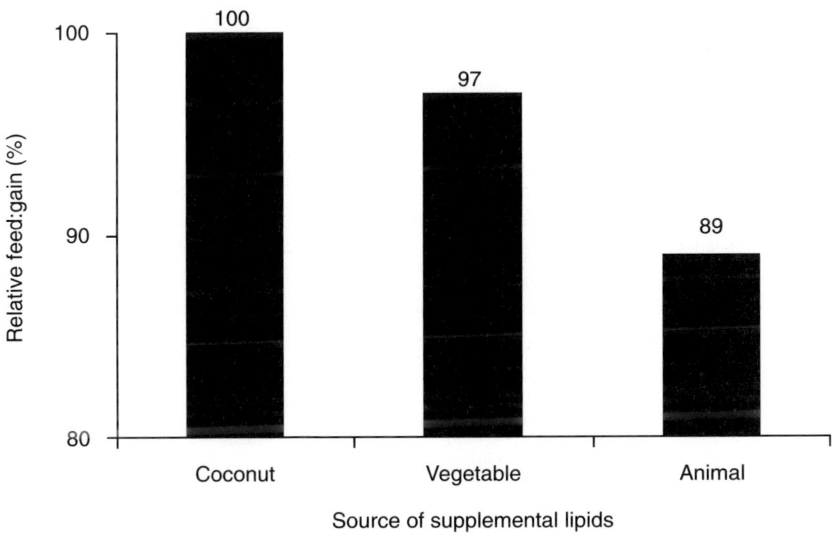

Fig. 2.3. Feed efficiency is affected by lipid source. (From Cera *et al.*, 1988b, 1989.)

It has recently been proposed (Morillo *et al.*, 2003) that supplemental lipids may be excluded from post-weaning diets because piglets do not utilize them very efficiently. Work by Campbell *et al.* (1975) clearly demonstrated, however, that growth in the young pig depends solely on energy intake (Fig. 2.4). Taking into account that recently weaned pigs will consume a fixed (but nevertheless variable) amount of feed regardless of its energy density (Black, 1995), it is reasonable to assume that increasing feed energy density will invariably increase energy intake and thus growth. To this end, high-energy diets are almost always recommended for weaned pigs, despite their reduced ability to use lipids. In evaluating trials where piglets fail to respond to supplemental energy sources, it is imperative to remember that during the first days post-weaning undernourished piglets expend body fat to cover energy needs, replacing it with water to maintain a relatively stable body mass (Whittemore *et al.*, 1978). It is most likely that when feed intake is low post-weaning, supplemental fats and oils will not enhance body weight growth, but rather aid in maintaining body composition.

Hypersensitivity to Soybeans

It is now common knowledge that soybean meal predisposes recently weaned piglets to digestive upsets and diarrhea. It has been clearly demonstrated (Newby *et al.*, 1985; Li *et al.*, 1990, 1991a,b) that weaned

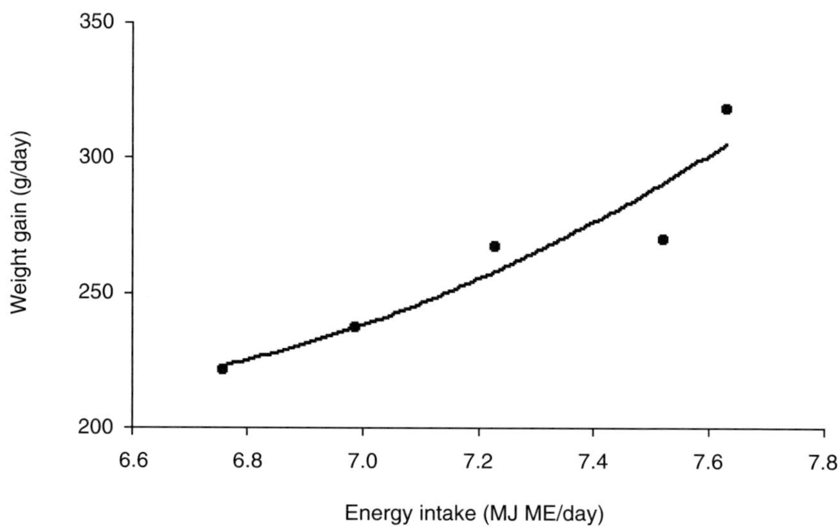

Fig. 2.4. In healthy young pigs, weight gain depends largely on energy (feed) intake (ME, metabolizable energy). (From Campbell *et al.*, 1975.)

piglets offered a soybean meal-based diet develop serum immunoglobulin G (IgG) antibodies specific for glycinin and β-conglycinin, the major storage proteins in soybeans. Such immunological response to dietary antigens is also associated with increased density of intestinal lympocytes, villous atrophy, and crypt cell hyperplasia; all indicative of gut health deterioration (Dreau *et al.*, 1994, 1995). This delayed-type hypersensitivity reaction to soybean antigens has been associated with depressed growth (Li *et al.*, 1990), and is often the cause of secondary diarrheas due to maldigestion and malabsorption (Miller *et al.*, 1984a,b).

Following initial exposure to dietary antigens, piglets develop tolerance with increasing age (Li *et al.*, 1990, 1991a,b). Thus, exposure to soybean protein during suckling via creep feeding may ameliorate post-weaning reaction to a soybean-based diet. To this effect, a substantial quantity of soybean protein must be consumed prior to weaning, however, for piglets to develop sufficient immunological tolerance (Hampson and Fu, 1988; Barnett *et al.*, 1989; Kelly, 1990). Such tolerance is almost never achieved in creep-fed piglets weaned before 25–28 days of age, due to insufficient consumption of creep feed. For early-weaned pigs, therefore, post-weaning diets must contain only minimal amounts of soybean proteins (not necessarily from soybean meal) to allow piglets to develop such tolerance (Tokach *et al.*, 2003) early on and transit easier to less complex diets with higher levels of soybean products. Delaying introduction to soybean proteins only postpones the onset of hypersensitivity reaction.

It has been suggested that dietary, social, environmental, and weaning stress factors compromise immunological status in young pigs, impeding thus their ability to discriminate between harmful and innocuous antigens (King *et al.*, 2003). It has also been proposed (McCracken *et al.*, 1995, 1998, 1999) that for dietary antigens to exert their negative effects on intestinal health, local inflammation must precede ingestion to enable antigens to pass through the epithelial barrier. Such inflammation is often caused by post-weaning depression in feed intake, and certain bacterial and viral diseases.

Feed Intake and Gut Health

Abrupt weaning at an early age has been associated with deterioration of gut health, as evidenced by alterations in gut epithelial morphology. Before weaning, intestinal villi (largely responsible for nutrient absorption) are thin and elongated, whereas after weaning they quickly become thick and short. Villus height has been shown to decrease about 75% during the first 24 h post-weaning (Hampson, 1986a; Cera *et al.*, 1988a). Similarly, depth of intestinal crypts (responsible for regeneration of villi) increases at weaning and continues during the first 2 weeks post-weaning (Hampson *et al.*, 1986a). Following recovery from weaning, villi become short and leaf-shaped similar to those found in adults.

The decrease in absorptive capacity in weaned pigs, coupled with reduction of enzymatic digestion (Miller *et al.*, 1984a,b), often lead to nutrient maldigestion and intestinal upsets causing diarrhea, depression of growth, and even death. Pluske *et al.* (1996) indicated that villus height is highly correlated with post-weaning growth and that the most important factor determining villus height post-weaning was the level of feed intake. Several other researchers have also confirmed the importance of high feed intake during the first week post-weaning on gut health (Kelly *et al.*, 1991; McCracken *et al.*, 1998; Zijlstra *et al.*, 1999).

It is now evident that it is not so much the type of diet offered post-weaning as the amount ingested that affects gut health. Pluske *et al.* (1996) in a classical study (Fig. 2.5) clearly demonstrated that weaned piglets offered cow's milk at levels below those achieved under *ad libitum* conditions exhibited reduced villus height and increased crypt depth, symptoms similar to those observed in piglets offered a solid diet. In contrast, when piglets were allowed to consume relatively high quantities of cow's milk, intestinal morphology parameters were similar to (or even better than) those observed prior to weaning.

Further evidence as to the pivotal role of feed intake on post-weaning gut health is furnished by a meta-analysis (Madec *et al.*, 1998), in which it was demonstrated that piglets consuming less than 140 g/day during the first week post-weaning were more prone to digestive disorders compared to piglets consuming at least 190 g/day.

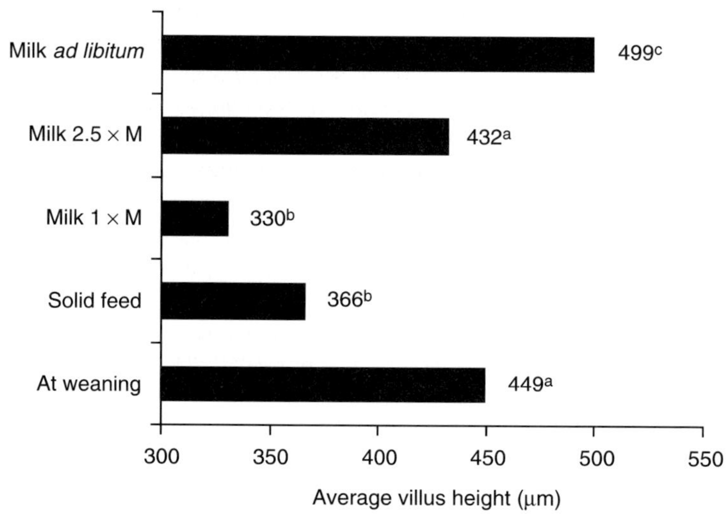

Fig. 2.5. Villus height and consequently gut health may be preserved by high levels of feed intake (M = maintenance) post-weaning ([a,b,c] bars with unlike superscript letters are different at $P < 0.05$). (From Pluske *et al.*, 1996.)

Finally, it should be noted that the abrupt increase in feed intake during the third to fifth day post-weaning, which is often associated with early weaning, is positively associated with digestive disorders and scours (Kamphues, 1987; cited by van Hees *et al.*, 2005). An overload of feed, especially of low digestibility, usually overwhelms the immature digestive system, especially if gastrointestinal health has been impaired due to anorexia during the first couple of days post-weaning. To this end, it is imperative to ensure piglets exhibit high levels of feed intake immediately post-weaning or their feed intake must be controlled during the first week.

Gut Immunity

Sow's colostrum provides the first wave of passive immunity through the absorption of intact immunoglobulins into the bloodstream (Aumaitre and Seve, 1978). This protective action of colostrum is only against pathogens to which the sow has been exposed. Mature milk is also a rich source of immunoglobulins, especially immunoglobulin A (IgA), which acts locally at the luminal level. Milk immunoglobulins provide a constant protective barrier against pathogenic invasion (Darragh and Moughan, 1998) and they also bind and inactivate antigens directly. The so-called 'mammary link' also ensures a rapid transfer of antigen-programed lymphocytes from the sow's gut directly to the mammary gland, where they produce relevant immunoglobulins immediately available for the suckling piglet (Gaskins and Kelley, 1995).

After weaning, the passive protection from sow's milk is withdrawn and the young piglet depends solely on any active (self) immunity developed during suckling. Active immunity develops slowly and depends on lactation length and level of exposure to pathogenic organisms. A change of environment and exposure to new pathogens virtually eliminate any benefits from active immunity acquired during suckling. At weaning, major alterations in intestinal immunity are observed during the first 24 h (McCracken *et al.*, 1999). The activation of the immune system at weaning is followed by systemic and local inflammatory reactions (McCracken *et al.*, 1995), which gear metabolism away from growth and development. Gastrointestinal inflammation also compromises the protective functions of the mucosal epithelial barrier and increases sensitivity to dietary antigens. Thus, minimizing activation of the immune system remains a major goal in early-weaning systems (King *et al.*, 2003).

Animal plasma is a rich source of immunoglobulins (up to 25%) and it is often included in post-weaning diets. It is now believed that its beneficial effects on feed intake are mediated through enhanced gut health and immunological protection (Touchette *et al.*, 1997), not unlike that conferred by sow's milk. To the same end, colostral- and egg-derived antibodies are also beneficial (see Chapter 7).

Intestinal Bacteria

The sterile gastrointestinal system of the newborn piglet is quickly colonized by a host of maternal and environmental bacteria (Kelly *et al.*, 1992). Nevertheless, the establishment of a healthy intestinal microflora is a gradual process affected by several ill-defined factors including nutrition and immunity status.

The presence of intestinal bacteria has significant effects on intestinal development and function. Compared to germ-free animals, the presence of a normal bacterial population in conventionally raised piglets increases gut mass, reduces villus height, and increases crypt depth (Clarke, 1975). Germ-free and antibiotic-treated animals also have greater digestive enzyme activity (Parker and Armstrong, 1987). The effects of intestinal bacteria on gut morphology and function appear to be superimposed on any adaptive responses to dietary changes (Kelly *et al.*, 1992), and thus maintaining piglets in a healthy environment will always reduce the impact of drastic dietary interventions.

Intestinal bacteria growth is always at the expense of the host. Thus, conventionally raised piglets exhibit reduced growth and efficiency of feed utilization (Yokata and Coates, 1982) compared to naïve animals. It is believed that this is due to a combination of: (i) reduced digestive and absorptive capacity; (ii) utilization of dietary nutrients for bacterial growth; and (iii) increased metabolic demand for a larger gut (Kelly *et al.*, 1992).

The presence of intestinal bacteria, however, is of paramount importance to the health of the host animal. Germ-free and antibiotic-treated animals are more susceptible to diseases (Kenworthy and Allen, 1966) because they lack the suppressive effect of a normal intestinal microflora on pathogenic organisms. To this end, the healthy intestinal microflora is often supplemented with substrates suitable for its proliferation (prebiotics). Preparations of live bacteria or spores (probiotics) are also used to augment the numbers of beneficial organisms at the expense of pathogens. Both dietary intervention strategies aim at the establishment of a healthy intestinal microflora to exclude any potential pathogens and maintain gut health.

References

Allee GL, Baker DH, and Leveille GA (1971) Fat utilization and lipogenesis in the young pig. *Journal of Nutrition* 101:1415–1422.

Aumaitre A and Seve B (1978) Nutritional importance of colostrum in the piglet. *Annales de la Recherche Veterinaire* 9:181–192.

Barnett KL, Kornegay ET, Risley CR, Lindemann MD, and Schurig GG (1989) Characterization of creep feed consumption and its subsequent effects on immune response, scouring index and performance of weanling pigs. *Journal of Animal Science* 67:2698–2708.

Black JL (1995) Modelling energy metabolism in the pig – critical evaluation of a simple reference model. In: *Modelling Growth in the Pig*, by Moughan PJ, Verstegen MWA, and Visser-Reyneveld MI (ed), 87–102. Wageningen Pers, Wageningen, The Netherlands.

Blok MC, Vahl HA, de Lange L, van de Braak AE, Hemke G, and Hessing M (2002) *Nutrition and Health of the Gastrointestinal Tract*. Wageningen Academic Publishers, Wageningen, The Netherlands.

Campbell RG, Taverner MR, and Mullaney PD (1975) The effect of dietary concentrations of digestible energy on the performance and carcass characteristics of early-weaned pigs. *Animal Production* 21:285–294.

Cera KR, Mahan DC, Cross RF, Reinhart GA, and Whitmoyer RE (1988a) Effect of age, weaning and postweaning diet on small intestinal growth and jejunal morphology in young swine. *Journal of Animal Science* 66:574–584.

Cera KR, Mahan DC, and Reinhart GA (1988b) Weekly digestibilities of diets supplemented with corn oil, lard or tallow by weanling swine. *Journal of Animal Science* 66:1430–1437.

Cera KR, Mahan DC, and Reinhart GA (1989) Apparent fat digestibilities and performance responses of postweaning swine fed diets supplemented with coconut oil, corn oil, or tallow. *Journal of Animal Science* 67:2040–2047.

Clarke RM (1975) Diet, mucosal architecture and epithelial cell production in the small intestine of specified-pathogen-free and conventional rats. *Laboratory Animals* 9:201–209.

Clemens ET, Stevens CE, and Southworth M (1975) Sites of organic acid production and pattern of digesta movement in the gastrointestinal tract of swine. *Journal of Nutrition* 105:759–768.

Cline TR, Coalson JA, Lecce JG, and Jones EE (1977) Utilization of fat by baby pigs. *Journal of Animal Science* 44:72–77.

Corring T and Saucier R (1972) Secretion pancreatique sur porc fistule. Adaptation a la teneur en proteines du regime. *Annales de Biologie Animal – Biochimie Biophysique* 12:233–241.

Corring T (1980) The adaptation of digestive enzymes to the diet: its physiological significance. *Reproduction, Nutrition, Development* 20:1217–1235.

Cranwell PD, Noakes DE, and Hill KJ (1968) Observations on the stomach contents of the sucking pig. *Proceedings of the Nutrition Society* 27:26A.

Cranwell PD, Noakes DE, and Hill KL (1976) Gastric secretion and fermentation in the suckling pig. *British Journal of Nutrition* 36:71–86.

Cranwell PD (1995) Development of the neonatal gut and enzyme systems. In: *The Neonatal Pig: Development and Survival*, by Varley MA (ed), 99–154. CAB International, Wallingford, UK.

Darragh AJ and Moughan PJ (1998) The composition of colostrum and milk. In: *The Lactating Sow*, by Verstegen MWA, Moughan PJ, and Schrama JW (ed), 3–21. Wageningen Pers, Wageningen, The Netherlands.

Dreau D, Lalles JP, Philouze-Rome V, Toullec R, and Salmon H (1994) Local and systemic immune responses to soybean protein ingestion in early-weaned pigs. *Journal of Animal Science* 72:2090–2098.

Dreau D, Lalles JP, Toullec R, and Salmon H (1995) B and T lymphocytes are enhanced in the gut of piglets fed heat-treated soyabean proteins. *Veterinary Immunology and Immunopathology* 47:69–79.

Eusebio JA, Hays VW, Speer VC, and McCall JT (1965) Utilization of fat by young pigs. *Journal of Animal Science* 24:1001–1007.

Friend DW, Gorrill DL, and MacIntyre TM (1970) Performance and proteolytic enzyme activity of the suckling piglet creep-fed at one or three weeks of age. *Canadian Journal of Animal Science* 50:349–354.

Gaskins HR and Kelley KW (1995) Immunology and neonatal mortality. In: *The Neonatal Pig: Development and Survival*, by Varley MA (ed), 39–55. CAB International, Wallingford, UK.

Geary TM, Brooks PH, Beal JD, and Campbell A (1999) Effect on weaner pig performance and diet microbiology of feeding a liquid diet acidified to pH 4 with either lactic acid or through fermentation with *Pediococcus acidilactici*. *Journal of the Science of Food and Agriculture* 79:633–640.

Graham PL, Mahan DC, and Shields RG, Jr (1981) Effect of starter diet and length of feeding regimen on performance and digestive enzyme activity of 2-week old weaned pigs. *Journal of Animal Science* 53:299–307.

Hampson DJ and Kidder DE (1986) Influence of creep feeding and weaning on brush border enzyme activities in the piglet small intestine. *Research in Veterinary Science* 40:24–31.

Hampson DJ (1986a) Alterations in piglet small intestine structure at weaning. *Research in Veterinary Science* 40:32–40.

Hampson DJ (1986b) Influence of creep feeding and dietary intake after weaning on malabsorption and occurrence of diarrhoea in the newly weaned pig. *Research in Veterinary Science* 41:63–69.

Hampson DJ and Fu ZF (1988) Pre-weaning supplementary feed and porcine post-weaning diarrhoea. *Research in Veterinary Science* 44:309–314.

Kelly D (1990) Effect of creep feeding on structural and functional changes of the gut of early weaned pigs. *Research in Veterinary Science* 48:350–356.

Kelly D, Smyth JA, and McCracken KJ (1991) Digestive development of the early-weaned pig: 1. Effect of continuous nutrient supply on the development of the digestive tract and on changes in digestive enzyme activity during the first week post-weaning. *British Journal of Nutrition* 65:169–180.

Kelly D, Begbie R, and King TP (1992) Postnatal intestinal development. In: *Neonatal Survival and Growth*, by Varley MA, Williams PEV, and Lawrence TLJ (ed), 63–79. Occasional Publication No. 15. British Society of Animal Production, Edinburgh, UK.

Kenworthy R and Allen WD (1966) Influence of diet and bacteria on small intestinal morphology with special reference to early-weaning and *Escherichia coli*. Studies on germ-free and gnotobiotic pigs. *Journal of Comparative Pathology* 76:291–296.

Kidder DE and Manners MJ (1978) *Digestion in the Pig*. Scientechnica, Bristol, UK.

King MR, Kelly D, Morel PCH, and Pluske JR (2003) Aspects of intestinal immunity in the pig around weaning. In: *Weaning the Pig – Concepts and Consequences*, by Pluske JR, Le Dividich J, and Verstegen MWA (ed), 219–257. Wageningen Academic Publishers, Wageningen, The Netherlands.

Koch F (2005) Organic acids in animal nutrition. *AminoNews* 6(1):11–18.

Lawrence NJ and Maxwell CV (1983) Effect of dietary fat source and level on the performance of neonatal and early weaned pigs. *Journal of Animal Science* 57:936–942.

Leibbrandt VD, Hays VW, Ewan RC, and Speer VC (1975) Effect of fat on performance of baby and growing pigs. *Journal of Animal Science* 40:1081–1084.

Li DF, Nelssen JL, Reddy PG, Blecha F, Hancock JD, Allee GL, Goodband RD, and Klemm RD (1990) Transient hypersensitivity to soybean meal in the early-weaned pig. *Journal of Animal Science* 68:1790–1799.

Li DF, Nelssen JL, Reddy PG, Blecha F, Klemm RD, and Goodband RD (1991a) Interrelationship between hypersensitivity to soybean proteins and growth performance in early-weaned pigs. *Journal of Animal Science* 69:4062–4069.

Li DF, Nelssen JL, Reddy PG, Blecha F, Klemm RD, Geisting DW, Hancock JD, Allee GL, and Goodband RD (1991b) Measuring suitability of soybean products for early-weaned pigs with immunological criteria. *Journal of Animal Science* 69:3299–3307.

Lindberg JE and Ogle B (2001) *Digestive Physiology of Pigs*. CAB International, Wallingford, UK.

Lindemann MD, Cornelius SG, Kandelgy SM, Moser RL, and Pettigrew JE (1986) Effect of age, weaning and diet on digestive enzyme levels in the piglet. *Journal of Animal Science* 62:1298–1307.

Madec F, Bridoux N, Bounaix S, and Justin A (1998) Measurement of digestive disorders in the piglet at weaning and related risk factors. *Preventive Veterinary Medicine* 35:53–72.

Manners MJ (1970) Milk replacers for piglets. *Journal of the Science of Food and Agriculture* 21:333–340.

McCracken BA, Gaskins HR, Ruwe-Kaiser PJ, Klasing KC, and Jewell DE (1995) Diet-dependent and diet-independent metabolic responses underlie growth stasis of pigs at weaning. *Journal of Nutrition* 125:2838–2845.

McCracken BA, Zijlstra RT, Donovan SM, Odle J, Lien EL, and Gaskins HR (1998) Neither intact nor hydrolyzed soy proteins elicit intestinal inflammation in neonatal piglets. *Journal of Parenteral and Enteral Nutrition* 22:91–97.

McCracken BA, Spurlock ME, Roos MA, Zuckermann FA, and Gaskins HR (1999) Weaning anorexia may contribute to local inflammation in the piglet small intestine. *Journal of Nutrition* 129:613–619.

Miller BG, Newby TJ, Stokes CR, and Bourne FJ (1984a) Influence of diet on postweaning malabsorption and diarrhoea in the pig. *Research in Veterinary Science* 36:187–193.

Miller BG, Newby TJ, Stokes CR, Hampson DJ, Brown PJ, and Bourne FJ (1984b) The importance of dietary antigen in the cause of postweaning diarrhea in pigs. *American Journal of Veterinary Research* 45:1730–1733.

Morillo TB, Carter SD, Genova S, Park JS, and Scneider JD (2003) Effects of reducing metabolizable energy concentration in diets containing spray-dried porcine plasma on weanling pig performance. *Journal of Animal Science* 81(Supplement 2):70.

Mroz Z (2003) Organic acids of various origins and physico-chemical forms as potential alternatives to antibiotic growth promoters for pigs. *Proceedings of 9th International Symposium on Digestive Physiology in Pigs (Volume 1)*, 267–293. University of Alberta, Canada.

Newby TJ, Miller B, Stokes CR, Hampson DJ, and Bourne FJ (1985) Local hypersensitivity response to dietary antigens in early weaned pigs. In: *Recent Developments in Pig Nutrition*, by Cole DJA and Haresign W (ed), 211–221. Butterworths, UK.

Odle J (1998) Medium-chain triglycerides: A unique energy source for neonatal pigs. *Pig News and Information* 20:25N–32N.

Parker DS and Armstrong DG (1987) Antibiotic feed additives and livestock production. *Proceedings of the Nutrition Society* 46:415–421.

Pluske JR, Williams IH, and Aherne FX (1996) Villous height and crypt depth in piglets in response to increases in the intake of cows' milk after weaning. *Animal Science* 62:145–158.

Polivoda DI, Derevins'kii VV, and Kudrik MA (1973) Shlunkove travleniya u porosyat pri rann'omu vidluchenni. *Svinovodstvo, Kiev* 26:68–73.

Shen WH and Liechty EA (2003) Digestion and absorption. In: *The Neonatal Pig: Gastrointestinal Physiology and Nutrition*, by Xu R-J and Cranwell P (ed), 157. Nottingham University Press, Nottingham, UK.

Shields RG, Ekstrom KE, and Mahan DC (1980) Effect of weaning age and feeding method on digestive enzyme development in swine from birth to ten weeks. *Journal of Animal Science* 50:257–265.

Smith HW and Jones JET (1963) Observations on the alimentary tract and its bacterial flora in healthy and diseased pigs. *Journal of Pathology and Bacteriology* 86:387–412.

Tokach MD, Dritz SS, Goodband RD, and Nelssen JL (2003) Nutritional requirements of the weaned pig. In: *Weaning the Pig – Concepts and Consequences*, by Pluske JR, Le Dividich J, and Verstegen MWA (ed), 259–299. Wageningen Academic Publishers, Wageningen, The Netherlands.

Touchette KJ, Allee GL, Newcomb MD, Pace LW, and Ellersieck MR (1997) Effect of feed intake and spray-dried plasma on nursery performance and intestinal morphology of weaned pigs. *Journal of Animal Science* 75(Supplement 1):198.

van Hees H, Vente-Spreeuwenberg M, and van Gils B (2005) Managing feed intake of weaned piglets: interactions between nutrition, ethology and farm management. In: *Animal Nutrition*, by Garnsworthy PC and Wiseman J (ed), 9–40. Nottingham University Press, Nottingham, UK.

Whittemore CT, Aumaitre A, and Williams IH (1978) Growth of body components in young weaned pigs. *Journal of Agricultural Science, Cambridge* 91:681–692.

Xu R-J and Cranwell P (2003) *The Neonatal Pig: Gastrointestinal Physiology and Nutrition*. Nottingham University Press, Nottingham, UK.

Yokata H and Coates ME (1982) The uptake of nutrients from the small intestine of gnotobiotic and conventional chicks. *British Journal of Nutrition* 47:349–356.

Zijlstra RT, McCracken BA, Odle J, Donovan SM, Gelberg HB, Petschow BW, Zuckermann FA, and Gaskins HR (1999) Malnutrition modifies pig small intestinal inflammatory responses to rotavirus. *Journal of Nutrition* 129:838–843.

3 Sow's Milk

Introduction

Sow's milk is widely accepted as the perfect nourishment (Fig. 3.1) for neonatal pigs (Darragh and Moughan, 1998). Thus, it is frequently used as the basis for developing milk replacer formulas and starter diets for piglets. The role of sow's milk, however, is not limited to nourishment of the piglet. Indeed, milk is a rich source of immunoglobulins that provide passive immunity against pathogens. It also contains a plethora of biopeptides that aid in the maturation and development of the gastrointestinal system and promote the establishment of a healthy microflora. Thus, to fully appreciate the biological significance of sow's milk it is imperative to understand its multiple roles and dynamic composition.

Colostrum

Colostrum is the first milk secreted during the first 24 to 48 h following birth. Its unique composition (Tables 3.1 and 3.2) is specifically suited to establish passive immunity and to nourish and sustain the suckling piglets. Colostrum contains about three times more proteins than mature (normal) milk, especially in the form of immunoglobulins, which are absorbed intact by the piglet during the first hours after parturition (King *et al.*, 2003).

The transition from colostrum to mature milk is gradual and is normally completed within the first week of lactation (Klobasa *et al.*, 1987). During this transition, the concentration of solids and proteins decreases and that of lactose and fat increases. Concurrently, the concentration of immuno-

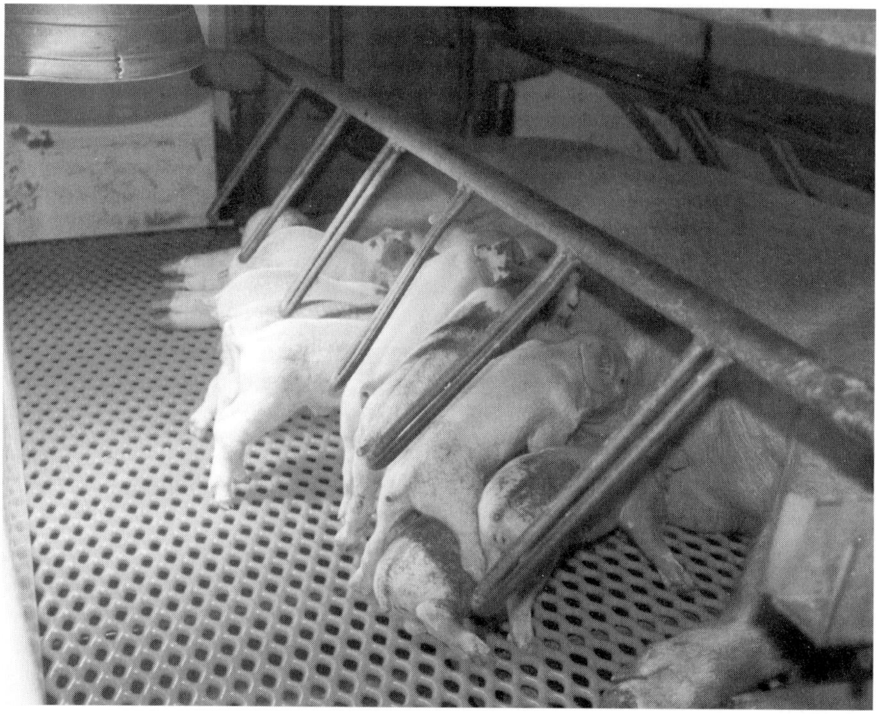

Fig. 3.1. Sow's milk remains the best nourishment for neonatal piglets.

globulins also decreases dramatically. Thus, the main role of (mature) milk becomes that of nourishment and secondary immunoprotection.

Piglets without a nursing sow may be reared artificially if they have access to colostrum during their first day of life (Veum and Odle, 2001). To this effect, bovine colostrum may be used, although porcine colostrum is preferred. Alternatively, a commercial immunoglobulin supplement may be an adequate replacement for natural colostrum if piglets will be reared under sanitary conditions. Ideally, piglets should be allowed to nurse a newly farrowed foster sow for a couple of hours before being placed in an artificial rearing scheme.

Nutrient Composition

Although the chemical composition of milk is in a dynamic state of change throughout the lactation, it becomes relatively stable after the first week (Klobasa *et al.*, 1987). Nutrient composition in mature milk is affected mainly by breed, nutrition, body condition, and health (Darragh and Moughan, 1998).

Table 3.1. Comparative composition of sow's colostrum and mature milk. (Compiled from Klobasa *et al.*, 1987; Csapo *et al.*, 1996; Darragh and Moughan, 1998.)

Component	Colostrum	Mature milk
Dry matter (%)	25	19
Protein (%, N × 6.25)	15	5.5
Fat (%)	6	7.5
Lactose (%)	3.5	5
Calcium (mg/100 ml)	68	163
Phosphorus (mg/100 ml)	102	118
Sodium (mg/100 ml)	68	39
Iron (mg/100 ml)	0.2	0.2
Potassium (mg/100 ml)	11	59
Vitamin A (mg/100 ml)	169	96
Vitamin E (mg/100 ml)	390	266
Vitamin C (mg/100 ml)	7	8

Table 3.2. Proteins in sow's colostrum and mature milk. (Compiled from Klobasa *et al.*, 1987; Csapo *et al.*, 1996; Darragh and Moughan, 1998.)

Component	Colostrum	Mature milk
Protein (%, N × 6.25)	15	5.5
Casein (%)	1.5	2.75
Whey (%)	15	2
IgA (mg/ml)	21	5
IgG (mg/ml)	96	1
IgM (mg/ml)	9	1.5

Ig, immunoglobulin.

Proteins

Sow's milk contains two predominant groups of protein, caseins and whey proteins. The ratio of casein to whey increases from 0.10 in colostrum milk to over 1.3 in mature milk (Table 3.2). This reflects the different role of each protein group. Whey proteins are predominantly associated with immune protection, whereas casein proteins are considered a primary source of amino acids (Jenness and Sloan, 1999).

Casein proteins are classified in several subtypes and are characterized by a higher concentration of glutamic acid, proline, and methionine (Gallagher *et al.*, 1997). Casein (from cow's milk) is over 95% digestible at terminal ileum (Rutherfurd and Moughan, 1998), depending on source and prior exposure to thermal treatment.

Whey proteins include albumin, α-lactalbumin, and β-lactoglobulin (Gallagher *et al.*, 1997). These proteins are also very digestible (Rutherfurd and Moughan, 1998) and appear to have a nutritional role similar to casein.

This is in contrast to whey immunoglobulins that provide passive immunity at the gastrointestinal level. Sow's milk contains IgA, IgG, and immunoglobulin M (IgM) (Table 3.2). Of these, IgA is predominant in mature milk, whereas colostrum is richer in IgG (Klobasa *et al.*, 1987). IgA acts mainly at the luminal epithelium level, whereas IgG is readily absorbed intact during the first few days after birth, providing systemic protection (King *et al.*, 2003). As a group, whey proteins are especially rich in cysteine, glycine, and threonine (Heine *et al.*, 1991) compared to caseins.

Lipids

The fat concentration in sow's milk is influenced primarily by breed (Fahmy, 1972; Alston-Mills *et al.*, 2000), although it tends to be different even among individual animals from the same breed (Perrin, 1955). For example, Meishan sows produce milk with 11% lipids compared to only 7–8% in milk from commercial Western breeds (Alston-Mills *et al.*, 2000). These differences in composition reflect an evolutionary adaptation in the Meishan breed to handle a larger litter (14–18 versus 9–11 pigs in Western sows) with lower birth weights (0.9 versus 1.4 kg/pig, respectively). This information could be used as an indication that smaller pigs may need diets richer in lipids (and calcium) to survive compared to larger littermates.

Fat concentration is also affected dramatically by sow nutrition, and especially by addition of dietary fat. From a comprehensive review of the literature (Pettigrew, 1981), it was estimated that sows consuming at least 1 kg fat (3–4% dietary fat when feed intake is about 2 kg/day) during the last two weeks before parturition give birth to more viable piglets and produce colostrum and milk with higher fat concentration. Feeding high-fat diets (8–10%) during lactation can also sustain higher levels of fat in milk to improve piglet growth and survivability (Pettigrew and Moser, 1991).

The main fatty acids in sow's milk are palmitic (37%), oleic (33%), and linoleic (8%) with trivial amounts of short-chain fatty acids (Csapo *et al.*, 1996). The fatty acid composition of milk fat is affected greatly by dietary fat source. For example (Hartmann and Holmes, 1989), beef tallow increases the concentration of oleic acid in milk, whereas corn oil increases linoleic acid. Medium-chain fatty acids such as palmitic acid are considered beneficial for young suckling piglets because they are more digestible than long-chain fatty acids (Odle, 1998). Sows on negative energy balance produce milk rich in long-chain fatty acids (Hartmann and Holmes, 1989).

Lactose

Mature milk contains about 5% lactose (Darragh and Moughan, 1998) and trivial amounts (<1%) of glucose, fructose, galactose, and other secondary metabolites of carbohydrate metabolism (Atwood and Hartmann, 1992). The ability of the sow to synthesize lactose is believed to be the major limit on milk yield (Mackenzie and Revell, 1998). For example, when lactose concentration in milk starts to decline (around the second week), milk yield increases dramatically, reaching its peak around the third week (Oftedal, 1984; cited by Darragh and Moughan, 1998).

The concentration of lactose in sow's milk is largely unaffected by nutrition. The only means of altering lactose concentration is by genetic manipulation. Indeed, researchers at the University of Illinois (Bleck *et al.*, 1998) have developed a genetically modified line of pigs that expresses the transgene of bovine α-lactalbumin, an integral component of lactose synthase, the enzyme that produces lactose. It has been reported that transgenic sows produce more milk with a higher concentration of lactose that results in significantly heavier piglets at weaning (Noble *et al.*, 2002).

Vitamins

The concentration of vitamins in mature milk declines as lactation advances, with the exception of vitamin C (Hidiroglou and Batra, 1995; Darragh and Moughan, 1998). Although pigs are able to synthesize ample quantities of vitamin C from the first week of life (Braude *et al.*, 1950), sow's milk is a rich source of vitamin C. In fact, sow's milk contains more vitamin C than milk from most species. For example, sow's and cow's milk contain about 8 and 2 mg vitamin C per 100 ml, respectively (Braude *et al.*, 1950; Csapo *et al.*, 1996). There is no logical explanation why sow's milk contains so much vitamin C, other than that of a rapid metabolism of vitamin C in neonatal pigs.

Sow's milk is a good source of vitamin D, but earlier reports (Hartmann and Holmes, 1989) indicated a possible deficiency in suckling piglets without access to sunlight. This is particularly important in production systems that practice late weaning in totally enclosed units with artificial lighting. In these cases, it is recommended that creep diets be fortified with superfluous quantities of vitamin D.

Minerals

The concentration of calcium in mature milk more than doubles compared with colostrum. The Ca/P ratio in mature milk is around 1.4, which is within the range recommended for most commercial solid diets (1.1–1.5). The relative bioavailability of phosphorus in cow's milk is very high (91%; NRC, 1998) and there is no evidence to indicate why it should not be at least as high in sow's milk.

Sow's colostrum and mature milk are both poor in iron (Table 3.1). This reflects an evolutionary adaptation to conditions where access to soil was not restricted. The same applies to milk from most species, and, for this reason, diets based on milk must always be fortified with iron. For the same purpose, commercially reared piglets should be provided with supplemental iron, either via injection or as an oral supplement, within the first week of life.

Digestibility of Sow's Milk

Sow's mature milk contains about 6.2 MJ gross energy (GE)/kg (Fowler and Gill, 1989). Whittemore (1998) used piglet growth as the basis to estimate that sow's milk contains about 5.4 MJ ME/kg. No studies are known regarding *in vivo* energy digestibility of sow's milk.

In an unpublished study (Livingstone *et al.*, 1959; cited by Lucas and Lodge, 1961), the total tract apparent digestibility of major nutrients in sow's milk was found to range from 92 to 98% (Table 3.3). These values are in close agreement with data generated from comparable studies using cow's milk (Wilson and Leibholz, 1981; Walker *et al.*, 1986).

In a more recent study (Mavromichalis *et al.*, 2001), the true digestibility of sow's milk was evaluated in piglets fitted with a simple T-cannula at the terminal ileum. Nitrogen and average amino acid digestibility values were 88 and 92%, respectively. These lower values represent the true digestibility of these nutrients without the confounding contributions of endogenous losses and hindgut microbial metabolism.

In the same study, amino acids found in abundance in whey proteins were less digestible than amino acids predominating in casein proteins. This reflects the resistant nature of immunoglobulins in whey proteins, which act primarily locally. Furthermore, when digestible amino acid concentrations in

Table 3.3. Apparent total tract digestibility of major nutrients in sow's milk[a]. (Adapted from Livingstone *et al.*, 1959; cited by Lucas and Lodge, 1961.)

	Digestibility (%) at 17–26 days of age	
	Pig 1	Pig 2
Dry matter	98	97
Protein	99	98
Lipids	99	98
Ash	96	93
Calcium	94	89
Phosphorus	98	97

[a] Piglets were fed 1 liter of milk daily from day 2 after birth.

sow's milk were expressed as ratios to digestible lysine, several amino acid ratios (threonine, tryptophan, and arginine) were lower than what has been considered optimal for maximal protein accretion (Table 3.4).

Biopeptides

Recently, our views regarding the many roles of sow's milk have expanded to include enhancement of gastrointestinal immunity against pathogenic microorganisms and, also, luminal nutrition from mature milk. Novel discoveries also indicate that milk affects the gastrointestinal microflora and aids in the establishment of healthy bacteria. Growth-promoting substances also have been reported in sow's milk, although their exact mode of action and significance (at least commercially) are still under investigation.

More specifically, sow's milk contains a number of peptides, hormones, and enzymes with a biological role capable of promoting maturation of the digestive system, modulating gut microflora, and inducing secretion of hormones and peptides in the gut (Lucas, 1986; James *et al.*, 1987). Such compounds include lactoferrin, lysozyme, protease inhibitors, lactoperoxidase, neurotensin, bombesin, thyroid hormones, prolactin, and insulin. In addition, several growth-stimulating substances such as insulin, epidermal growth factor, and insulin-like growth factors have been identified in sow's milk (Jaeger *et al.*, 1987).

The presence of insulin-like growth factors (IGF-I and IGF-II) in milk has received considerable attention because these compounds have been shown (Odle *et al.*, 1996; Burrin, 1997) to increase villus height and enhance maturation of the gastrointestinal tract. It is also believed that absorption of these factors might enhance development of body organs and promote muscle growth (Xu *et al.*, 1994). Today, there is considerable interest in the commercial aspects of using such compounds in milk replacers and other nutritional supplements for neonatal and weaned pigs.

Table 3.4. True ileal digestibility of amino acids in sow's milk. (Adapted from Mavromichalis *et al.*, 2001.)

	Total		True ileal digestible	
	%	Lysine = 100%	%	Lysine = 100%
Protein (N × 6.25)	4.80		88	
Lysine	2.09	100	92	100
Tryptophan	0.32	15	96	16
Threonine	1.24	59	84	54
Methionine	0.64	31	99	33
Cystine	0.53	25	84	23
Leucine	2.55	122	91	121
Isoleucine	1.15	55	90	54
Valine	1.62	78	87	73

Is Sow's Milk the Perfect Feed?

Milk has traditionally been considered the ideal feed for neonatal animals (Lucas and Lodge, 1961). Indeed, neonatal pigs fed on sow's milk alone can double their birth weight twice in 3 weeks. Without doubt, milk is the optimal nourishment for piglets within its evolutionary context, but questions have risen regarding its suitability for commercially raised piglets (Pluske and Dong, 1998).

As described in Chapter 1, artificially raised piglets (Hodge, 1974; Harrell *et al.*, 1993) are capable of growing at rates well beyond those possible by natural suckling. Thus, the quantity of sow's milk is a limiting factor by itself in determining piglet growth. For example, it has been suggested (Harrell *et al.*, 1993) that sows must produce over 18 kg milk/day, by day 21 of lactation, for piglets to achieve their genetic potential for growth. Obviously, this is more than currently possible in commercial farms.

Furthermore, sow's milk is rich in lipids and consequently energy. This results in a low protein/energy ratio (9–10 g/MJ GE), which favors fat instead of lean deposition in the neonatal piglet. Naturally, rapid fat deposition during the first weeks of life would favor survivability in wild pigs exposed to unfavorable environmental conditions, as pigs are born with extremely low body fat reserves (1–2%; Mellor and Cockburn, 1986). Under controlled (indoor) commercial conditions, however, excess lipid deposition might be unnecessary. Thus, sow's milk might be considered as deficient in protein for modern production practices. Williams (1995) indicated that sow's milk should contain around 50% more protein to maximize lean deposition and minimize lipid retention in piglets.

Finally, sow's milk (like milk from most farm animal species) is poor in iron, copper, and vitamin D (Darragh and Moughan, 1998). Under natural conditions, these nutrients were easily secured from contact with soil and exposure to sunlight and, thus, their presence in milk became evolutionarily redundant. Under modern commercial practices, however, piglets must be supplied with at least supplemental iron pre-weaning, and the full complement of all vitamins and minerals immediately after weaning.

In conclusion, it appears that sow's milk is not the perfect feed for neonatal pigs raised under commercial conditions. Its supply is limited and its composition does not favor lean deposition. To this end, nutritional supplements for suckling piglets and (or) nutritional intervention strategies for sows might be of benefit in terms of early piglet growth.

References

Alston-Mills B, Iverson SJ, and Thompson MP (2000) A comparison of the composition of milks from Meishan and crossbred pigs. *Livestock Production Science* 63:85–91.

Atwood CS and Hartmann PE (1992) Collection of fore and hind milk from the sow and the changes in milk composition during suckling. *Journal of Dairy Research* 59:287–298.

Bleck GT, White BR, Miller DJ, and Wheeler MB (1998) Production of bovine α-lactalbumin in the milk of transgenic pigs. *Journal of Animal Science* 76:3072–3078.

Braude R, Kon SK, and Porter JWG (1950) Studies in vitamin C metabolism of the pig. *British Journal of Nutrition* 4:185–199.

Burrin DG (1997) Is milk-borne insulin-like growth factor-1 essential for neonatal development? *Journal of Nutrition* 127:975S–979S.

Csapo J, Martin TG, Csapo-Kiss ZS, and Hazas Z (1996) Proteins, fats, vitamin and mineral concentrations in porcine colostrum and milk from parturition to 60 days. *International Dairy Journal* 6:881–902.

Darragh AJ and Moughan PJ (1998) The composition of colostrum and milk. In: *The Lactating Sow*, by Verstegen MWA, Moughan PJ, and Schrama JW (ed), 3–21. Wageningen Pers, Wageningen, The Netherlands.

Fahmy MH (1972) Comparative study of colostrum and milk composition of seven breeds of swine. *Canadian Journal of Animal Science* 52:621–627.

Fowler VR and Gill BP (1989) Voluntary food intake in the young pig. In: *The Voluntary Food Intake of Pigs*, by Forbes JM, Varley MA, and Lawrence TJ (ed), 51–60. Occasional Publication No. 13. British Society of Animal Production, Edinburgh.

Gallagher DP, Cotter PF, and Mulvihill DM (1997) Porcine milk proteins: a review. *International Dairy Journal* 7:99–118.

Harrell RJ, Thomas MJ, and Boyd RD (1993) Limitations of sow milk yield on baby pig growth. *Cornell Nutrition Conference for Feed Manufacturers*, 156–164. Cornell University, Ithaca, NY.

Hartmann PE and Holmes MA (1989) Sow lactation. In: *Manipulating Pig Production II. Proceedings of the Australasian Pig Science Association*, by Barnett JL and Hennessy DP (ed), 72–97. Australasian Pig Science Association, Werribee, Australia.

Heine WE, Klein PD, and Reeds PJ (1991) The importance of α-lactalbumin in infant nutrition. *Journal of Nutrition* 121:277–283.

Hidiroglou M and Batra TR (1995) Concentrations of vitamin C in milk of sows and in plasma of piglets. *Canadian Journal of Animal Science* 75:275–277.

Hodge RW (1974) Efficiency of food conversion and body composition of the preruminant lamb and the young pig. *British Journal of Nutrition* 32:113–126.

Jaeger LA, Lamar CH, Bottoms GD, and Cline TR (1987) Growth stimulating substances in porcine milk. *American Journal of Veterinary Research* 48:1531–1533.

James PS, Smith MW, Tivey DR, and Wilson TJG (1987) Epidermal growth factor selectively increases maltase and sucrase activities in neonatal piglet intestine. *Journal of Physiology* 393:583–594.

Jenness R and Sloan RE (1999) The composition of milks of various species: a review. *Dairy Science Abstracts* 32:599–612.

King MR, Kelly D, Morel PCH, and Pluske JR (2003) Aspects of intestinal immunity in the pig around weaning. In: *Weaning the Pig – Concepts and Consequences*, by Pluske JR, Le Dividich J, and Verstegen MWA (ed), 219–257. Wageningen Academic Publishers, Wageningen, The Netherlands.

Klobasa F, Werhahn E, and Butler JE (1987) Composition of sow milk during lactation. *Journal of Animal Science* 64:1458–1466.

Lucas A (1986) Breast feeding and gut hormones. In: *The Breastfed Infant – A Model for Performance*, by Filer LJ and Fomon SJ (ed), 73–83. Ross Laboratories, Columbus, OH.

Lucas IAM and Lodge GA (1961) *Nutrition of the Young Pig*. Technical Bulletin No. 22. Commonwealth Agricultural Bureaux, Farnham Royal, UK.

Mackenzie DDS and Revell DK (1998) Genetic influences on milk quantity. In: *The Lactating Sow*, by Verstegen MWA, Moughan PJ, and Schrama JW (ed), 97–112. Wageningen Pers, Wageningen, The Netherlands.

Mavromichalis I, Parr TM, Gabert VM, and Baker DH (2001) True ileal digestibility of amino acids in sow's milk for 17-day-old pigs. *Journal of Animal Science* 79:707–713.

Mellor DJ and Cockburn F (1986) A comparison of energy metabolism in the newborn infant, piglet and lamb. *Quarterly Journal of Experimental Physiology* 71:361–379.

Noble MS, Rodriguez-Zas S, Bleck GT, Cook JS, Hurley WL, and Wheeler MB (2002) Lactational performance of first parity transgenic gilts expressing bovine α-lactalbumin in their milk. *Journal of Animal Science* 80:1090–1096.

NRC (1998) *Nutrient Requirements of Swine* (10th edn). National Academy Press, Washington, DC.

Odle J, Zijlstra RT, and Donovan SM (1996) Intestinal effects of milkborne growth factors in neonates of agricultural importance. *Journal of Animal Science* 74:2509–2522.

Odle J (1998) Medium-chain triglycerides: a unique energy source for neonatal pigs. *Pig News and Information* 20:25N–32N.

Perrin DR (1955) The chemical composition of the colostrum and milk of the sow. *Journal of Dairy Research* 22:103–107.

Pettigrew JE (1981) Supplemental dietary fat for peripartal sows: a review. *Journal of Animal Science* 53:107–117.

Pettigrew JE and Moser RL (1991) Fat in swine nutrition. In: *Swine Nutrition*, by Miller ER, Ullrey DE, and Lewis AJ (ed), 133–146. Butterworth-Heinemann, Stoneham, MA.

Pluske JR and Dong GZ (1998) Factors influencing the utilization of colostrum and milk. In: *The Lactating Sow*, by Verstegen MWA, Moughan PJ, and Schrama JW (ed), 45–70. Wageningen Pers, Wageningen, The Netherlands.

Rutherfurd SM and Moughan PJ (1998) The digestible amino acid composition of several milk proteins: application of a new bioassay. *Journal of Dairy Science* 81:909–917.

Veum TL and Odle J (2001) Feeding neonatal pigs. In: *Swine Nutrition* (2nd edn), by Lewis AJ and Southern LL (ed), 671–690. CRC Press LLC, Boca Raton, FL.

Walker WR, Maxwell CV, Owens FN, and Buchanan DS (1986) Milk versus soybean protein sources for pigs: I. Effects on performance and digestibility. *Journal of Animal Science* 63:505–512.

Whittemore CT (1998) *The Science and Practice of Pig Production* (2nd edn). Blackwell Science Ltd, Oxford, UK.

Williams IH (1995) Sow milk as a major nutrient source before weaning. In: *Manipulating Pig Production V*, by Hennessy DP and Cranwell PD (ed), 107–113. Australasian Pig Science Association, Werribee, Australia.

Wilson RH and Leibholz J (1981) Digestion in the pig between 7 and 35 d of age. 3. The digestion of nitrogen in pigs given milk and soyabean proteins. *British Journal of Nutrition* 45:337–346.

Xu R-J, Mellor DJ, Birtles MJ, Breier BH, and Gluckman PD (1994) Effects of oral IGF-I or IGF-II on digestive organ growth in newborn piglets. *Biology of the Neonate* 66:280–287.

4 Feed Intake and Management

Introduction

Low feed intake – or, more appropriately, inadequate feed intake – is the main theme in young pig nutrition. There is a myriad of reasons why piglets will not eat enough to fully express their genetic potential for early growth. Not only commercial husbandry practices hinder development of early appetite, but also management inadequacies often exaggerate the problem. Growth in suckling pigs is often limited by inadequate milk yield and generally poor intake of creep feed. Weaned pigs usually go through an initial phase of anorexia, as they are abruptly switched from sow's milk to solid feed, followed by abnormal patterns of feed intake for the first couple of weeks post-weaning. Following this adjustment period, feed intake increases markedly, but never reaches potential maximum because of restrictions in physical gut capacity and competition among pen mates. Thus, nutritional and management interventions with the potential of increasing feed intake are always in high demand.

Why Young Pigs Do Not Eat Enough

To better understand the problem of inadequate early feed intake under standard commercial conditions, it is beneficial to consider the natural development of appetite for solid feed in the young wild pig (see also Brooks and Tsourgiannis, 2003).

Under natural conditions, piglets remain in the nest until about 10 days of age, receiving sow's milk as their only source of nutrients and water (Jensen and Redbo, 1987). Following their introduction to the herd, young pigs gradually start to root and forage as they imitate the behavior of their mother (primarily) and that of other experienced pigs (Jensen, 1986). With increasing experience in foraging, intake of solid feed naturally increases in a gradual pattern. By the end of the fourth week of age, milk yield starts to decline and the sow ceases to lie down to milk her litter, forcing piglets to drink while standing (Boe, 1991). This restricts intake of milk, which in turn encourages further foraging behavior. Weaning in the wild is a gradual process starting between 4 and 8 weeks of age (Jensen and Recen, 1989) as pigs become progressively more dependent on foraging than sow's milk. Although some litters may receive an occasional drink of milk up to 20 weeks of age, most pigs are weaned completely by the end of the 16th week of age (Boe, 1991).

The natural process of gradual weaning enables the young pig to learn how and when to forage and what to eat as dependence on sow's milk declines over a period of many weeks. It also allows for adaptation of the digestive system to handle feed of a form and composition quite distinctive from that of milk. Additionally, until complete weaning, milk continues to offer some immunological (passive) protection as piglets develop their own active immune system (Miller and Slade, 2003).

Under commercial conditions, young pigs remain with their mother until about 3 weeks of age. In some areas of the world, weaning takes place as early as 10 days of age, whereas in others it is delayed until pigs are 42 days of age or older (Mavromichalis and Varley, 2003). Nevertheless, in most if not all cases, weaning is an abrupt event taking place spontaneously as piglets are separated from their dams. Following weaning in intensive production systems, piglets are faced with behavioral, nutritional, and immunological challenges that culminate in depressed feed intake, poor health, and weak growth performance (Fig. 4.1).

Without considerable experience in consuming creep feed, weaned pigs are unlikely to associate dry diets offered in unfamiliar self-feeders with acceptable nourishment (Aherne *et al.*, 1982; Kelly, 1990). For this reason, weaning over 21 days of age is believed to reduce the negative impact of weaning on feed intake, as it generally allows pigs at least some experience with creep feed (see Chapter 10). To the same end, liquid diets and milk replacers are also considered more acceptable forms of nourishment for early-weaned pigs (see Chapter 11), as their composition and physical form are not as unfamiliar as those of dry feed. Finally, it has been shown that the natural rooting instinct can be easily exploited to the benefit of the pig when feed is spread on the floor or an appropriate floor-mat (Mavromichalis and Baker, 2000).

Following early weaning, piglets are additionally required not only to recognize an unusual diet as nourishment but also to decide when and how much to eat. Before weaning, feeding was a communal event initiated usually by the sow (Lewis and Hurnik, 1986). After weaning, piglets must satisfy their hunger at their own accord. At the same time, they must

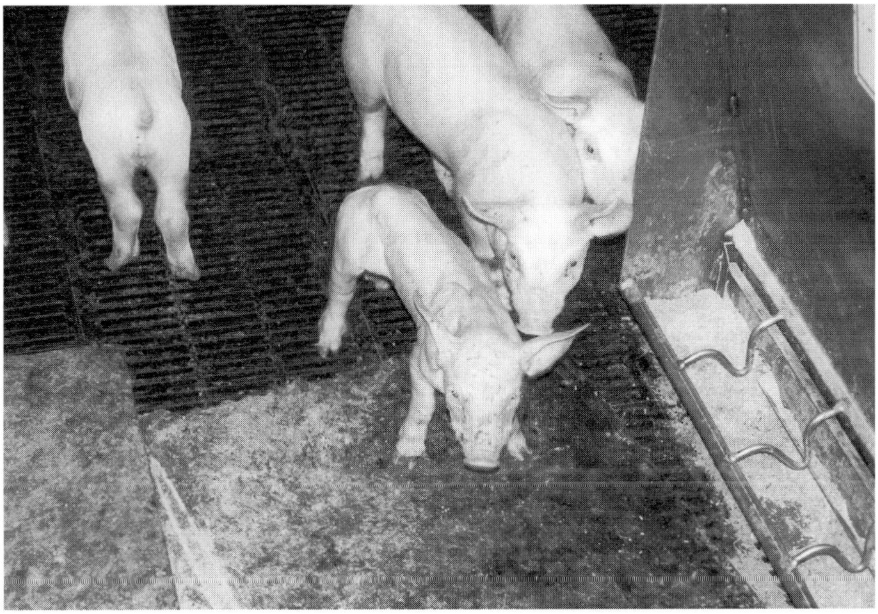

Fig. 4.1. Pigs that fail to establish vigorous eating patterns during the early post-weaning period often end up sick.

distinguish thirst from hunger and learn how to fulfill these needs via separate media, as water is no longer an integral part of their feed. In this aspect, it is obvious that liquid diets offer clear advantages over solid diets in terms of development of early appetite (see Chapter 11).

Nutritional challenges come not only from differences in form (dry versus liquid), but also in the nutrient composition of feed. Sow's milk is extremely rich in highly digestible fat (40% in DM), protein (25% in DM), and lactose (25% in DM). In contrast, most piglet diets are rather low in fat (usually below 10%) and extremely rich in starch (often over 60%), which is not as digestible as lactose. To this effect, most high-quality piglet feeds are fortified with lactose, easily digestible oils, specialty proteins, and cooked cereals (Cole and Sprent, 2001). It is remarkable, however, how rapidly the digestive system adapts to changes in dietary nutrient composition. For example, ingestion of starch induces secretion of sufficient quantities of amylolytic enzymes from the gastrointestinal tract within 4 days (Kidder and Manners, 1978). For such rapid digestive adaptation, however, feed intake must be relatively higher than usually achieved currently under most commercial conditions.

Immunological challenges at weaning are usually complicated by the transition from passive immunity (from sow's milk) to active (from self) immunity. It is well established that passive immunity starts to decline rapidly, reaching its minimum about the third week after birth. In contrast, active immunity builds up slowly and the process is not complete until pigs are several months old (King *et al.*, 2003). Thus, segregated early weaning, which takes place before the third week of age, offers the benefits of high levels of passive immunity (Nelssen *et al.*, 1999). In contrast, however, late weaning offers benefits from enhanced levels of active immunity. Currently, the balance is believed to be between the third and fourth week of age (Whittemore and Green, 2001).

When pigs are transferred to a nursery facility with a host of microorganisms against which they have no chance of acquiring passive immunity or developing their own active immunity, the system is activated to deter these novel pathogens (Williams *et al.*, 1997a). Under these conditions, feed intake is depressed invariably through the release of pro-inflammatory cytokines that alter metabolism and induce muscle protein degradation (Klasing, 1988). To this end, ensuring high standards of hygiene is the best way of maximizing feed intake and growth performance in piglets.

In conclusion, it appears that depressed feed intake after abrupt weaning under commercial conditions is nothing but a 'natural' response to challenges against which pigs did not have enough evolutionary time to adapt! Thus, unless weaning age increases considerably to match the pig's biological profile, current management and nutritional interventions can only alleviate the negative effects of early weaning, as some loss of growth potential appears unavoidable at the moment.

General Factors that Limit Feed Intake

Apart from the negative effects of abrupt weaning on feed intake and growth, there are several other factors that can depress feed intake throughout the nursery period.

Although factors that depress growth invariably reduce feed intake (e.g. disease), there is still considerable debate whether factors that depress feed intake by itself may be negated by increased nutrient intake (e.g. through increased dietary nutrient density). This leads to the puzzling question whether pigs grow because they eat or eat because they desire to grow; a clear answer to which remains currently elusive. It is evident, however, that when management-imposed restrictions on feed intake (e.g. limited feeder space) are removed, feed intake increases proportionally and pigs grow faster (Hyun *et al.*, 1998). It is also unequivocal that when feed or nutrient intake is artificially increased (e.g. by gavage feeding or nutrient-dense diets), pigs fail to respond in terms of increased growth if they are sick or stressed by crowding (Murray and Murray, 1979).

It is suggested here that there are factors that limit feed intake (mostly external) with obvious negative consequences on growth, and factors that limit growth (mostly internal) with ensuing depression of feed intake. In the former case, growth is hampered by lack of nutrients and remedy of the limiting factor usually improves feed intake and growth. In the latter case, feed is not consumed because excess nutrients constitute at best a burden and at worst a toxicant for the challenged organism. Restoration of feed intake follows removal of the causative factor that limits growth.

Competition for feed

Inappropriate management decisions usually reduce feed intake due to restricted access to the feeder. Such management decisions generally involve group size for facilities/equipment used, stocking density, pen design, and feeder/drinker placement and design (Wolter *et al.*, 2000; Brumm and Gonyou, 2001). Frequent handling and mixing may also increase aggression among unfamiliar pigs that could result in some pigs (subordinate or injured) being denied free access to feed for many days. Multiple stress factors have additive effects on growth and feed intake, and by one estimate (Hyun *et al.*, 1998) may reduce performance by about 10% each.

Temperature

It is well known that growing-finishing pigs and sows adjust their feed intake according to seasonal patterns of temperature (Whittemore, 1998). Pigs raised under their lower critical temperature eat more to generate metabolic heat that keeps them warm. In contrast, pigs under heat stress reduce their feed intake to curtail generation of metabolic heat.

Because piglets do not have the physical capacity to indiscriminately increase feed intake to compensate for reduced environmental temperature, they use dietary energy to keep warm. During the late stages of the nursery period (usually over 12 kg body weight), pigs are often capable of moderate increases in feed intake in response to moderate declining room temperature (Brumm *et al.*, 1995).

Pigs require approximately 0.015 MJ ME/kg $BW^{0.75}$ for each degree Celsius below their thermoneutral zone (Whittemore and Fawcett, 1976). Thus, a piglet kept at 2°C under its comfort zone throughout the nursery period (6–25 kg) diverts energy from about 600 g feed just to keep warm (assuming dietary ME density is 16 MJ/kg and a growth curve similar to that presented in Chapter 1). With an expected feed/gain ratio of around 1.5, it is obvious that exit weight will be about 400 g less unless pigs manage to eat more throughout the nursery period.

Gut capacity

Limited gut capacity is one of the main reasons restricting feed intake in pigs below 50 kg body weight (Black *et al.*, 1986). Feed intake that approximates gut capacity may be roughly calculated at around four times maintenance needs when diets of low fiber content are used, but it may be estimated more precisely by (Whittemore, 1998):

$$\text{Gut capacity (kg/day)} = 0.14 \times \text{BW}^{0.75}. \tag{4.1}$$

More intricate estimates may be obtained by allowing for differences in digestibility of dietary organic matter, reflecting largely fiber concentration and its water-holding capacity. Thus, the following equation has also been suggested (Whittemore, 1998):

$$\text{Gut capacity (kg/day)} = (0.013 \times \text{BW})/(1 - \text{digestibility coefficient}). \tag{4.2}$$

For example, according to Equation 4.1, gut capacity in pigs weighing 10, 20, or 30 kg is estimated around 0.79, 1.32, or 1.79 kg/day, respectively. Assuming 80% overall feed digestibility, gut capacity is predicted at 0.65, 1.30, or 1.95 kg/day, respectively, by Equation 4.2. According to the same equation, if digestibility increases from 80 to 85% (+6.25%), estimated gut capacity increases by 33% and actually doubles when digestibility reaches 90%. This reflects the tremendous potential in enhanced growth performance by offering highly digestible diets to young pigs.

Gastrointestinal fill

Gastrointestinal fill differs from gut capacity in that it reflects the amount of feed and digesta present in the gastrointestinal system at a given time. In the young pig, this figure is highly variable but it is commonly estimated at 5% of body weight (Lawrence and Fowler, 1997). Naturally, gut fill is strongly associated with dietary fiber, because fiber increases the volume and weight of the digesta by attracting water (Mosenthin *et al.*, 1991). Excess dietary fiber (usually over 3–4%) also reduces overall nutrient digestibility, resulting in even more gut fill (Wenk, 2001). Thus, when dietary fiber is in excess of 4%, gut fill may be estimated by the following equation (Lawrence and Fowler, 1997):

$$\text{Gut fill (\%)} = 5 + 0.4 \times [\text{crude fiber (\%)} - 4]. \tag{4.3}$$

Diurnal feeding patterns also affect gut fill because feed intake is generally reduced during the night and peaks in the morning hours (Gonyou *et al.*, 1998). Gut fill may be an important confounding factor in trials comparing feeds or ingredients of different fiber concentration.

Health status

Pigs are continuously exposed to pathogenic and non-pathogenic microorganisms through their interaction with the environment and other animals. Even though disease may not always prevail, chronic exposure to antigens constantly triggers the immune system and causes subclinical disease symptoms that are difficult to identify and quantify (Johnson *et al.*, 2001). Antigenic stimuli activate the immune system and cause the release of pro-inflammatory cytokines that modulate the immune response and alter intermediate metabolism (Klasing, 1988). The most important cytokines are IL-1, IL-6, and TNF-α that are produced in massive amounts during immunological stress (Johnson, 1997). These cytokines, which are considered essential for the defense of the host, also reduce appetite, increase muscle protein degradation, reduce muscle protein synthesis, and divert nutrients to the synthesis of components of the immune system such as acute-phase proteins (Spurlock, 1997; Mitchell *et al.*, 2001). Thus, overall metabolism is switched from anabolism and growth in the healthy pig to catabolism and muscle loss in the challenged pig. The negative effects of chronic activation of the immune system (i.e. subclinical disease) in pigs reared under immunological stress are illustrated in Table 1.2. From this study (Williams *et al.*, 1997b), it is apparent that pigs of high health status consume more feed, grow faster, and are more efficient than pigs under constant immunological stress. Healthy pigs also deposit more protein and proportionally less fat than challenged pigs. It is clearly evident that increasing dietary lysine to counteract the negative effects of reduced feed intake in immunologically challenged pigs does not increase growth or protein deposition rate.

Energy density

Fiber in diets for young pigs not only decreases nutrient digestibility but it also dilutes energy density, as benefits from fermentation at the hindgut level are extremely limited in young pigs. In general, increasing fiber concentration in piglet feeds usually results in reduced ingestion of nutrients, unless diets are balanced to account for reduced feed intake. It is well established that growth in piglets is dependent on energy intake (Campbell *et al.*, 1975) and since feed intake is not responsive to energy density, high-energy diets are strongly recommended to enhance growth in young pigs.

Imbalanced diets

A slight imbalance in the energy to protein (amino acids) ratio does not cause significant changes in feed intake, although feed efficiency is likely to deteriorate. Severe amino acid imbalances and (or) deficiencies, however, are expected to markedly suppress feed intake and consequently growth (D'Mello, 1994). Pigs are not expected to compensate by eating more when offered a diet with an imbalanced protein profile.

Palatability

It is often assumed that pigs will consume more of a given feed when a certain flavor is added to their diet. Indeed, pigs consume more of a flavored diet when given free choice alongside a similar diet without flavor. When not given a choice, however, pigs will consume similar amounts of each feed regardless of the presence of flavor (Wahlstrom *et al.*, 1974). Despite the fact that comprehensive research projects and numerous literature reviews have clearly demonstrated the ineffectiveness of flavors in pig diets, commercial practice defies such knowledge.

It is also well known that pigs prefer a fresh to a stale diet. For example, when rancidity increases due to prolonged storage feed intake drops dramatically (DeRouchey *et al.*, 1999). Pigs also prefer a sweet or sour diet as they seem to consume readily diets based on bakery products or liquid dairy products. There is limited evidence indicating that recently weaned pigs may benefit from sweet diets, especially those supplemented with a high-intensity sweetener (Purser *et al.*, 2000), but more research is needed to clarify in which type of diet (complex versus simple) such products may be most beneficial.

Flavors are often used to mask off-flavors from certain unpalatable ingredients, usually of generally lower quality, or from specific medications or other supplements used in high concentrations. But the greatest benefit of aromas and sweeteners is their marketing appeal to human operators in pig facilities.

Water intake

In general, pigs consume water according to their feed intake (usually in ratio of 3:1). In young pigs, however, the reverse is actually observed as feed intake is markedly driven by availability of easily accessible water (Brooks, 1998). Thus, ensuring that weaned pigs locate and learn how to use drinkers is of paramount importance to the establishment of a healthy early appetite, as is availability of drinker spaces and flow rate. It is commonly suggested that young pigs are encouraged to drink more from open-surface containers (bowls and turkey drinkers) than nipple-type drinkers (see Chapter 12).

Prediction of Feed Intake

It is rather difficult, if not impossible, to predict feed intake in piglets without a good knowledge of the above factors and historical records. Nevertheless, several authorities have risked empirical expressions to predict feed intake, at least past the phase of post-weaning anorexia that lasts about 2 weeks post-weaning.

For all practical purposes, optimal feed intake for piglets under non-limiting conditions may be estimated with reasonable accuracy by the equation proposed by Whittemore (1983):

$$\text{Feed intake (g/day)} = 120 \times \text{BW}^{0.75}. \quad (4.4)$$

This equation approaches maximum gut capacity (see Equation 4.1). It is notable, however, that dietary energy concentration is not taken into account in the above estimate of feed intake, as the pig's ability to adjust feed intake based on dietary energy density is not prevalent until pigs reach 20–30 kg body weight (Black *et al.*, 1986). Nevertheless, Cole *et al.* (1967) proposed the following equation that may be used to predict energy intake in young pigs with reasonable accuracy:

$$\text{Digestible energy intake (MJ/day)} = 2.4 \times \text{BW}^{0.68}. \quad (4.5)$$

Likewise, NRC (1988) proposed an empirical equation for 5–15 kg pigs based on body weight:

$$\text{Digestible energy intake (MJ/day)} = 1.93 \times \text{BW} - 0.0407 \times \text{BW}^2 - 6.4. \quad (4.6)$$

Based on the these equations, predicted feed intake is presented in Fig. 4.2 for pigs between 5 and 30 kg body weight consuming a diet with 16 MJ digestible energy (DE)/kg. Clearly, the first two equations overestimate feed intake during the initial phases of the nursery period, whereas the third equation assumes suboptimal intake during the final phases.

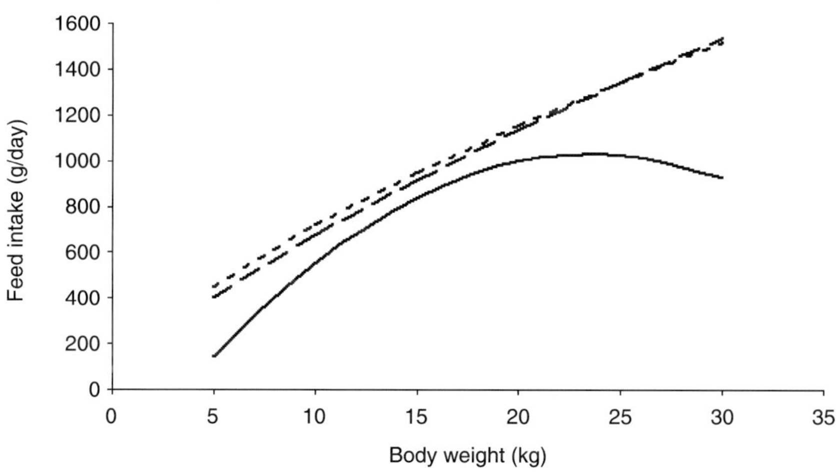

Fig. 4.2. Maximum feed intake as limited by gut capacity in young pigs (– – –, Equation 4.4; - - -, Equation 4.5; ——, Equation 4.6; see text for equations).

Intake of Sow's Milk

On average, pigs grow about 250 g/day during the course of a typical 3-week lactation period, whereas small litters or litters on very productive sows may reach or even exceed 300 g/day. If lactation exceeds 3 weeks, piglet growth is greatly influenced by the consumption of creep feed, as sows reach their maximum milk yield around this time. Typical growth rates for 4-, 5-, and 6-week lactation periods are around 275, 300, and 325 g/day, respectively, always depending on the success of the creep-feeding program and the sow's milking ability.

For maintenance purposes, piglets require about 0.44 MJ ME/kg $BW^{0.75}$ (NRC, 1998). Assuming that sow's milk contains around 5.4 MJ ME/kg (Whittemore, 1998), it is calculated that a 6-kg piglet requires daily at least 310 g milk only for maintenance during the third week post-weaning. An additional (250×4) 1000 g milk are needed to grow at 250 g/day (Whittemore, 1998), bringing the total to 1310 g/day or about 250 g DM. This is roughly equivalent to 280 g solid (creep) feed, giving a theoretical feed/gain of about (280/250) 1.10. For pigs weaned beyond the third week of age, intake of creep feed must make up the difference in growth targets, especially with declining milk production.

Intake of Creep Feed

Intake of creep feed is highly variable and largely unpredictable as variability exists not only among but also within litters (Appleby *et al.*, 1992). In general, intake of creep feed increases and becomes more predictable as age at weaning is delayed.

Most authorities agree that creep feeding is beneficial mainly in production systems where pigs are weaned beyond the third week of age (Pluske *et al.*, 1995). Pigs weaned before the third week of age concentrate their efforts in stimulating milk production by the sow (Brooks and Tsourgiannis, 2003), rather than supplementing their diet with solid creep feed. It is notable that neonatal pigs will not consume a highly digestible and palatable creep diet even though they have the genetic potential of almost doubling their growth rate. Even liquid milk replacers enhance pre-weaning growth rate to a limited degree (Azain *et al.*, 1996) when pigs are weaned before the third week of lactation. Nevertheless, some pigs start sampling creep feed by the second week of age, and a few become regular eaters consuming substantial quantities of feed. On average, however, consumption is extremely limited and rarely exceeds 10 g/day per piglet (Metz and Gonyou, 1990; Pajor *et al.*, 1991).

Intake of creep feed becomes substantial, yet still insufficient to fully cover nutrient needs for genetic potential, in the fourth week of lactation. During this time, the majority of pigs consume at least some creep feed, whereas a small proportion may consume large quantities regularly (up to 500 g/day). On average, creep feed intake in pigs weaned around 4 weeks of age is about 100 g/day per piglet (Metz and Gonyou, 1990).

For pigs weaned later than 4 weeks of age, creep feed intake increases almost linearly and may reach up to 1 kg/day in pigs weaned at 8 weeks of age (Boe and Jensen, 1995). However, variation remains extremely high even at this late age, and greatly affects piglet growth rates. For example, in pigs weaned at 8 weeks of age (Boe and Jensen, 1995), intake of creep feed ranged from 0 to almost 1600 g/day per piglet during the last week of lactation, with pigs weighing from 6 to 27 kg in body weight at the time of weaning.

Substantial intake of creep feed confers the benefits of heavier pigs at weaning and the digestive experience of solid feed. Heavier pigs at weaning not only grow faster throughout market age, but also require less complex diets during the post-weaning period (see Chapter 1). Pigs with sufficient experience in consuming solid feed during lactation suffer less from post-weaning anorexia. Thus, their growth is penalized less by the weaning event, and their digestive system remains healthier. It has been suggested that at least 500 g feed must be consumed before weaning (Pluske *et al.*, 1995; English, 1999) for young pigs to truly benefit from creep feeding. Consumption of insufficient quantities of solid feed (less than 500 g/pig) triggers an enteric allergenic reaction to certain dietary antigenic proteins (as in soybean meal), but it does not allow for education of the digestive immune system to handle such proteins at weaning (Hampson, 1986). For these reasons, creep feeding for pigs weaned at 3 weeks of age or less is practically ineffective.

Feed Intake during the First Week Post-weaning

It is accepted today that pigs experience minimal nutritional challenge at weaning if they manage to sustain their pre-weaning growth rate during the first week post-weaning. To illustrate how much feed must be consumed to sustain a growth rate of 250 g/day, the following assumptions must be made (NRC, 1998; Whittemore, 1998):

- Energy requirements for maintenance are 0.44 MJ ME/kg $BW^{0.75}$.
- Weight gain requires 16 MJ ME/kg (less fat deposited compared to suckling pigs).
- A 21-day-old piglet weighs about 6.5 kg at weaning.
- Pigs do not catabolize body fat to support protein deposition or maintenance.
- Post-weaning diet contains 16.5 MJ ME/kg and is balanced for all nutrients.

Based on these assumptions, it is calculated that 1.8 MJ ME are required for maintenance and 4 MJ ME for growth daily, for a total of 5.8 MJ ME/day.

Thus, if pigs were to catabolize no body fat for maintenance, they would need to consume about (1.8/16.5 × 100) 109 g feed per day simply to sustain body weight and its composition. To grow at 250 g/day, another (4/16.5 × 1000) 242 g feed would be required, bringing total feed intake to just over 350 g/day.

It is evident that to grow at a similar growth rate (250 g/day), a weaned pig must consume more dry matter (feed) than a suckling pig. In the above examples, 350 g feed or 57% more feed was required to sustain similar growth, but of different composition, enjoyed by a suckling pig consuming the equivalent of roughly 280 g feed (milk solids converted to 90% DM in feed). This, of course, reflects the higher energy density in milk (25.6 versus 16.5 MJ ME/kg on 90% DM) and the disposition of suckling piglets to deposit fat.

Based on these calculations, feed efficiency (feed/gain) should be (350/250) 1.4. This is remarkably higher compared to current commercial performance records, where it is not uncommon for feed/gain to be around 1 during the first week post-weaning. This apparent paradox is explained by the fact that commercially raised pigs actually lose fat and gain protein and water during the first couple of weeks post-weaning (Whittemore *et al.*, 1978).

If we were to allow for about 50 g body fat to be catabolized daily for energy, 1.67 MJ ME would be generated, assuming that catabolized body fat yields 33.4 MJ ME/kg. This is the equivalent of roughly 100 g feed (16.5 MJ ME/kg), which would lower daily feed intake requirements to 250 g, giving the familiar (250/250) 1:1 feed/gain ratio. Indeed, it has been observed that post-weaned pigs may lose at least 50 g or more fat per day during the first week (or even longer) post-weaning in substitution for water retention (Whittemore *et al.*, 1978). Thus, in severe cases of fat depletion, apparent feed efficiency may be even lower than 1:1, but this is an indication of reduced appetite rather than improved feed digestibility.

The above calculations assume the use of a high-energy (i.e. high-fat) diet. Because young pigs cannot adjust feed intake to maintain constant energy intake when dietary energy decreases (Black *et al.*, 1986), it is imperative they have constant access to high-energy diets to ensure maximal energy intake. It is apparent that more feed is required to sustain growth if dietary energy concentration is reduced (Fig. 4.3). However, young pigs do not utilize fat very efficiently (Cera *et al.*, 1989) and, thus, they often fail to respond to high-fat diets, especially when factors that limit their growth potential are present (e.g. disease).

Under most commercial conditions, feed intake rarely exceeds 200 g/day on average during the first week post-weaning for pigs weaned before the fourth week of lactation. In fact, feed intake may often be well below 100 g during the first couple of days post-weaning, whereas individual piglets may actually starve for as long as 5 to 7 days (Fig. 4.4). Exceptional levels of early feed intake are achieved usually in high-health operations and

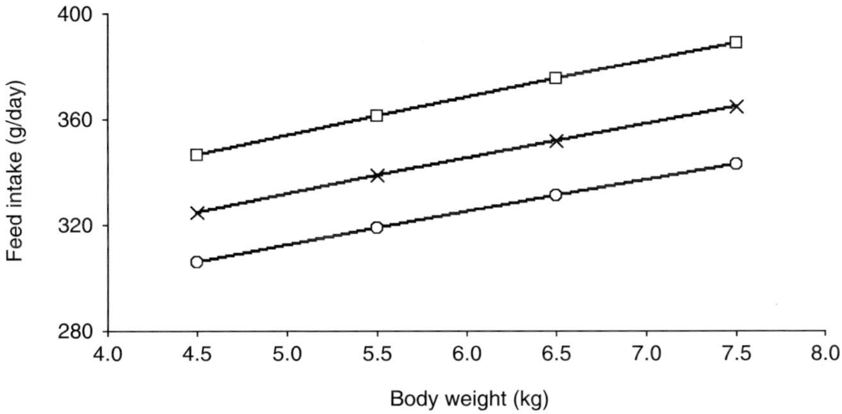

Fig. 4.3. Feed intake to gain 250 g/day during the first week post-weaning on diets with different of dietary energy concentration (—□—, 15 MJ metabolizable energy (ME)/kg; —×—, 16 MJ ME/kg; —○—, 17 MJ ME/kg).

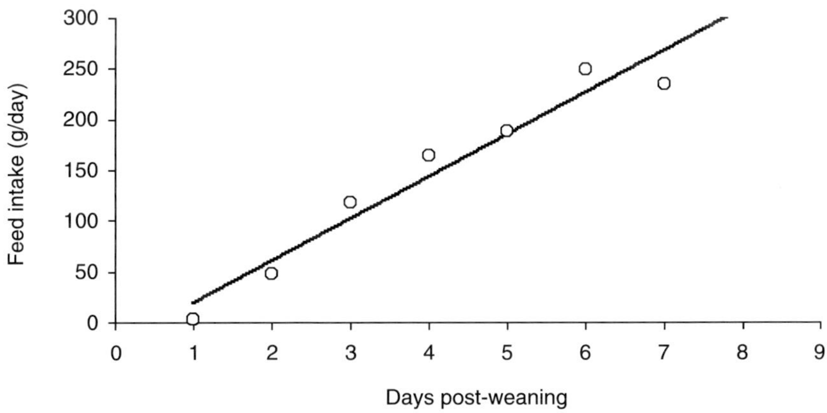

Fig. 4.4. Actual mean feed disappearance of 12 pens of pigs (six pigs per pen) during the first week post-weaning: Intake (g/day) = 41 × day – 23, $r^2 = 0.95$. (From Mavromichalis and Baker, 2000.)

with appropriate diets and feeding management techniques (Fig. 4.5). Naturally, longer lactation periods confer the benefit of familiarity with solid feed and, thus, feed intake is relatively higher post-weaning, although some anorexia is evident even in pigs weaned at 6 weeks of age.

Ways to Enhance Feed Intake Post-weaning

From the above discussion, it is evident that under most commercial conditions, weaned pigs are expected to experience some degree of appetite

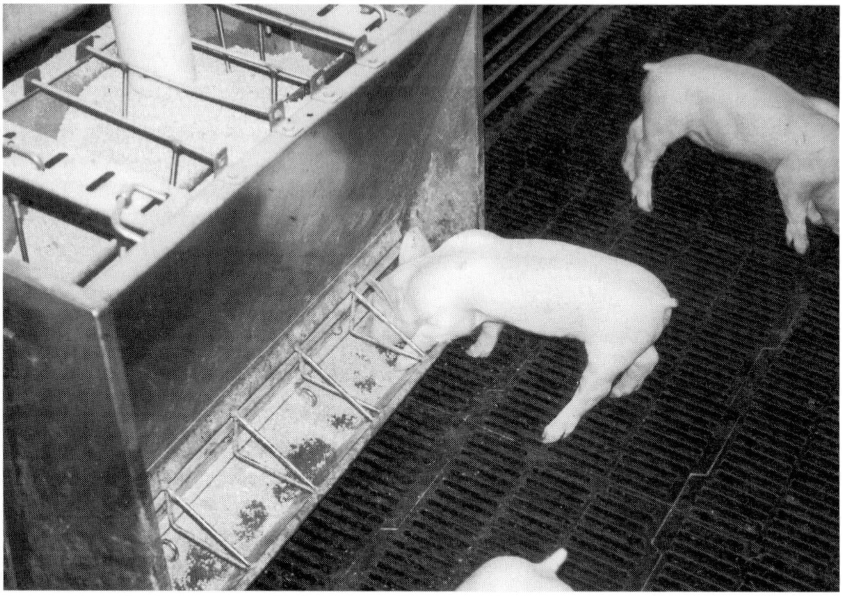

Fig. 4.5. A strong appetite is the best criterion in evaluating post-weaning diets.

depression. This invariably increases cost of production and hampers performance throughout the finishing stage. In addition, starving pigs are prone to succumb to disease, requiring expensive veterinary interventions. To enhance feed intake immediately after weaning, the following measures are employed in many well-managed nurseries with substantial success.

Health management

The importance of hygiene and overall management in creating an environment for maximal weaning performance cannot be overemphasized. Increased biosecurity measures, disease prevention schemes, improved pig/human flow, and staff training are essential steps to increase health status and awareness of the importance of properly managing young pigs.

Temperature

Although pigs should be kept comfortably warm (to avoid catabolism of fat for thermogenesis), keeping piglets too warm may not be in the best interest as far as feed intake is concerned. Best results are obtained when pigs are kept at temperatures around their lower critical temperature zone. Alternatively, temperature may be reduced during night hours (Brumm *et al.*, 1995). This way pigs look more eagerly for feed.

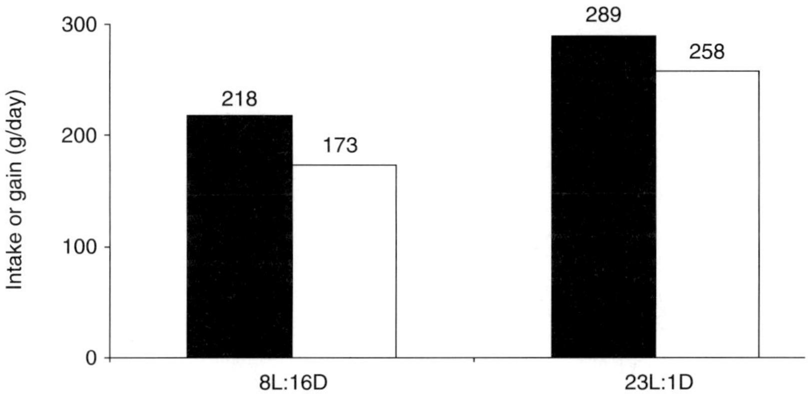

Fig. 4.6. Increased photoperiod improves growth performance (■, intake (g/day); □, gain (g/day)) in early-weaned pigs. (From Bruininx *et al.*, 2001.)

Lighting

Recent evidence suggests that providing continuous lighting during the first two weeks post-weaning reduces the time pigs take to start eating solid feed (Bruininx *et al.*, 2001), because during dark periods piglets prefer to remain in the safety of the group instead of venturing out for feed. In general, increased photoperiod during the first couple of post-weaning weeks has been shown to improve growth performance (Fig. 4.6).

Diet digestibility

It is well established that feed intake increases with increasing nutrient digestibility (see above). For this reason, nursery diets fortified with cooked cereals, milk proteins, specialty proteins, fishmeal, and simple sugars such as lactose and sucrose, are readily consumed by young pigs.

Light versus heavy pigs

High-quality diets are very helpful in promoting growth performance, but advantages can be easily lost if fed for too long or at the wrong level for each weight class of pigs. A properly designed feed budget not only allows for greater quantities of complex diets for lightweight pigs, but it also provides enough of these diets for heavyweight pigs. Heavy pigs are accustomed to consuming large quantities of milk and, thus, they tend to take longer than lightweight pigs to adapt to dry diets (Bruininx *et al.*, 2001).

Additives

Antimicrobial agents, zinc oxide, copper sulfate, organic acids, and sources of immunoglobulins (e.g. plasma protein) markedly improve post-weaning feed intake, mostly through increases in weight gain. An improvement of 10 to 50% in performance can be easily realized when the proper combination of such ingredients is used, but the response is more intense when health, facilities, and management are suboptimal (van Dijk *et al.*, 2001). These ingredients are not easily interchangeable because their mode of action is not similar, thus requiring different formulation profiles. For example, antibiotics are effective in high-protein diets, but organic acids need low-protein diets to exert their beneficial effects.

Appetizers

These are commercial products that entice piglets to explore and ingest solid feed based on aroma and texture. Based on anecdotal evidence and commercial practice, it appears they can be very successful in enhancing appetite during the first few days post-weaning. Such products are usually in meal/powder form and they are rich in milk products and highly digestible oils to promote digestion along with appetite. About 100 g/pig are usually enough to start pigs on solid feed.

Milk replacers

Nursery pigs readily consume a liquid milk replacer of the proper temperature and composition (Azain *et al.*, 1996). However, pigs drinking large amounts of milk replacer may fail to relate to dry feed. For this reason, a milk replacer must be combined with a high-quality solid diet. Good sanitation and frequent feeding are essential to prevent spoilage and attract pigs to drink.

Gruel feeding

A gruel (50:50) of feed and water or liquid milk replacer is often offered to fallback and light pigs in bowl feeders during the first two to three days post-weaning to improve feed intake and overall condition. This practice prevents not only starvation but also dehydration. Unless the gruel is gradually thickened, piglets may fail to adapt easily to dry feeding.

Liquid feeding

Research and experience indicate dramatic increases of dry matter intake during the first week post-weaning when piglets are offered a liquid diet combining dairy by-products and dry feed (Brooks *et al.*, 1999). Fermented liquid feeding offers additional advantages in terms of increased gut acidity and lactobacteria that improve gastrointestinal health (Scholten *et al.*, 1999).

Water supplements

Nutrients and additives delivered via the water system reach even pigs that fail to consume (enough) dry feed post-weaning. Ingredients commonly used are organic acids (citric acid), plasma protein-based products, hyperimmunized egg proteins, water-soluble probiotics and nucleotide preparations, and of course medications. These practices have the theoretical potential of reducing scouring and enhancing feed intake and growth rates post-weaning, but results are almost invariably product- and farm-specific. Some supplements are also likely to reduce variability in growth rates among the most underprivileged piglets (Borg *et al.*, 1999).

Mat-feeding

A practical and cost-effective way to increase feed intake is to spread a small quantity of feed on floor-mats. This practice encourages piglets to rut and ingest solid feed. In controlled trials (Mavromichalis and Baker, 2000), newly weaned pigs (5.5 kg) had more than double daily weight gain when offered feed on floor-mats during the first 3 days post-weaning compared to control pigs (Fig. 4.7). Performance of pigs during the subsequent period (days 4 to 7) was similar across treatments, whereas overall weight gain for the entire 7-day period was improved by about 25%.

Weaned pigs require about 3 days of mat-feeding before they become accustomed to eating from regular feeders, but some producers offer feed on mats only the first day post-weaning to save on labor. Feeding on floor-mats

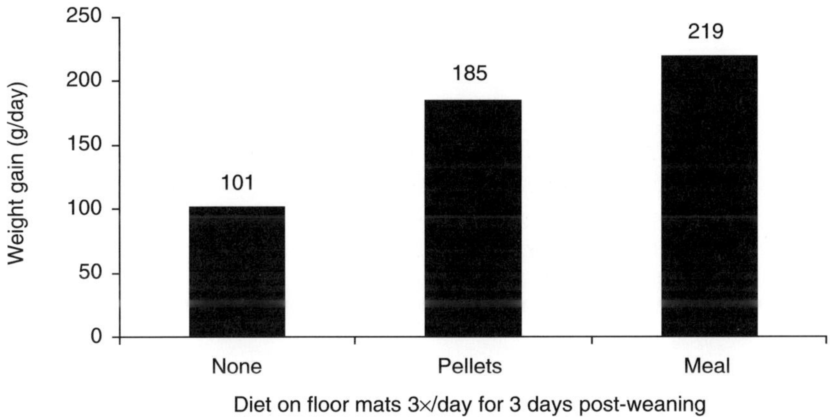

Fig. 4.7. Mat-feeding improves growth performance in weaned pigs. (From Mavromichalis and Baker, 2000.)

for more than 3 days or feeding more than three times per day may satisfy hunger and prevent piglets from exploring feed offered in typical self-feeders. Some producers prefer to mat-feed just the fallback piglets that fail to thrive on typical diets, whereas others feed all piglets on floor-mats (Fig. 4.8). The diet used on floor-mats may be the same diet used in self-feeders or just an appetizer.

The most common problem with mat-feeding is feed wastage. Placing mats away from corners and drinkers keeps mats clean, whereas placing mats near self-feeders promotes feeding behavior. Frequent feedings of small quantities is also helpful in keeping waste to a minimum. As a general guide, enough feed should be placed on mats for pigs to consume in a single feeding episode of about 20–30 min. Large floor-mats, with at least 1-cm rims and grooves, reduce feed wastage markedly. Mats without rims should not be combined with pelleted diets because pigs enjoy rolling pellets off the edge. In solid-floor systems, fouling may distract piglets from consuming feed spread on the floor and, thus, a shallow feeder with a large surface area is recommended (e.g. a large lock-down bowl).

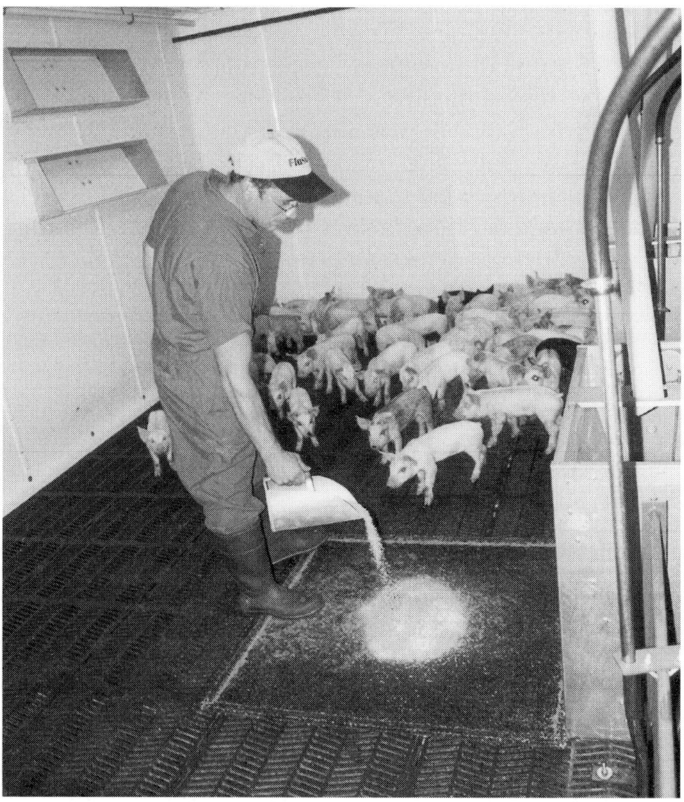

Fig. 4.8. Mat-feeding greatly enhances performance post-weaning.

Feed Intake Targets for the Nursery Period

Under commercial conditions, a rough estimate of expected feed intake for a specific period of time is often required in order to place an order for feed or schedule manufacturing on the farm. Although records of feed intake are useful in estimating expected feed intake, such knowledge should always be combined with records of growth rate and calculated feed efficiency. In young pigs, feed intake rarely responds to minor changes in nutrient composition, especially when pigs are already consuming feed well below their expected target levels. In contrast, growth rate and feed efficiency are extremely sensitive to changes in feed quality, especially early in life. Weekly targets proposed in Table 4.1 are for well-managed, high-health pigs. Pigs of average health or under poor management may be expected to eat up to 25% less feed.

In addition, feed intake may be indirectly estimated from expected feed efficiency for a specific weight range, based on historical records and (or) practical experience. To this end, expected feed intake in pigs receiving highly digestible diets is presented in Table 4.1. For example, if expected feed efficiency for 10–20 kg pigs is around 1.5, pigs should require about 15 kg feed (10 kg gain × 1.5) for this phase.

Pigs growing according to targets outlined in Table 4.1 should reach 30 kg body weight around 70 days of age, with a feed efficiency of 1.6 (or less) and overall growth rate of over 450 g/day. Of course, first-class units will outperform these targets, whereas other units will have difficulty reaching them.

It is recommended that a feed intake curve be constructed for each specific nursery facility based on actual data. Based on such a graph, feed requirements can then be easily estimated. Seasonal graphs are even more useful when the environment inside the barn is difficult to control at pig

Table 4.1. Example weekly feed intake targets and expected growth performance[a].

Week of age	Body weight (kg)	Feed intake (g/day)	Feed (kg/week)	Estimated feed/gain	Expected growth rate (g/day)
3	4–6	250	1.75	1.00	227
4	6–8	350	2.45	1.25	280
5	8–10	450	3.15	1.40	321
6	10–13	600	4.20	1.50	400
7	13–16	750	5.25	1.60	469
8	16–20	950	6.65	1.70	559
9	20–25	1150	8.05	1.80	639
10	25–30	1400	9.80	1.90	737
		Avg = 734	Total = 41 kg	Avg = 1.62	Avg = 454

[a] For high-health and well-managed piglets. Other factors also affect intake (see text for details).

comfort level throughout the year. Examples of feed intake curves are presented in Figs 4.9 and 4.10 for dry and liquid feeding, respectively.

Target feed intake figures in Table 4.1 assume minimal post-weaning depression of performance. In reality, pigs experiencing severe post-weaning anorexia may take longer to reach optimal levels of feed intake. In some cases, feed intake and growth rate appear to increase during the last phase of the nursery period. However, in most cases this represents increased gut fill, enlargement of internal organs, and fat deposition (see Chapter 1 for discussion on compensatory growth).

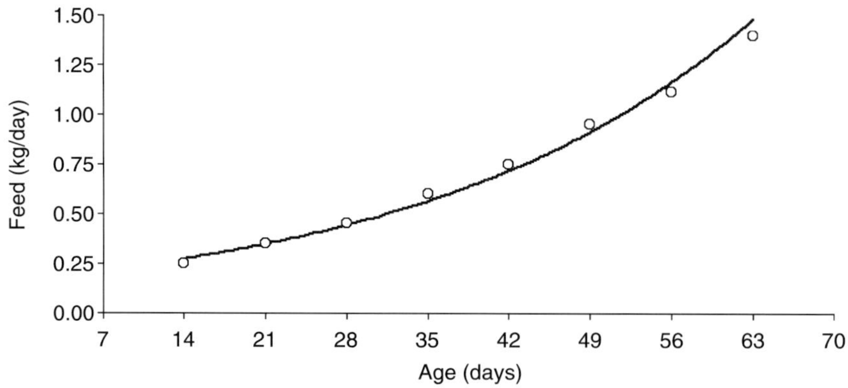

Fig. 4.9. Example of a commercial feed intake curve based on actual data: Intake (kg/day) = $0.1678 \times e^{0.0346 \times BW}$, $r^2 = 0.99$. (From the author's records.)

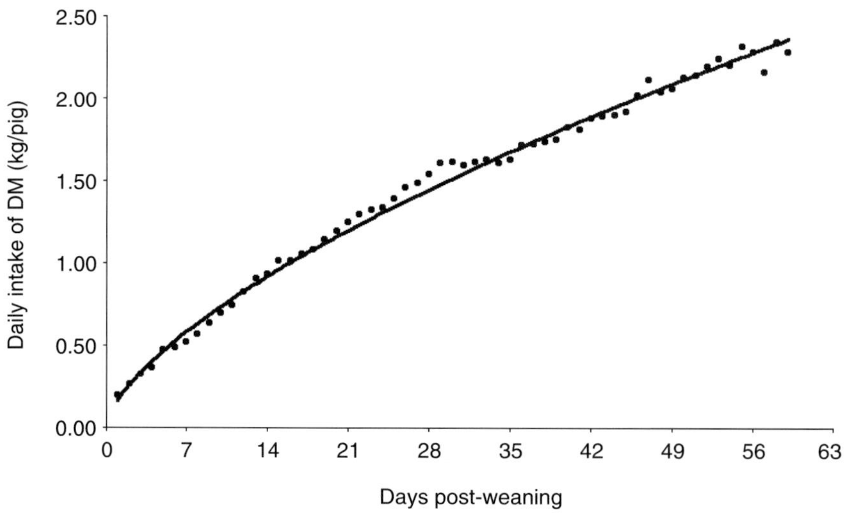

Fig. 4.10. Example of a dry matter (DM) intake curve from a commercial farm feeding liquid diets: DM intake (kg/day) = $0.1634 \times day^{0.6551}$, $r^2 = 0.99$. (From the author's records.)

Feed Efficiency and How to Improve It

The efficiency of feed utilization is properly defined as weight gain per unit of feed intake (gain/feed), but in practice the reverse term (feed required per a unit of weight gain, or simply feed/gain) is more popular. Regardless of the term used to express it, feed efficiency is an important figure in assessing success of a nutrition program. For the purposes of this book, the commonly used term of feed/gain will be used. Feed efficiency is influenced by the following major factors.

Nutrient digestibility

Higher nutrient digestibility supports better feed efficiency, because more nutrients are extracted for growth per unit of feed. In turn, digestibility is affected by ingredient selection and processing, and by exogenous modifiers such as antimicrobial agents, enzymes, and acidifiers.

Particle size

Research has clearly demonstrated that reducing the particle size of the cereal portion of a diet improves feed efficiency, due to improved nutrient digestibility. For example, for every 100-μm reduction in particle size of maize, feed efficiency improves approximately by 1.3% (Hancock and Behnke, 2001). To further illustrate this point, assume a complete diet based on maize that supports feed efficiency of 1.5 (feed/gain). If maize is ground 200 μm finer (e.g. from 900 to 700 μm), feed efficiency is expected to improve by 2.6% and be around 1.45. This is a substantial difference for commercial purposes, as pigs growing from 6 to 30 kg body weight will require approximately 1 kg less feed of the same (but finer) diet. The effects of reducing particle size of the protein sources (e.g. soybean meal) are less pronounced (Fastinger and Mahan, 2001).

Gut health

Pigs suffering from diarrhea are obviously not digesting feed as efficiently as healthy pigs. However, looseness is not always an indication of diarrhea and may not affect feed efficiency. Damage to the gastrointestinal villi architecture, by starvation and transient starvation, also reduces digestive capacity with negative effects on feed efficiency (McCracken *et al.*, 1999; Zijlstra *et al.*, 1999).

Feed intake

Rapid passage of digesta through the gut reduces digestibility and feed efficiency (Kidder and Manners, 1978). This is one of the many reasons why nutrients in high-fiber diets are less digestible than nutrients in diets with normal levels of fiber (Wenk, 2001).

Growth rate

For practical purposes, measurement of (overall) feed efficiency does not differentiate between feed consumed for maintenance needs versus that consumed for growth. Thus, increased growth rates generally improve feed efficiency as maintenance needs become a lesser fraction of total needs.

Nutrient balance

A diet with a lysine/energy imbalance will reduce feed efficiency as pigs will either consume more feed to cover their needs and discard nutrient excesses, or simply reduce their feed intake and growth rate to avoid protein overload (D'Mello, 1994). An imbalance among amino acids has similar effects, as pigs cannot properly utilize all nutrients for growth.

Fat versus lean

Depositing 1 kg of fat requires approximately 2.5 times more energy than depositing 1 kg of lean tissue, which has over 80% water (Whittemore, 1998). Thus, when pigs deposit more fat than lean tissue (mainly because of serious imbalances between the energy and protein/amino acid components of the diet), feed efficiency deteriorates rapidly.

Feed wastage

Feed efficiency accounts for feed disappearance from feeders and not actual feed ingestion. Thus, wasted feed is normally included in feed efficiency estimates. Excessive wastage (more than 2–3%) can negatively affect profitability and it should be controlled. Obviously, reducing feed wastage improves feed efficiency by an equal percentage.

Feed Allowance Budgets

Development of a farm-specific feeding program for nursery pigs involves establishment of: (i) dietary specifications; (ii) number and time of diet changes; and (iii) amount of each diet to be fed per pig. The first issue is examined in detail in Chapter 5, whereas the next two issues are examined here.

A proper feed-management plan prevents overfeeding of expensive diets without sacrificing performance or animal health and welfare. Most commercial pigs, today, are fed on a phase-feeding program that employs complex starter diets early post-weaning to prevent growth depression and simpler diets during the later stages of the nursery period to ensure maximal profitability.

Changing diets

The best criterion for determining when to switch pigs from one diet to another of lower nutrient specifications is the actual weight of pigs, because all diets are formulated to meet nutrient requirements for a specific range of body weight. This practice, however, requires frequent weighing of a representative sample of pigs for each group, and thus it is rarely followed. To avoid this arduous task, many nutritionists and producers assess body weight growth based on time.

Feed intake curve

Establishment of a meaningful feed intake curve for a specific farm requires at least weekly feed intake records from a relatively large number of pigs throughout the entire nursery period (Figs 4.6 and 4.7). Because feed intake is highly variable during the nursery phase, a representative curve should be based on several groups of pigs of similar health status and genetic background, raised throughout the course of an entire year to allow for seasonal effects on performance. Because measurement of feed intake is rather complicated under commercial conditions, many nutritionists and producers calculate expected feed intake using a standard growth curve (see Chapter 1) with estimated or historical feed efficiency records to calculate expected feed intake.

Time budgets

A more practical feed-management plan calls for diet changes based on time. Such programs are usually developed based on practical experience and assumptions regarding feed intake and growth patterns. In that, they are simplified versions of a feed intake curve. Time-based feed programs require a low level of management and are easy to implement and follow. Their greatest disadvantage, however, is that small pigs do not receive enough of the complex diets and, thus, their performance is not maximized, whereas larger pigs receive more than they actually need to thrive. This method is best for small batches of pigs and continuous-flow nurseries. An example of such a time-based program is outlined in Table 4.2.

Feeding weaners according to body weight

All weaned pigs within a group are often fed a fixed amount of feed based on expected average weaning weight. Within each group, however, large

Table 4.2. Example detailed time budgets (days/diet) according to weaning age[a].

	Average weaning age (days)[c]						
Diet[b]	18	21	24	27	30	33	36
1	4	3	2				
2	6	4	2	2	2		
3	7	7	7	7	7	7	7
4	14	14	14	14	14	14	14
5	21	21	21	20	17	16	13

[a] These budgets are more applicable in continuous-flow nurseries. For fewer phases combine days and diets.
[b] Diets of decreasing ingredient complexity and nutrient specifications (see Chapter 5).
[c] For pigs weaned over 3 weeks of age, provide creep feed for at least 1 week before weaning.

variation in body weight exists at weaning. For example, pigs weaned at 3 weeks of age are expected to weigh at least 6 kg on average. However, a significant number of these pigs (2.3%) are expected to be less than 4 kg, whereas an equal percentage will be over 8 kg, based on a normal distribution pattern of natural variation (Table 4.3).

To allow for proper nutrition for all pigs, the first couple of diets post-weaning may be distributed according to body weight after pigs are distributed in predetermined weight classes (Table 4.4). To develop a farm-specific feed budget based on weight classes, the average weaning weight and its standard deviation are first calculated from historical records. Although average weaning weight is quite variable and farm-specific, its standard deviation is less variable and may be assumed to be around 1 kg. This information is used to calculate the number of pigs that are expected to fall in different weight groups around the average.

For example, in a batch of 1000 weaned pigs with an average weaning weight of 6 kg and SD of 1 kg, 68% of the pigs are expected to be between 5 and 7 kg (weight ± SD), whereas 16% of the pigs are expected to be less than 5 kg and another 16% above 7 kg. Table 4.3 may be used to establish more groups based on total number of pigs per batch and available facilities, but three weight groups are the norm in the industry. As a rule of thumb, the larger the batch of pigs and the smaller the number of pigs per pen, the more the weight categories that can be established, but then the more labor is required to manage an elaborate feed budget.

Working example

A feed-management plan for the above group of 1000 weaners is calculated in Table 4.5 for the first diet post-weaning (Mavromichalis, 1999). To begin with, weight groups that correspond to a 6-kg average weaning weight are

Table 4.3. Normal (statistical) distribution (percentage of pigs falling within each weight group) of weaning weights with a standard deviation of 1.0 kg.

	Average weaning weight (kg)				
Weight (kg)	4.0	5.0	6.0	7.0	8.0
<2	2.3				
2–3	13.6	2.3			
3–4	34.1	13.6	2.3		
4–5	34.1	34.1	13.6	2.3	
5–6	13.6	34.1	34.1	13.6	2.3
6–7		13.6	34.1	34.1	13.6
7–8			13.6	34.1	34.1
8–9				13.6	34.1
9–10				2.3	13.6
>10					2.3

Table 4.4. Example feed budgets (kg/pig) according to weaning weight[a].

		Average weaning weight (kg)[e]					
Diet[b,c]	Body weight (kg)[d]	<4	4–5	5–6	6–7	7–8	8–9
1		2	1.5	1	0.5		
2		3	2.5	2	1.5	1	
3	9–12	5	5	5	5	5	5
4	12–22	15	15	15	15	15	15
5	22–32	20	20	20	20	20	20

[a] These budgets were developed assuming ~1.65 overall feed/gain for piglets weighing 30 kg at 70 days of age.
[b] Diets of decreasing ingredient complexity and nutrient specifications (see Chapter 5).
[c] For programs with fewer phases combine diets and amount of feed.
[d] The first two diets should be adjusted as needed to allow pigs to reach about 9 kg body weight.
[e] For pigs weaned over 3 weeks of age, allow creep feeding for at least 1 week before weaning.

copied from Table 4.3 to column A in Table 4.5. Then, the number of pigs falling in each group is calculated in column B by multiplying the percentages from Table 4.3 by 1000 (number of pigs in batch). Then, a decision is made to establish four working weight groups (column C): one for light (<4 kg), one for heavy (>7 kg), and two for pigs of medium weight (4 to 5 kg and 5 to 6 kg). The two medium groups could be merged in only one large group, but the size of this batch is large enough to justify management of these two sizable groups. Again, this step is subjective and depends entirely on how many separate weight groups can be handled successfully at each farm. In column D, the total number of pigs for each working weigh group is summed

Table 4.5. Example worksheet for developing a detailed feed-management plan for 1000 6-kg weaned pigs[a].

Body weight range (kg) A	Pigs B	Groups[b] (kg) C	Pigs/group D	Feed/pig (kg) E	Feed/group (kg) F	Bags/group[c] (25 kg/bag) G	Pens/group (20 pigs/pen) H	Feed/pen (kg) I
<4	23							
4–5	136	<5	159	1.5	239	10	8	30
5–6	341	5–6	341	1.0	341	14	17	20
6–7	341	6–7	341	0.5	170	6	17	10
7–8	136	>7	159	–[d]			8	
>8	23							
Total	1000		1000	0.75	750	30	50	

[a] Only for the first diet post-weaning. Similar calculations should be applied for subsequent diets.
[b] The two medium-weight groups are often combined into one large group (see text for explanation).
[c] When feed allotment is based on number of bags, it is suggested to err towards overfeeding the lighter pigs.
[d] These pigs may start on the second available diet. Alternatively allow around 100 g/pig of the first diet.

up. Column E is basically transferred from Table 4.4, and these figures are used to calculate total feed allowance by group in column F. If the size of feed bags is known (here set to 25 kg), then the number of bags needed for each group can be determined easily (column G). In the same worksheet, the number of pens required for each group (column H) can be calculated by dividing the number of pigs in each group by the desired pen density (here it is set to 20 pigs/pen). Pen density could be adjusted based on weight of each group. Finally, the amount of feed that needs to be delivered in each pen (column I) is calculated by dividing the total feed per group (column F) by the number of pens per group (column H).

The above is solely an example and it should be modified to accommodate variation in weaning weight and farm-specific recommendations of feed allowances.

Feed Intake under Disease Stress

The release of pro-inflammatory cytokines in response to exposure to antigenic stimuli activates the immune system and dramatically alters metabolism (Klasing, 1988). Activation of the immune system reduces appetite with catastrophic effects on productivity because normal growth is closely associated to a constant supply of nutrients. Anorexia, however, is an integral part of the overall host acute-phase response to immunological stress, at least initially, because it (Langhans, 2000):

1. Reduces feeding activity and, thus, reserves energy for immune system functions;
2. Prevents proliferation of the pathogenic agents by reducing nutrient availability;
3. Minimizes the negative side-effects of the acute-phase response; and
4. Increases plasma glucagon levels (glucagon is a potentiator of the immune system).

Pigs are continuously exposed to a myriad of pathogenic and non-pathogenic microorganisms through their interaction with the environment and other animals. Even though disease may not always prevail, chronic exposure to antigens triggers the immune system to release pro-inflammatory cytokines that reduce appetite as part of their function as modulators of the immune system response. Vaccinations present antigens to the immune system, causing a mild inflammation reaction.

Under experimental conditions, force-feeding infected animals increased mortality and reduced survival time, further illustrating the beneficial effects of anorexia (Murray and Murray, 1979). However, long-term anorexia is equally detrimental because restricted food intake beyond the first seven to ten days of disease outbreak greatly decreases the chances of a rapid recovery (Langhans, 2000) and depresses overall growth performance.

A common intervention strategy to counteract the negative effects of anorexia during an immunological challenge is to increase dietary nutrient density to oversupply nutrients that potentially limit growth. However, increasing lysine (Williams *et al.*, 1997a,b,c) or protein concentration (van Heugten *et al.*, 1994) or treating pigs with porcine somatotropin, an anabolic agent (Evock-Clover *et al.*, 1997), failed to increase protein deposition and overall growth rates in pigs experiencing a high level of immune system activity. These findings are supported by similar evidence with other species (Webel *et al.*, 1998).

Post-weaning anorexia is strongly associated with damage to the gastrointestinal tract and allergenic reactions to antigens from legumes, both of which invariably lead to nutritional diarrhea (King *et al.*, 2003). When starving pigs suddenly start eating (usually between the second and fifth day post-weaning), the already challenged digestive system is overloaded with partially digested feed that promotes microbial proliferation and diarrhea. Thus, abnormal feed intake patterns are always associated with digestive upsets post-weaning.

Vaccinations and feed intake

Vaccination regimens for nursery pigs require administration at times that ensure maximal development of immunity. Protection against pathogens is of paramount importance in pigs weaned at or before 3 weeks, because at this age both passive (i.e. antibodies from sow's milk) and active (i.e. antibodies produced by the pig itself) immunity are very low (King *et al.*, 2003). Therefore, it is often recommended that the primary immunization be administered 1 to 2 weeks before weaning followed by a booster immunization 1 to 2 weeks after weaning.

Many producers, however, prefer to administer vaccinations at weaning to save labor and time, and to decrease animal stress due to double handling. Immunity, however, develops at least 1 week after initial vaccination, and, therefore, postponing vaccinations until after weaning increases the risk of infection. Furthermore, mild local and systemic reactions to vaccination from the vigorous stimulation of the immune system following the initial vaccination may further depress appetite at the most critical time.

In a field study (Mavromichalis, 2001) the side-effects of a vaccination regimen were investigated. Injections were given 1 week before (as recommended by the manufacturer) or at the time of weaning (21 days of age). Results indicated that feed intake was depressed during days 4 and 5 post-weaning in pigs vaccinated at weaning (Fig. 4.11) but not in pigs vaccinated 1 week before weaning. Thus, the success of any nutrition program should be always assessed along other management intervention strategies that affect feed intake.

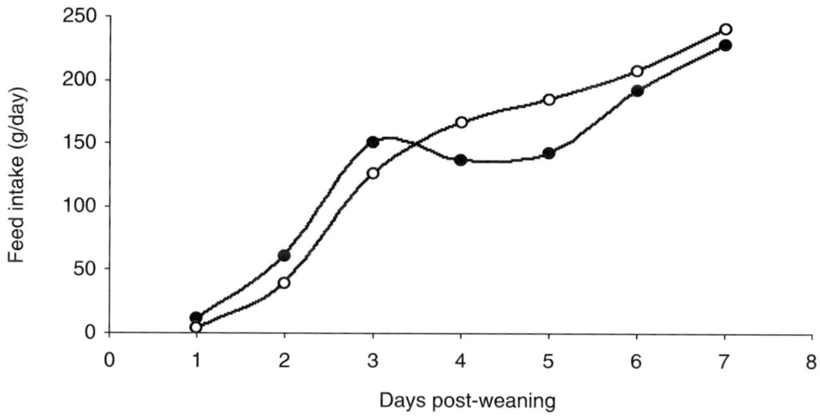

Fig. 4.11. Effect of vaccinations given 1 week before (—○—) or at weaning (—●—) on feed intake during the first week post-weaning. (From Mavromichalis, 2001.)

Controlling Feed Wastage

Feed wastage is usually around 5% under most commercial conditions. However, as pigs get heavier and if adjustment of the feed-release mechanism in self-feeders is neglected, wastage may easily exceed 10% (Gadd, 1996; Hutson and Dickenson, 1997). The easiest way to control feed wastage is to select an appropriate feeder design that has a proven record of minimizing feed wastage. Adjustment of feeder gates is the second most powerful management tool in controlling feed wastage (Fig. 4.12). Finally, feeder placement away from corners minimizes fouling of feed and reduces rejected feed during clean-up.

Proper adjustment of feeders is a labor- and time-intensive task, albeit an essential one in that it markedly reduces feed wastage, especially during the nursery period when diets are most expensive. Below is a list to ensure minimal feed wastage (from hopper-type self-feeders), yet provide *ad libitum* access to feed for maximal growth (Mavromichalis, 2003).

- Feeders must be cleaned thoroughly before filling with the first diet post-weaning. Feeders must be filled with gates (or other feed-releasing mechanism) closed and then gates adjusted to proper height while feeders are lightly shaken in place.
- When switching from pellets to meal, care should be taken to ensure that feed flow is enhanced. Meal diets rich in milk products tend to bridge in feeders more often than simpler diets based on cereals and vegetable proteins. Thus, another round of feeder adjustment may be required when diet complexity is reduced.
- Meal diets flow better when particle size is increased (optimal at 700–900 μm), but this practice reduces feed efficiency and increases nutrient load in excreta.

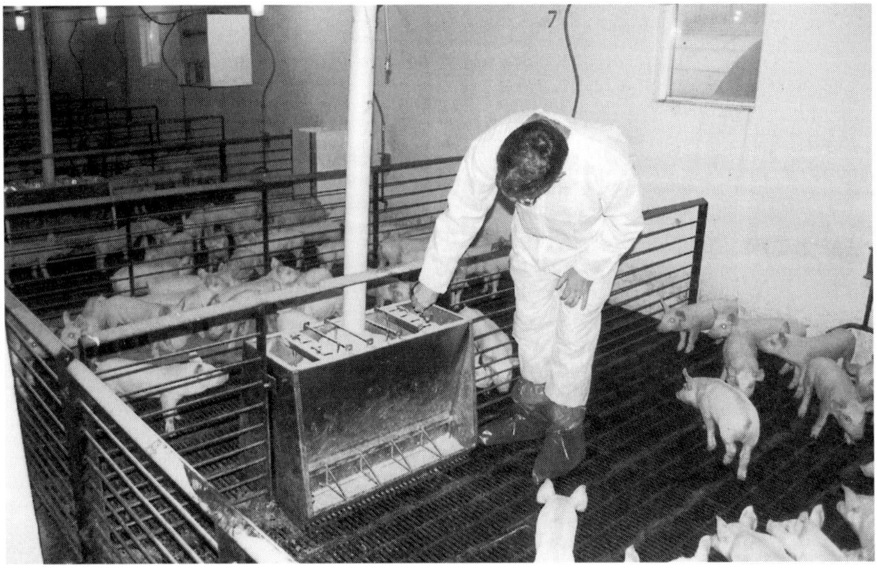

Fig. 4.12. Proper adjustment of self-feeders is crucial to avoid wastage.

- Feeders should be inspected, adjusted, and cleaned if necessary on a daily basis. Fouled feed and accumulated fines must be removed as frequently as possible.
- Pig behavior should be routinely observed while they are eating. If pigs must shake the feeder or lick feed underneath gate openings then they have restricted access to feed. If they freely play with feed then the gates need to be tightened.
- Feed around feeders and underneath slats is an indication of feed wastage.
- Moistened feed from environmental moisture and pig saliva tends to stick on gate openings, reducing feed flow. Thus, flow must be increased accordingly as pigs get heavier.
- Feed tends to bridge more during periods of increased temperature and humidity.
- During the first week post-weaning, two-thirds of the feeder pan should be covered with feed to attract pigs. It is best to err towards feed wastage during this crucial period rather than be restrictive in feed allowances.
- In the following weeks of the nursery period, no more than a third of the feeder pan should be covered with feed, especially when meal is fed.
- Tube feeders that require pigs to rotate a propeller to release feed must be adjusted for easier operation during the first week post-weaning. If pigs are constantly at the feeder but they look skinny, feed intake is restricted.

References

Aherne FX, Danielson V, and Nielsen HE (1982) The effects of creep feeding on pre- and post-weaning pig performance. *Acta Agricultura Scandinavia Section A* 32:155–160.

Appleby MC, Pajor EA, and Fraser D (1992) Individual variation in feeding and growth of piglets: effects of increased access to creep food. *Animal Production* 55:147–152.

Azain MJ, Tomkins T, Sowinski JS, Arentson RA, and Jewell DE (1996) Effect of supplemental pig milk replacer on litter performance: seasonal variation in response. *Journal of Animal Science* 74:2195–2202.

Black JL, Campbell RG, Williams IH, James KJ, and Davies GT (1986) Simulation of energy and amino acid utilization in the pig. *Research and Development in Agriculture* 3:121–146.

Boe K (1991) The process of weaning in pigs – when the sow decides. *Applied Animal Behaviour Science* 30:47–59.

Boe K and Jensen P (1995) Individual-differences in suckling and solid food-intake by piglets. *Applied Animal Behaviour Science* 42:183–192.

Borg BS, Campbell JM, Russell LE, Thomson DU, and Weaver EM (1999) Effects of water soluble globulin on the performance of weanling pigs. *Journal of Animal Science* 77(Supplement 1):193.

Brooks PH (1998) Realising the growth potential of newly weaned pigs. *Pig Progress* 14(1):6–8.

Brooks PH, Geary TM, Morgan DT, and Campbell A (1999) New developments in liquid feeding. *Pig Journal* 36:43–64.

Brooks PH and Tsourgiannis CA (2003) Factors affecting the voluntary feed intake of the weaned pig. In: *Weaning the Pig – Concepts and Consequences*, by Pluske JR, Le Dividich J, and Verstegen MWA (ed), 81–116. Wageningen Academic Publishers, Wageningen, The Netherlands.

Bruininx EMAM, van der Peet-Schwering CMC, Schrama JW, Vereijken PFG, Vesseur PC, Everts H, den Hartog LA, and Beynen AC (2001) Individually measured feed intake characteristics and growth performance of group-housed weanling pigs: effects of sex, initial body weight, and body weight distribution within groups. *Journal of Animal Science* 79:301–308.

Brumm MC, Shelton DP, and Dahlquist JM (1995) Interaction of diet composition and a reduced nocturnal temperature regimen in weanling pigs. *Journal of Animal Science* 73:2518–2523.

Brumm MC and Gonyou HW (2001) Effects of facility design on behavior and feed and water intake. In: *Swine Nutrition* (2nd edn), by Lewis AJ and Southern LL (ed), 499–518. CRC Press LLC, Boca Raton, FL.

Campbell RG, Taverner MR, and Mullaney PD (1975) The effect of dietary concentrations of digestible energy on the performance and carcass characteristics of early-weaned pigs. *Animal Production* 21:285–294.

Cera KR, Mahan DC, and Reinhart GA (1989) Apparent fat digestibilities and performance responses of postweaning swine fed diets supplemented with coconut oil, corn oil, or tallow. *Journal of Animal Science* 67:2040–2047.

Cole DJA, Duckworth JE, and Holmes W (1967) Factors affecting voluntary feed intake in pigs. *Animal Production* 9:141–148.

Cole M and Sprent M (2001) Protein and amino acid requirements of weaner pigs. In: *The Weaner Pig – Nutrition and Management*, by Varley MA and Wiseman J (ed), 45–63. CABI Publishing, Wallingford, UK.

D'Mello JPF (1994) Amino acid imbalances, antagonisms, and toxicities. In: *Amino Acids in Farm Animal Nutrition*, by D'Mello JPF (ed), 63–97. CAB International, Wallingford, UK.

DeRouchey JM, Hancock JD, Maloney CA, Park JS, Lee DJ, Cao H, Dean DW, and Hines RH (1999) Effects of rancidity in choice white grease on growth performance in nursery pigs. *Journal of Animal Science* 77(Supplement 1):195.

English P (1999) The importance of a high weaning weight and milk intake. *Pig Progress* 15(1):27–30.

Evock-Clover CM, Myers MJ, and Steele NC (1997) Effects of endotoxin challenge on growth performance, carcass accretion rates and serum hormone and metabolite concentrations in control pigs and those treated with recombinant porcine somatotropin. *Journal of Animal Science* 75:1784–1790.

Fastinger ND and Mahan DC (2001) Effects of soybean meal particle size on amino acid and energy ileal digestibilities in grower-finisher swine. *Journal of Animal Science* 79(Supplement 2):83.

Gadd J (1996) Optimize resources and watch out for that waste. *PIGS-Misset* 12(6):35–37.

Gonyou HW, Beltranena E, Whittington DL, and Patience JF (1998) The behaviour of pigs weaned at 12 and 21 days of age from weaning to market. *Canadian Journal of Animal Science* 78:517–523.

Hampson DJ (1986) Influence of creep feeding and dietary intake after weaning on malabsorption and occurrence of diarrhoea in the newly weaned pig. *Research in Veterinary Science* 41:63–69.

Hancock JD and Behnke KC (2001) Use of ingredient and diet processing technologies to produce quality feeds for pigs. In: *Swine Nutrition* (2nd edn), by Lewis AJ and Southern LL (ed), 469–497. CRC Press LLC, Boca Raton, FL.

Hutson GD and Dickenson LG (1997) Impact of feeding surface design on feeding behaviour and feed wastage by grower pigs. In: *Manipulating Pig Production VI*, by Cranwell P (ed), 312. Australasian Pig Science Association, Werribee, Australia.

Hyun Y, Ellis M, Riskowski G, and Johnson RW (1998) Growth performance of pigs subjected to multiple concurrent environmental stressors. *Journal of Animal Science* 76:721–727.

Jensen P (1986) Observations on the maternal-behavior of free-ranging domestic pigs. *Applied Animal Behaviour Science* 16:131–142.

Jensen P and Redbo I (1987) Behavior during nest leaving in free-ranging domestic pigs. *Applied Animal Behaviour Science* 18:355–362.

Jensen P and Recen B (1989) When to wean – observations from free-ranging domestic pigs. *Applied Animal Behaviour Science* 23:49–60.

Johnson RW (1997) Inhibition of growth by pro-inflammatory cytokines: an integrated view. *Journal of Animal Science* 75:1244–1255.

Johnson RW, Escobar J, and Webel DM (2001) Nutrition and immunology of swine. In: *Swine Nutrition* (2nd edn), by Lewis AJ and Southern LL (ed), 545–562. CRC Press LLC, Boca Raton, FL.

Kelly D (1990) Effect of creep feeding on structural and functional changes of the gut of early weaned pigs. *Research in Veterinary Science* 48:350–356.

Kidder DE and Manners MJ (1978) *Digestion in the Pig*. Scientechnica, Bristol, UK.
King MR, Kelly D, Morel PCH, and Pluske JR (2003) Aspects of intestinal immunity in the pig around weaning. In: *Weaning the Pig – Concepts and Consequences*, by Pluske JR, Le Dividich J, and Verstegen MWA (ed), 219–257. Wageningen Academic Publishers, Wageningen, The Netherlands.
Klasing KC (1988) Nutritional aspects of leukocytic cytokines. *Journal of Nutrition* 118:1436–1446.
Langhans W (2000) Anorexia of infection: current prospects. *Nutrition* 16:996–1005.
Lawrence TLJ and Fowler VR (1997) *Growth of Farm Animals*. CAB International, Wallingford, UK.
Lewis NJ and Hurnik JF (1986) An approach response of piglets to the sows nursing vocalisation. *Canadian Journal of Animal Science* 66:537–539.
Mavromichalis I (1999) Phase-feed plans for the nursery. *Pig Progress* 15(6):24–27.
Mavromichalis I and Baker DH (2000) Floor-feeding enhances early appetite of weaned pigs. *Journal of Animal Science* 78(Supplement 1):52.
Mavromichalis I (2001) How much should weaners eat. *Pig International* 31(11):21–24.
Mavromichalis I (2003) 12 rules for adjusting a self-feeder. *Pig International* 33(2):17.
Mavromichalis I and Varley MA (2003) Transition feeding systems for weaned pigs. In: *Perspectives of Pig Science*, by Wiseman J, Varley MA, and Kemp KBF (ed), 405–456. Nottingham University Press, Nottingham, UK.
McCracken BA, Spurlock ME, Roos MA, Zuckermann FA, and Gaskins HR (1999) Weaning anorexia may contribute to local inflammation in the piglet small intestine. *Journal of Nutrition* 129:613–619.
Metz JHM and Gonyou HW (1990) Effect of age and housing conditions on the behavioural and haemolytic reaction of piglets to weaning. *Applied Animal Behaviour Science* 27:299–309.
Miller HM and Slade RD (2003) Digestive physiology of the weaned pig. In: *Weaning the Pig – Concepts and Consequences*, by Pluske JR, Le Dividich J, and Verstegen MWA (ed), 117–144. Wageningen Academic Publishers, Wageningen, The Netherlands.
Mitchell AD, Scholz AM, and Mersmann HJ (2001) Growth and body composition. In: *Biology of the Domestic Pig* (2nd edn), by Pond WG and Mersmann HJ (ed), 225–308. Cornell University Press, Ithaca, NY.
Mosenthin R, Hambrecht E, and Sauer WC (1999) Utilization of different fibers in piglet feeds. In: *Recent Advances in Animal Nutrition*, by Garnsworthy PC and Wiseman J (ed), 227–256. Nottingham University Press, Nottingham, UK.
Murray MJ and Murray AB (1979) Anorexia of infection as a mechanism of host defense. *American Journal of Clinical Nutrition* 32:593–596.
Nelssen JL, Dritz SS, Tokach MD, and Goodband RD (1999) Nutritional programs for segregated early weaning. In: *Diseases of Swine* (8th edn), by Straw BE, D'Allaire S, Mengeling WL, and Taylor DJ (ed), 1045–1055. Iowa State University, Ames, IA.
NRC (1998) *Nutrient Requirements of Swine* (10th edn). National Academy Press, Washington, DC.
Pajor EA, Fraser D, and Kramer DL (1991) Consumption of solid food by suckling pigs: individual variation and relation to weight gain. *Applied Animal Behaviour Science* 32:139–155.
Pluske JR, Williams IH, and Aherne FX (1995) Nutrition of the neonatal pig. In: *The Neonatal Pig: Development and Survival*, by Varley MA (ed), 187–235. CAB International, Wallingford, UK.

Purser KW, Ward TL, and Felisa D (2000) Effect of high intensity sweetener level on nursery pig performance. *Journal of Animal Science* 78(Supplement 2):56.

Scholten RHJ, van der Peet-Schwering CMC, Verstegen MWA, den Hartog LA, Schrama JW, and Vesseur PC (1999) Fermented co-products and fermented compound diets for pigs: a review. *Animal Feed Science and Technology* 82:1–19.

Spurlock ME (1997) Regulation of metabolism and growth during immune challenge: an overview of cytokine function. *Journal of Animal Science* 75:1773–1783.

van Dijk AJ, Everts H, Nabuurs MJA, Margry RJCF, and Beynen AC (2001) Growth performance of weanling pigs fed spray-dried animal plasma: a review. *Livestock Production Science* 68:263–274.

van Heugten E, Spears JW, and Coffey MT (1994) The effect of dietary protein on performance and immune response in weanling pigs subjected to an inflammatory challenge. *Journal of Animal Science* 72:2661–2669.

Wahlstrom RC, Hauser LA, and Libal GW (1974) Effects of low lactose whey, skim milk and sugar on diet palatability and performance of early weaned pigs. *Journal of Animal Science* 38:1267–1271.

Webel DM, Johnson RW, and Baker DH (1998) Lipopolysaccharide-induced reductions in food intake do not decrease the efficiency of lysine and threonine utilization for protein accretion in chickens. *Journal of Nutrition* 128:1760–1766.

Wenk C (2001) The role of dietary fibre in the digestive physiology of the pig. *Animal Feed Science and Technology* 90:21–33.

Whittemore CT and Fawcett RH (1976) Theoretical aspects of a flexible model to simulate protein and lipid growth in pigs. *Animal Production* 22:87–96.

Whittemore CT, Aumaitre A, and Williams IH (1978) Growth of body components in young weaned pigs. *Journal of Agriculture Science, Cambridge* 91:681–692.

Whittemore CT (1983) Development of recommended energy and protein allowances for growing pigs. *Agricultural Systems* 11:156–186.

Whittemore CT (1998) *The Science and Practice of Pig Production* (2nd edn). Blackwell Science Ltd, Oxford, UK.

Whittemore CT and Green DM (2001) Growth of the young weaned pig. In: *The Weaner Pig – Nutrition and Management*, by Varley MA and Wiseman J (ed), 1–15. CAB International, Wallingford, UK.

Williams NH, Stahly TS, and Zimmerman DR (1997a) Effect of chronic immune system activation on body nitrogen retention, partial efficiency of lysine utilization, and lysine needs of pigs. *Journal of Animal Science* 75:2472–2480.

Williams NH, Stahly TS, and Zimmerman DR (1997b) Effect of level of chronic immune system activation on the growth and dietary lysine needs of pigs fed from 6 to 112 kg. *Journal of Animal Science* 75:2481–2496.

Williams NH, Stahly TS, and Zimmerman DR (1997c) Effect of chronic immune system activation on the rate, efficiency, and composition of growth and lysine needs of pigs fed from 6 to 27 kg. *Journal of Animal Science* 75:2463–2471.

Wolter BF, Ellis M, Curtis SE, Parr EN, and Webel DM (2000) Group size and floor-space allowance can affect weanling-pig performance. *Journal of Animal Science* 78:2062–2067.

Zijlstra RT, McCracken BA, Odle J, Donovan SM, Gelberg HB, Petschow BW, Zuckermann FA, and Gaskins HR (1999) Malnutrition modifies pig small intestinal inflammatory responses to rotavirus. *Journal of Nutrition* 129:838–843.

5 Dietary Specifications

Introduction

Dietary specifications or nutrient allowances are the interface between animal requirements and nutrients available in ingredients. Dietary specifications not only cover requirements for maintenance and growth, but they also include safety margins.

Feed intake is the major link between daily nutrient requirements (absolute amounts per day) and dietary specifications, which are commonly expressed in relative terms (percentage or amount per kilogram of feed). For example, at a feed intake level of 800 g/day, a daily requirement of 10 g lysine translates to 1.25% dietary lysine (or 12.5 g lysine/kg feed). However, at a feed intake level of 600 g/day, a dietary lysine specification of 1.67% is required to furnish 10 g lysine. It is thus imperative to distinguish between animal requirements (independent of feed intake) and dietary specifications (dependent on feed intake).

Variable safety margins are added to dietary specifications when feeds are designed to be used under a wide array of commercial conditions. Safety margins not only increase feed cost but also contribute to environmental pollution if excess nutrients are not utilized properly by animals.

Requirements

Many scientific groups periodically review nutrient requirement studies. Among the most comprehensive reviews, the following have been taken into consideration in combination with commercial experience in deriving practical recommendations for this book:

- UK: *Nutrient Requirement Standards for Pigs* (BSAS, 2003).
- France: *Tables d'alimentation pour les porcs* (ITP, 2002).
- USA: *Nutrient Requirements of Swine* (NRC, 1998).

Of course, many other publications are available and they should be consulted for specific local conditions. Differences among published values are a reflection of the differences in production methods, ingredients, research approaches, and statistical methods used in the original reports that formed the basis of each review. Most commercial nutritionists regard these estimates as the starting point in the process of establishing practical dietary specifications under commercial conditions.

Factorial versus empirical requirements

The most appropriate method of estimating nutrient requirements is the factorial approach that considers separately daily expenditures for maintenance and growth. For example, the calculated daily lysine requirement of a 10-kg piglet is 0.25 g for maintenance and 8.03 g for protein deposition (55 g), for a total of 8.28 g (NRC, 1998). With a known or estimated feed intake of 635 g/day, this calculated requirement translates to 1.3% dietary lysine.

Most published requirement estimates for young pigs, however, are based on empirical evidence from dose-titration experiments. In these trials, requirements were related to maximal body weight gain to derive recommendations. However, nutrient requirements for maximal growth do not necessarily support optimal performance in terms of feed efficiency, tissue metabolite concentrations, and bone development. For example, maximal bone strength and ash content are maximized at calcium and phosphorus levels considerably higher than those required for maximal weight gain (at least 10% higher; NRC, 1998). Likewise, optimal efficiency of feed utilization is achieved at amino acid concentrations much higher than those required for maximal weight gain.

Expressing requirements and specifications

Typically, requirements and dietary specifications are both expressed in relative terms as percentages or amount per kilogram (e.g. g/kg) feed, because references to daily requirements are not practical outside the sphere of research or academic discussion.

Most nutrient requirements have been determined on a total nutrient basis. The term 'total' refers to the amount of a nutrient that can be determined without taking into account any interactions with the animal organism. This is acceptable as long as practical formulations do not deviate much from those used in the original experiments; a rare finding under commercial conditions.

Expressing requirements and dietary specifications on a digestible basis (total minus nutrients excreted in feces) is strongly recommended to ensure adequate supply of nutrients for maximal performance. Unfortunately, existing digestibility coefficients for most ingredients are derived from studies with growing-finishing pigs and, thus, their value in formulating diets for young pigs is at best questionable. Plus, digestibility coefficients are not available for all ingredients used today in piglet diets. Nevertheless, many nutritionists use digestibility values on a constant basis.

For certain nutrients (minerals, vitamins, and even amino acids) bioavailability values can be found in the literature. The term bioavailability is often confused with the term digestibility. Bioavailability refers to that portion of an ingested nutrient that is metabolically available to the animal for maintenance and (or) growth, whereas digestibility refers to that portion of ingested nutrient that disappears from the lumen of the gastrointestinal tract. Not all of a digested nutrient becomes available for metabolic use because of inherent metabolic inefficiencies, although digestibility is an adequate measure of bioavailability for most ingredients. In certain cases, however, as with amino acids in overprocessed protein ingredients, digestibility is clearly an inadequate estimate of bioavailability (van Barneveld *et al.*, 1991).

Bioavailability is determined as relative availability. Using *in vivo* assays, the availability of a specific nutrient is compared to the availability of the same nutrient from a standard source, which is arbitrarily taken as 100%. In maize, for example, phosphorus is 14% as bioavailable (NRC, 1998) as phosphorus in monosodium phosphate (standard). Yet, only 88% of phosphorus in monosodium phosphate is actually digestible (de Blas *et al.*, 2003). Relative bioavailability is the preferred methodology in evaluating or comparing mineral and vitamin sources. For formulation purposes, however, digestibility values are recommended by most authorities (ITP, 2002; BSAS, 2003).

For amino acids, the use of terminal ileum digestibility values is clearly more accurate than fecal digestibility values, because the latter include bacterial protein synthesis in the large intestine that contributes little if anything to the protein nutrition of the animal. A step further, deduction of endogenous amino acid losses yields true ileal digestibility, which is of course more representative than apparent ileal digestibility. Apparent ileal amino acid digestibility values tend to underestimate low-protein ingredients as they tend to increase with increasing dietary protein concentration (NRC, 1998).

For most commercial piglet diets, the following rules of thumb may be used to navigate between amino acid digestibility values (NRC, 1998):

- From total to true ileal, multiply by 0.90.
- From total to apparent ileal, multiply by 0.82.
- From true ileal to apparent ileal, multiply by 0.94.

Factors affecting requirements

Nutrient requirements for piglets depend on maintenance needs, and the rate and composition of body weight gain. In young pigs, maintenance needs are only a trivial fraction of total requirements, under thermoneutral conditions. For example, the lysine requirement for maintenance is less than 2% of total lysine requirements (NRC, 1998). Also, the composition of growth in young pigs is relatively constant because of limited appetite that usually restricts growth under commercial conditions (Whittemore and Green, 2001). It is, therefore, difficult to produce overly fat piglets with well-balanced diets. In conclusion, it appears that growth rate alone largely determines nutrient requirements.

Growth rate in young pigs is affected mainly by genotype, gender, disease pressure, environmental conditions and their management, and body weight. Of course, nutrition (the scope of this book) can drastically affect growth rate by limiting or allowing expression of genetic potential.

Genotype

Despite the fact that modern genotypes are leaner and grow faster than traditional genotypes of 20 years ago, the absolute lysine requirements of young pigs do not appear to have changed considerably (Auldist *et al.*, 1997). This is a reflection of the fact that modern pigs have similar physiological maturity at lighter body weight compared to past genotypes. Nevertheless, fast-growing pigs require greater dietary nutrient concentrations compared to slower-growing pigs at similar feed intake levels.

Gender

It has been reported (Cromwell *et al.*, 1996) that gilts are likely to grow about 5% faster than barrows. It is most likely, however, that gilts are also more aggressive eaters (Bruininx *et al.*, 2001) and, thus, they tend to grow faster. In practice, it is widely accepted that gender does not appear to significantly affect nutrient requirements for pigs less than 20–30 kg, perhaps because protein deposition rates do not differ substantially between genders in this weight range.

Health status

Health status and disease pressure are major determinants of growth rate as they clearly cap growth potential. Healthy pigs, reared off-site under strict biosecurity conditions, are expected to have higher growth rates and, thus, higher nutrient requirements, than pigs of lower health status (Williams *et al.*, 1997a,b,c). A common, but faulty, approach in feeding disease-challenged animals is to increase dietary nutrient density. It has been clearly demonstrated that such practice cannot restore growth depression from disease pressure (Webel *et al.*, 1998).

Environment

Adverse environmental conditions, inappropriate management, and social stress can markedly depress growth rate and reduce absolute nutrient requirements (Hyun *et al.*, 1998). In accord with responses under disease stress, increasing dietary nutrient density is not an effective measure against mediocre management practices.

Body weight

It is apparent that absolute nutrient requirements increase with increasing body weight because maintenance and growth needs also increase, although not proportionately. Dietary nutrient specifications, however, tend to decrease with age, because appetite increases faster than rate of protein deposition (NRC, 1998).

Safety Margins

Most nutrient requirement studies have been conducted under experimental conditions that are generally deemed more favorable than current commercial conditions. In such experiments, diets are carefully prepared from ingredients of known chemical composition, and they are fed shortly after mixing to avoid nutrient losses. Thus, most commercial nutritionists add a margin of safety over published nutrient requirement estimates, based on experience and limited experimental work, to account for variables that are hard or impossible to control or even predict during feed preparation and use. The following is a non-exclusive list of cases that call for margins of safety.

- *Label guarantees*. By definition, in least-cost formulations the probability for any nutrient to be below target is always 50%. Thus, formulas may be slightly overfortified to meet declared concentrations in feed labels as required by law.
- *Nutrient variability*. Certain ingredients can be highly variable in terms of nutrient composition. Agro-industrial products of unknown quality and origin can be highly problematic if they are not assayed frequently, especially if they make up a substantial part of a diet.
- *Formulation basis*. Diets formulated on total rather than digestible nutrient basis are often overfortified to account for unknown variability in nutrient digestibility, especially in low-quality and novel ingredients.
- *Nutrient losses*. Several nutrients (e.g. amino acids and vitamins) are susceptible to destruction during thermal processing (pelleting, expanding,

flaking), and also during prolonged storage, where significant losses of bioavailability may occur.

- *The 'average' pig*. Published nutrient requirements usually refer to the 'average' pig, which in reality does not exist. This definition of convenience leaves half the pigs in a group undernourished while the other half is overfed. Production systems that place emphasis on rapid turnover require high rates of growth that can only be sustained by diet overfortification to allow for proper nutrition of most pigs.

Minimizing unknown factors and monitoring quality in ingredients and finished diets obviously reduces the need for excessive safety margins. If animal performance (weight gain and feed intake) is known from records, then a feeding program with minimal safety margins that closely meets requirements can be easily designed by a qualified nutritionist. Nevertheless, it is always beneficial to challenge dietary specifications in specific pig production systems that manage to monitor performance. To this end, margins may be gradually increased (or decreased) in 5–10% increments and animal performance evaluated. This exercise should cover a long-term period and a wide range of conditions.

Typical margins of safety range from 5 to 30%, depending on the gravity of the factors taken into consideration. As a rule of thumb, a 5–10% safety margin over requirements is adequate when a quality control program closely monitors incoming ingredients and finished products. Higher safety margins are needed when significant variations in nutrient composition are expected due to ingredient selection, processing conditions, storage, and animal performance (Table 5.1).

But, not all nutrients require the same safety margins. For example, if a considerable fraction of the variability in lysine concentration is due to destruction by the Maillard reaction (see Chapter 8), then lower safety

Table 5.1. Recommended margins of safety (%) for dietary lysine specifications in piglet diets[a].

Criteria	With quality control	Without quality control
Minimal feed storage[b]		
Pellets[c]	10	15
Meal	5	10
Prolonged feed storage		
Pellets[c]	15	20
Meal	10	15

[a] Reduced feed intake requires increased margins of safety to ensure adequate supply of nutrients.
[b] When storage does not exceed 30 days under moderate environmental conditions.
[c] Includes any other thermal processing method (e.g. extrusion, expansion).

margins can be justified for the rest of the indispensable amino acids that are more stable during thermal processing. This can be easily achieved by: (i) using a 'dummy' lysine dietary specification to estimate other amino acids based on an ideal protein profile; or (ii) calculating specifications based on an ideal protein profile and then applying different safety margins separately to each amino acid.

Several vitamins are extremely prone to destruction during thermal processing, prolonged storage, and mixing with choline chloride and (or) trace minerals. Thus, they are usually added at concentrations that exceed requirements (e.g. tenfold increases is common industry practice for certain vitamins; BSAS, 2003). In this case, stabilized vitamin forms and organic minerals greatly reduce the need for large safety margins.

Energy

Energy is the most expensive 'nutrient' in a piglet diet. Although energy is a physical property and not a chemically distinctive compound, it is often regarded as such for simplicity. Dietary energy is provided by: (i) sugars, such as starch and lactose; (ii) lipids, which contain about 2.5 times more energy than most carbohydrates; (iii) proteins, although there is a negative balance when proteins are used for energy; and (iv) some forms of fermentable fiber, such as hemicellulose and pectins. Energy in the body is used for: (i) maintenance, to sustain basic functions and moderate activity; (ii) growth, in terms of protein and lipid deposition; and (iii) thermogenesis, when ambient temperature falls below the thermoneutral zone.

Selection of energy system

Energy requirements in pigs are described in scientific reports mostly in terms of metabolizable energy, which accounts not only for fecal (i.e. digestible energy) but also for energy losses in urine. In contrast, most available information regarding energy density in feedstuffs is in terms of digestible energy (Le Dividich and Seve, 2001). Nevertheless, the net energy (NE) system is considered the most accurate, and it enjoys widespread approval but limited use. The net energy system has been validated extensively in growing-finishing pigs and it appears that it is also valid for young pigs (Beattie *et al.*, 1998).

According to international standards, the correct unit for measuring energy is the joule (J). Nevertheless, the calorie (cal) is still very popular in nutrition textbooks and, thus, dietary energy concentrations are often expressed in both megajoules (MJ) and kilocalories (kcal). The MJ is used as the unit of energy in this book, but conversions to kcal may be easily obtained by multiplying MJ by 239.

Energy in feedstuffs

The average energy content of most common ingredients and practical diets used in commercial conditions can be estimated from their chemical composition:

$$GE = [4143 + (56 \times \%EE) + (15 \times \%CP) - (44 \times \%Ash)]/239 \; (r^2{=}0.98;\ \text{NRC, 1998}) \quad (5.1)$$

$$DE = [4151 + (38 \times \%EE) + (23 \times \%CP) - (122 \times \%Ash) - (64 \times \%CF)]/239 \; (r^2{=}0.90,\ \text{Noblet and Percz, 1993}) \quad (5.2)$$

$$ME = DE \times [1.003 - (0.0021 \times \%CP)] \; (\text{Noblet and Perez, 1993}) \quad (5.3)$$

$$NE = [(0.703 \times DE) + (15.8 \times \%EE) + (4.7 \times \%Starch) - (9.7 \times \%CP) - (9.8 \times \%CF)]/239 \; (r^2 = 0.97;\ \text{Noblet } et\ al.\text{, 1994}), \quad (5.4)$$

where EE = ether extract, CP = crude protein and CF = crude fiber. This is particularly useful in evaluating new varieties or sources of ingredients that deviate somewhat in chemical composition from reference material. For most practical diets and ingredients, metabolizable energy can be assumed to be roughly 96% of digestible energy (NRC, 1998). A more accurate estimate, however, would take into account dietary protein content, which in excess of requirements requires energy for catabolism and excretion in urine as urea. Therefore, low-protein diets, well balanced for all amino acids, contain more metabolizable energy than diets with higher protein and the same digestible energy concentrations, at least theoretically. Similarly, the net energy concentration in most ingredients and practical diets is about 71% of digestible energy or 74% of metabolizable energy (ITP, 2002).

Energy requirements

Energy requirements for maintenance and moderate activity are expressed on a metabolic body weight basis ($BW^{0.75}$), because this accounts for changes in the relationship between weight and body surface, which increases as pigs grow.

The daily metabolizable energy requirement for maintenance (ME_m) is 0.44 MJ ME/kg $BW^{0.75}$ (NRC, 1998). This is equivalent to about 0.46 MJ DE/kg $BW^{0.75}$ or 0.36 MJ NE/kg $BW^{0.75}$ (Noblet *et al.*, 1994). Energy used for maintenance does not produce, obviously, any profit-yielding product (i.e. growth in nursery pigs) and it is, thus, considered an undesirable, yet unavoidable, expense. The relative contribution of maintenance to total energy requirements increases as pigs grow heavier and decreases as pigs grow faster. For example, a 5-kg pig requires daily 1.5 MJ ME for maintenance and about 4 MJ ME for 250 g of growth. In this scenario, ME_m is about 27% of total energy requirements, but had growth rate been double, ME_m would have been only 16% of total. In contrast, a 30-kg pig requires 5.6 MJ ME for maintenance and 6.4 MJ ME to grow at 400 g per day. In this heavier pig, ME_m is almost half of total energy needs (47%), but with a double growth rate this figure falls to 30%. Because fast-growing pigs require fewer days to reach a specific body weight target, fast growth is very efficient in early life as maintenance requirements are minimized.

For growth, pigs require about 44 MJ ME per kg deposited protein, and approximately 55 MJ per kg deposited lipid (NRC, 1998). Assuming that 1 kg lean tissue contains about 20% protein (Whittemore, 1998), it is evident that depositing 1 kg of fat is energetically more expensive than 1 kg of lean tissue. Thus, efficiency of feed utilization is always improved when pigs deposit more lean tissue than fat tissue. This is another reason why growth in early life, which is primarily lean gain, is so desirable and profitable. Young pigs require about 16 MJ ME/kg body weight gain, assuming 1:1 protein to lipid ratio in weight gain (Whittemore, 1998).

Young pigs kept under their lower critical temperature zone will spend a considerable amount of dietary energy to maintain body temperature. Of course, this expenditure is deducted from energy available for growth, unless pigs are able to consume more feed. In young pigs, however, increases in feed intake due to exposure to cold ambient temperature are not likely to occur, especially during the early stages of the nursery period. On average, pigs require approximately 0.015 MJ ME/kg $BW^{0.75}$ for each degree Celsius below the thermoneutral zone (Whittemore and Fawcett, 1976). For example, if 10-kg pigs are kept 2°C under their comfort zone, they use approximately 0.17 MJ from daily metabolizable energy intake for thermogenesis. Thus, pigs would grow 11 g/day less to spare energy for thermogenesis, or increase feed intake by 11 g/day (16 MJ ME/kg feed), with the latter being rather unlikely.

Dietary energy density

In general, pigs given diets with different energy density try to maintain similar energy intake by adjusting feed intake. Of course, when diets are too dilute so that pigs reach their physical gut capacity before they meet their energy needs, or too dense so that pigs cannot satiate hunger, then energy intake cannot be controlled. However, the ability of pigs to compensate for decreasing dietary energy concentration is related to pig size (Black *et al.*, 1986).

Therefore, piglets of high genetic merit growing below their potential for lean gain (as a result of limited voluntary feed intake) are not able to adjust their energy intake when presented with low-energy diets. It appears that, in general, modern pigs of less than 50 kg in body weight cannot regulate energy intake efficiently (Whittemore and Green, 2001). In this light, it has been suggested that dietary energy densities below 15.5 MJ ME/kg may reduce energy intake in pigs less than 15 kg (Fowler and Gill, 1989). A minimum of 14 MJ ME/kg is also suggested for pigs over 15 kg, as each MJ ME below this threshold is most likely to reduce daily energy intake by at least 1.5 MJ (NRC, 1987).

Recommended dietary energy concentrations in Table 5.2 should be used as a guideline only, because ingredient selection and availability of added fats and oils should determine upper thresholds in dietary energy density.

Nutrient to energy ratios

When pigs become able to regulate their energy intake, it is advisable to provide all other nutrients in a constant proportion to energy to ensure similar intake at variable dietary energy densities. Because weaned piglets are expected to consume only a small amount of feed regardless of dietary energy density, it is only logical to assume that growth should be accelerated by high-energy diets. In this case, the concentration of other nutrients, and specifically of amino acids, must be proportionately increased to support growth.

For small-scale production systems that use one or at most two diets during the whole nursery phase, a ratio of 1 g total lysine per MJ digestible energy has been suggested as a convenient rule of thumb (Cole and Sprent, 2001). In more complex phase-feeding programs, however, gradual reductions in dietary energy density are more suitable (Table 5.3) to reduce feed cost and nitrogen excretion.

It follows that the concentration of all amino acids must be in proportion to lysine according to the ideal protein concept (see below). There is no scientific evidence to indicate that mineral and vitamin concentrations should not be similarly adjusted to reflect energy density, although this is not practiced often; perhaps because these nutrients are always supplied in excesses. Finally, it should be noted that certain additives and medications are not adjusted to reflect energy density as their concentration is often regulated by law.

Starch

In sow's milk, lactose (25% of DM) and lipids (40% of DM) are the major sources of energy. In a typical cereal-based diet, however, starch (70% of DM) is the major source of energy because of cost considerations. Only in

Table 5.2. Recommended dietary energy specifications (MJ/kg) for piglet diets[a].

Body weight (kg)	Digestible energy	Metabolizable energy	Net energy
4–6	17.5	16.5	12.5
6–8	17.0	16.0	12.0
8–12	16.5	15.5	11.5
12–20	16.0	15.0	11.0
20–30	15.5	14.5	10.5

[a] 1 MJ = 239 kcal.

Table 5.3. Recommended dietary true ileal digestible lysine to energy ratios (g/MJ) for piglet diets[a].

Body weight (kg)[b]	Lys/DE	Lys/ME	Lys/NE
4–6	0.90	0.95	1.25
6–8	0.85	0.90	1.20
8–12	0.80	0.85	1.15
12–20	0.75	0.80	1.10
20–30	0.70	0.75	1.05

DE, digestible energy; ME, metabolizable energy; NE, net energy.
[a] 1 MJ = 239 kcal.
[b] For other weight ranges use average of adjacent values.

early post-weaning or creep diets does lactose (20–30%) become a substantial source of energy, but its contribution declines rapidly.

Thermally processed cereals provide more readily digested starch, but their value is debatable. Although enzymatic ability to digest raw starch is induced rapidly to high levels post-weaning (Wiseman *et al.*, 2001), cooked cereals are deemed beneficial for young pigs when feed intake is problematic (Mavromichalis and Varley, 2003).

It should be noted, however, that growth performance does not respond in any consistent pattern to increasing starch gelatinization (Hongtrakul *et al.*, 1998). In fact, overcooking may render a portion of the starch resistant to digestion and eventually increase its availability for bacterial proliferation in the large intestine (Annison and Topping, 1994). From a practical perspective, however, gelatinization values proposed in Table 5.4 may be used as rough guidelines.

Lactose

Lactose is an integral part of most commercial piglet diets because of its well-documented beneficial effects on growth performance post-weaning (Krider *et al.*, 1949; Graham *et al.*, 1981). The most common sources of

Table 5.4. Typical gelatinization values for major cooked cereals. (From S. Tibble, SCA Iberia SA, 2004, personal communication.)

Cereal	%
Maize	65
Wheat	70
Oats	60
Barley	75
Rice	45

lactose are skim milk (50% lactose) and dried whey (70% lactose). Other dairy products that may be less expensive yet equally effective in supplying lactose include crystalline lactose, deproteinized whey, whey permeate, milk chocolate product, cheese powder, and whey protein concentrate.

Pigs less than 8–10 weeks old cannot utilize starch very effectively (Kidder and Manners, 1978), but the starch digestive enzymes can be rapidly induced by dietary substrates (Kelly *et al.*, 1991a,b). Nevertheless, weaning stress accompanied by low feed intake prolong physiological maturation of the digestive system (Wiseman *et al.*, 2001), and for this reason, simple sugars and cooked cereals are generally more digestible than raw cereals (Veum and Mateo, 1981; Carter and Leibholz, 1991). It is, thus, widely accepted that piglets benefit from readily digestible carbohydrates until their digestive system is fully capable of utilizing raw starch.

Diets based on cereals and vegetable protein sources can support greater growth performance when supplemented with milk products such as dried whey and skim milk. Inclusion of 10–20% dried whey in simple diets (corn, soybean meal, and oat groats) has consistently improved growth performance by at least 15% in pigs weaned at 3 weeks of age (Tokach *et al.*, 1989; Lepine *et al.*, 1991; Mahan and Newton, 1993). Other dairy products are equally effective in enhancing post-weaning growth performance (Giesting *et al.*, 1985; Nessmith *et al.*, 1997a,b), although they are usually more expensive.

Initially, the effectiveness of dairy products was attributed to increased palatability and protein digestibility (Wahlstrom *et al.*, 1974; Graham *et al.*, 1981). However, it has been demonstrated since then that lactose and not the protein fraction of whey is responsible for improved feed intake and weight gain during the first weeks post-weaning (Mahan, 1992). In these trials, lactose supplementation restored growth performance in diets devoid of dried whey, whereas lactalbumin supplementation failed to improve performance (Table 5.5).

It should be remarked that supplementation with a highly digestible source of protein or crystalline amino acids was essential for lactose to elicit its beneficial effects in whey-free diets. In the same studies (Mahan, 1992), it was demonstrated that after the first 2 weeks post-weaning, piglets responded more to protein supplementation, an indication of a rapidly maturing digestive system and increased need for highly digestible protein.

Lactose specifications

Several studies have investigated dietary lactose concentrations that support maximal growth performance in weaned pigs (Dritz *et al.*, 1993; Touchette *et al.*, 1995b; Bertol *et al.*, 2000; Mahan *et al.*, 2004). These data suggest that: (i) high concentrations of lactose are needed immediately post-weaning; (ii) lactose concentrations can be reduced rapidly afterwards; and

Table 5.5. Effects of whey components (lactose and lactalbumin) on performance in young pigs. (Adapted from Mahan, 1992.)

Item g/day	Maize + soybean meal	+ 20% whey	+ lactalbumin and starch	+ lactose and amino acids	+ lactalbumin and lactose
Weight gain	210[a]	233[b]	208[a]	251[b]	243[b]
Feed intake	341[a]	395[b]	371[a]	398[b]	388[b]
Gain/feed	616[a]	590[b]	561[b]	631[a]	626[a]

A total of 420 pigs (6.8 kg) in 14 replicates per treatment were used in a 21-day growth assay.
[a,b] Values within a row with unlike superscript letters are significantly different ($P < 0.05$).

(iii) piglets heavier than 10–12 kg in body weight do not benefit greatly from supplemental lactose. Although responses to lactose have been variable, due to basal diet composition, genetics, environment, and health conditions, most experiments report similar lactose requirements for nursery pigs. Therefore, practical recommendations for dietary lactose specifications are presented in Table 5.6.

Addition of animal plasma may lower lactose requirements because it promotes feed intake post-weaning (Touchette *et al*., 1995a). For example, pigs fed diets with 6.75% plasma protein required about 15% added lactose for maximal growth performance during the first week post-weaning. In contrast, when plasma protein was replaced with extruded soy protein concentrate, performance peaked between 30 and 45% dietary lactose. It appears that when feed intake is high, lower levels of dietary lactose are

Table 5.6. Recommended dietary specifications for lactose equivalents (%) in piglet diets[a].

Body weight (kg)	Minimum[b]	Optimum[c]	Maximum[d]
Sow's milk		25[e]	
4–6	20	30	40
6–8	10	20	30
8–12	5	10	15
12–20	0	0	5
20–30	0	0	0

[a] Lactose equivalents include lactose and other simple sugars such as dextrose and sucrose.
[b] Minimum concentrations for acceptable growth performance in low-cost production systems.
[c] Optimum concentrations for balanced diet cost and growth performance.
[d] Maximum concentrations for accelerated growth performance.
[e] On a 90% dry matter equivalent basis.

needed, perhaps because feed intake is closely related to digestive system maturation (Kelly *et al.*, 1991a,b).

Lactose equivalents

Earlier studies indicated that although weaned pigs prefer lactose over starch, they can also use other forms of simple sugars (Kidder and Manners, 1978). Monosaccharides (e.g. glucose, fructose, and maltose) and oligosaccharides (e.g. sucrose and maltodextrins) can be as effective as lactose in supporting growth performance (Lee *et al.*, 2000; Mavromichalis *et al.*, 2001). Therefore, the term 'lactose equivalent' is proposed as more appropriate to express dietary specifications for simple sugars (Mavromichalis, 2000a), as piglets do not have a requirement for lactose *per se*. Lactose equivalent values for several sources of simple sugars that can replace lactose are given in Table 5.7.

Several concerns arise, however, with the replacement of lactose by other simple sugars in pelleted diets. For example, sucrose may increase pellet hardness as it 'burns' easily in the Maillard reaction during pelleting (see Chapter 8). Also, dextrose and other reducing sugars may readily destroy amino acids during pelleting. For these reasons, lower pelleting temperatures or even cold pelleting are recommended for diets rich in reducing sugars.

Simple sugars also differ considerably in sweetness, and, therefore, changes in diet palatability should be taken into consideration when using lactose alternatives. Pigs prefer simple sugars in the following order: sucrose > fructose > maltose = lactose > glucose > galactose (Glaser *et al.*, 2000).

Excessive concentrations of simple sugars are also known to predispose pigs to secretory diarrhea. For instance, by changing the amount of sugars

Table 5.7. Sources of lactose equivalents for piglet diets. (Adapted from Mavromichalis, 2000a.)

Ingredient	Dry matter (%)	Main simple sugar(s)	Lactose equivalents (%)
Lactose	95	Lactose	90
Dextrose, anhydrous	98	Glucose	95
Dextrose, monohydrate	90	Glucose	85
High-fructose corn syrup	75	Fructose	50
Regular corn syrup	85	Glucose and fructose	45
Molasses	75	Sucrose, glucose, fructose	45
Table sugar	98	Sucrose	95

(sucrose and corn syrup solids), dietary osmolality was manipulated between 250 and 700 mOsm/kg (Case *et al.*, 1981). Absorption of water and carbohydrates from the small intestine in piglets increased, and thus chances for diarrhea were minimized, as osmolality increased at similar dietary electrolyte balance. Maltodextrin was shown to increase water absorption, whereas glucose increased water secretion in the gastrointestinal tract (Weber and Ehrlein, 1998), indicating that sugar oligomers are more effective than monomers in preventing secretory diarrhea.

Fiber

The non-digestible fraction of dietary carbohydrates has been characterized traditionally by crude fiber analysis, a term widely recognized as imprecise (NRC, 1998). Alternative and more inclusive terms, such as non-starch polysaccharides and dietary fiber, have been suggested as more informative, but crude fiber remains the choice term of reference. This is a reflection of the fact that analytical values for crude fiber are readily available for most ingredients. Certainly, it does not help that certain feed labeling laws require 'fiber' to be declared as crude fiber.

Non-digestible carbohydrates can be fermented by the intestinal microflora to produce volatile fatty acids, which in turn can be absorbed and used as an energy source (Kidder and Manners, 1978). But, such contribution to the energy nutrition of the young pig is rather insignificant (NRC, 1998), and usually ignored. In contrast, fiber dilutes dietary energy, increases feed bulkiness, and reduces overall nutrient digestibility (NRC, 1998). It has been estimated (ARC, 1981) that each 1% dietary crude fiber decreases energy digestibility by 1.3%, feed efficiency by 3%, and growth by 2% in growing pigs (the effects are expected to be more pronounced in piglets). Thus, with the exception of certain oligosaccharides, which might have beneficial effects on gastrointestinal health (Davis *et al.*, 2002), non-starch polysaccharides are considered undesirable in piglet diets (Pluske *et al.*, 2001). Nevertheless, a limited amount of fiber is considered essential to allow for proper gastrointestinal motility (Bolduan *et al.*, 1988).

Although conclusive dose-titration studies are not available to derive practical recommendations, commercial practice indicates that for pigs below 10–12 kg in body weight diets should contain around 2–3% crude fiber to avoid feed intake depression. For heavier pigs, up to 5% crude fiber may be added in low-cost diets, but feed intake is likely to be less than maximal.

Lipids

Apart from a relatively small requirement for linoleic acid (0.1 g/MJ NE; NRC, 1998), which is easily met in most practical diets, pigs do not have a physiological need for lipids. Nevertheless, the use of animal fats and vegetable oils in piglet diets has consistently drawn the attention of scientists and producers (for a review see Mavromichalis, 2000b) because lipids:

- are good sources of energy, having as much as 2.5 times more than most cereals;
- may be less expensive as a source of energy under certain conditions;
- reduce feed-borne dust, especially when diets are fed in meal form; and
- aid in the pelleting process by lubricating the die.

In many parts of the world, animal fats and vegetable oils are usually included in high-nutrient-density diets because piglets are considered to be in a continual energy-deficient state (Fenton *et al.*, 1985). An energy deficit early in life usually results in considerable losses of body fat reserves, which is especially undesirable during the post-weaning period (Whittemore *et al.*, 1978). Therefore, high-energy diets, well balanced for all nutrients, are strongly recommended for young pigs to allow maximum expression of genetic potential for growth (Campbell *et al.*, 1975). To this effect, many creep and post-weaning diets contain as much as 10–12% total lipids, when contributions from natural ingredients and added lipid sources are considered together. Diets for the later nursery period usually contain 3 to 6% total lipids.

Fat utilization

As noted in Chapter 2, weaned piglets are rather restricted in their ability to digest animal and vegetable lipids during the early nursery period. Two main factors affect digestibility of lipids in piglets: age and source. In the work conducted by Cera *et al.* (1988, 1989, 1990) it was clearly demonstrated that weaned piglets benefit more from supplemental lipids with increasing age, whereas vegetable oils are more digestible than animal fats, with coconut oil being the best source of lipids for post-weaning diets.

Fat instead of antibiotics?

A research team from Denmark (Dierick *et al.*, 2002) investigated the role of medium-chain fatty acids as an antibiotic replacement in controlling intestinal microbiota. In an *in vitro* test, lipids rich in medium-chain fatty acids were incubated with a lipase enzyme under conditions that simulated digestion at the gastrointestinal tract. The lipase released up to 20% medium-chain fatty acids. In a subsequent test, it was found that a minimal concentration of 0.35% (wt/wt) or 25 mM medium-chain fatty acids in incubation fluid was enough to exert a tenfold suppression of the intestinal microbial population. Although these results are very promising, it should be noted that this was a pilot study. Medium-chain fatty acids are absorbed rapidly in the stomach and, thus, they may have minimal effects in the small intestine where they are needed most.

Protein

Protein (amino acids) is the second most expensive nutrient after energy in piglet diets. Not only are amino acids used as building blocks for protein deposition, but also certain amino acids have other physiological roles. For example, tryptophan is involved in the regulation of feed intake (Lynch *et al.*, 2000), whereas glutamine is involved in enteric immunity (Hernandez *et al.*, 2000).

Among the ten essential amino acids, the most likely to become limiting in low-protein piglet diets are lysine, methionine, threonine, tryptophan, isoleucine, and valine (Mavromichalis *et al.*, 1998). In contrast, histidine, phenylalanine, leucine, and arginine are not problematic in most practical diets. Glutamine supplementation in early nursery diets may be also warranted on grounds of gut health (Wu *et al.*, 1996; Burrin and Stoll, 2003), but no specific requirement has been established.

Crystalline forms of lysine, methionine, threonine, and tryptophan are commercially available, although tryptophan cost is almost prohibiting in all but the most complex piglet diets. As a general rule, it is recommended to limit individual additions of crystalline amino acids to 0.5% in piglet diets to prevent unbalancing the ideal protein profile, especially for non-essential and essential amino acids that are not included in diet formulation. In reality, however, up to 0.75% is added in antibiotic-free diets that must be low in crude protein to avoid digestive upsets.

Lysine

Pigs require lysine for maintenance and protein deposition in lean-tissue gain. For maintenance, 36 mg true ileal digestible lysine are required daily per kilogram metabolic weight ($BW^{0.75}$; Fuller *et al.*, 1989). For protein deposition, 120 mg true ileal digestible lysine are needed per gram protein, reflecting the average concentration of lysine in muscle protein (70 mg/g) and the marginal efficiency (58%) of converting true ileal digestible lysine to muscle protein-bound lysine (Bikker *et al.*, 1994).

Assuming that weight gain in piglets is 16% protein (Whittemore, 1998), a factorial approach may be used in determining requirements and dietary specifications with known feed intake. For example, a 10-kg pig growing 400 g/day on 600 g feed requires 0.2 and 7.7 g digestible lysine for maintenance and protein deposition, respectively. Therefore, a diet with at least 1.3% digestible lysine (without allowing for any margins of safety) would be needed to cover the daily requirement for lysine. Had actual feed intake been 750 g/day, dietary digestible lysine concentration should have been only 1.05%; a remarkable 20% reduction! This example illustrates the importance of appropriate estimates of actual feed intake before setting dietary lysine specifications for a specific farm or group of pigs.

Factors that prevent pigs from attaining their genetic potential for growth (see Chapter 1) also affect lysine requirement, because: (i) maintenance requirement is trivial (even at 30 kg body weight it is only 0.5 g/day); and (ii) protein deposition in young pigs increases linearly with increasing weight gain and feed intake. Health status is perhaps the most important determinant of growth during the nursery phase, because piglets of high health status have greater biological capacity for protein deposition.

Healthy pigs, such as those reared off-site under segregated early-weaning management protocols, are expected to grow faster, and thus have higher lysine requirements, than pigs of lower health status. In the classical studies of Williams *et al.* (1997a,b,c), healthy pigs required 25% more lysine to maximize performance compared to challenged pigs that did not benefit from increasing dietary lysine concentrations. Interestingly, the efficiency of lysine utilization for protein accretion between these two groups of pigs was similar.

For feed formulation purposes, dietary lysine specifications should be determined based on the lysine to energy ratios, examples of which are in Table 5.3. These values include a moderate margin of safety and should allow for optimal growth performance under good management conditions. Nevertheless, a qualified nutritionist should be consulted to adapt such guidelines to specific local conditions.

Ideal protein profile

An evaluation of dose-titration studies and composition of sow's milk and body tissue reveals that pigs require amino acids in a specific balance or pattern (ideal protein profile) that remains constant regardless of the magnitude of absolute requirements (ARC, 1981; NRC, 1998). Although the amino acid balance is different for maintenance and growth (Fuller *et al.*, 1989), a single profile is satisfactory for nursery pigs because maintenance needs represent a rather small fraction of total requirements up to 20–30 kg body weight. The ideal protein profile is not affected by gender, genetics, dietary energy density, feed intake, rate or composition of gain, and environmental conditions that determine, nonetheless, absolute requirements (Boisen *et al.*, 2000).

The ideal protein profile concept relates the requirement for all amino acids to a reference amino acid for easier diet formulation (Cole and van Lunen, 1994). Lysine is the most common reference amino acid because:

- it is the first-limiting amino acid in most practical diets;
- its requirement is better established than the requirements for other amino acids;
- it is used exclusively for protein synthesis; and
- its chemical analysis is relatively simple.

Diet formulation using an ideal protein profile requires first the establishment of a lysine specification, which is available through dose-titration studies. Then, dietary specifications for other essential amino acids are calculated based on the ideal protein profile (Table 5.8). In this way, the need for dose-titration studies for each amino acid for every possible weight range and condition is eliminated.

For example, a diet for 10-kg piglets would require 1.32% digestible lysine at 11.5 MJ NE (Tables 5.2 and 5.3) and 0.25% digestible tryptophan (1.32 × 0.19) based on a 19% tryptophan to lysine ratio (Table 5.8). Likewise, a diet for 25-kg pigs would require 1.1% digestible lysine and 0.21% digestible tryptophan (1.1 × 0.19). Even though pigs differ in body weight and require different levels of dietary lysine and tryptophan, the ratio between the two amino acids remains constant at 19%. The ideal protein profile concept is of paramount importance in formulating low-protein diets with increasing concentrations of crystalline amino acids.

The ideal protein concept was originally developed based on the theory that providing amino acids closer to actual requirements would enhance performance, because excess amino acids would not have to be catabolized at an energy cost for the animal (Baker, 1997). Yet, there is no scientific evidence to support that pigs fed practical diets cannot handle slight excesses of amino acids (Edmonds *et al.*, 1987), which are unavoidable when diets are balanced on the first-limiting amino acid. Growth performance, however, is affected when an amino acid is supplied in toxic

Table 5.8. Ideal amino acid profiles for piglet diets.

Amino acids	Recommended	Sow's milk[a]	USA (NRC, 1998)	France (ITP, 2002)	UK (BSAS, 2003)
Lysine	100	100	100	100	100
Methionine[b]	30	33	26	30	30
Methionine + cysteine	60	56	56	60	59
Threonine	65	55	64	65	65
Tryptophan	19	16	18	19	19
Isoleucine	58	55	54	–	58
Valine	70	73	68	–	70

[a] Adapted from Mavromichalis *et al.* (2001).
[b] Methionine can cover cystine requirements with an efficiency of 81% (i.e. 1 g Met = 0.81 g Cys).

concentrations or in excess of its requirement when a more limiting amino acid is deficient. For example, growth depression caused by 0.2% added methionine was alleviated by the addition of only 0.2% lysine, which was limiting (Wahlstrom and Libal, 1974).

Limiting amino acids

Because all sources of amino acids are expensive, dietary excesses are always against profitability. The amino acid present in the least amount relative to its specification is referred to as the first-limiting amino acid (Baker, 1997) and dictates performance. When the specification for the first-limiting amino acid is met, the next amino acid with the least concentration relative to its specification becomes second-limiting and dictates performance.

The order by which each amino acid becomes limiting depends entirely on ingredient selection and adopted ideal protein profile. Thus, isoleucine becomes limiting in diets rich in blood products (Kats *et al.*, 1994), histidine in diets based on barley (Fuller *et al.*, 1979), and tryptophan in diets based on maize and meat meals (Batterham, 1970). In such diets, supplementation with specific crystalline amino acid(s) and (or) higher levels of protein-rich ingredients becomes essential to meet specifications. It is therefore suggested that specifications for all essential amino acids are included in diet formulation to eliminate the risk of potential deficiencies when using novel ingredients.

In most practical piglet diets, lysine is clearly the first-limiting amino acid (Mavromichalis *et al.*, 1998). In low-protein diets, however, other amino acids rapidly become limiting as protein level decreases. When dietary protein concentration is decreased by 2–4 percentage units, methionine, threonine, and tryptophan are most likely to become limiting (Russell *et al.*, 1987), with valine and isoleucine becoming limiting with more severe reductions in crude protein concentration (Baker and Mavromichalis, 2000).

Tryptophan

The role of tryptophan lies beyond protein synthesis to appetite regulation and control of sleep via its metabolite serotonin. Because tryptophan is rather expensive in its crystalline form, an accurate estimate of tryptophan requirement is essential in balancing growth performance and cost of production. European researchers (Lynch *et al.*, 2000) evaluated the tryptophan requirement of pigs between 10 and 30 kg body weight. A basal diet formulated with cereals, peas, whey, and fishmeal was fortified with increasing doses of crystalline tryptophan to achieve tryptophan to lysine ratios between 15 and 25%. Results indicated that growth rate and feed efficiency were maximized at a ratio between 19 and 21% for pigs between

10 and 20 kg body weight, whereas growth from 10 to 30 kg was optimized at about 19%. These results are also supported by Canadian researchers (Lorschy and Patience, 1999), who found the digestible tryptophan and lysine requirements for protein deposition to be 16.8 and 89.8 mg/g, respectively, giving a ratio of tryptophan to lysine of 19%.

Low-protein diets

Reduction of dietary protein in nursery diets is currently deemed beneficial for improving animal health and reducing environmental pollution (Lenis and Jongbloed, 1999). Low-protein diets are formulated to meet amino acid specifications with the least amount of crude protein (nitrogen). Thus, such diets are naturally more digestible than conventional diets because crystalline amino acids (100% digestible) and (or) protein sources of higher biological value are used in greater proportions. In result, less undigested protein remains for bacterial proliferation and excretion to the environment.

It has been shown (Prohaszka and Baron, 1980) that piglets fed diets low in crude protein are more resistant to digestive upsets from *E. coli* infection. Low-protein diets have been shown also to reduce nitrogen excretion by 30–50%, depending on original specifications, ingredient selection, and magnitude of reduction in dietary protein concentration. In general, for each percentage unit reduction in dietary crude protein, nitrogen excretion is expected to be lower by approximately 8% (Kerr and Easter, 1995).

As dietary protein concentration is reduced, several unique concerns arise in diet formulation. First, the balance between essential and non-essential amino acids is disturbed. This ratio should be around 50:50 to allow optimal nitrogen retention and utilization (Lenis *et al.*, 1999). Second, the importance of predicting lysine requirement increases because the more expensive crystalline amino acids supply a larger fraction of the total. Third, it is often recommended that the net energy system be used in formulating low-protein diets based on true ileal amino acid digestibilities (Boisen *et al.*, 2000). Fourth, amino acid antagonisms may develop if arginine becomes excessive compared to the lysine concentration or leucine compared to the sum of isoleucine and valine concentrations (D'Mello, 1994). Fifth, sodium bicarbonate additions may be needed to buffer the acidic effect of excessive amounts of free amino acids in diets past the post-weaning period.

Taking into account benefits and challenges of a low-protein nutrition approach for piglets, it appears that a moderate reduction (2%) in dietary protein is quite feasible. A more drastic reduction (3–4%) requires a higher degree of accuracy in diet formulation, and perhaps changes in ingredient selection and nutrient matrices. Reducing protein beyond 4% is expected to reduce performance in commercial production systems.

D-Amino Acids

With few exceptions, animals require dietary amino acids in the L-enantiomer form. Proteins with even small amounts of D-amino acids are poorly digested because they impair the activity of endogenous exopeptidases. Additionally, the absorption of free or oligopeptide-bound D-amino acids is slower compared to their L-enantiomers. The apparent ileal digestibility of most D-amino acids is lower than 40%, although they are readily utilized by gut microbiota (de Vrese *et al.*, 2000).

In natural ingredients, the vast majority of amino acids are present in the L-enantiomer form. Processing, particularly heat and (or) alkaline conditions, increases the concentration of D-amino acids via racemization (Vargane-Visi *et al.*, 2004). Overheated ingredients and diets, by-products of the alcohol industry, and NaOH-treated products may, therefore, contain excessive amounts of D-amino acids and be of lower biological value. With the exception of DL-methionine, which is 100% digestible, all commercial crystalline amino acids are available in their L-enantiomer form (for example, L-lysine HCl, L-threonine, and L-tryptophan).

Macro Minerals

Minerals required in concentrations exceeding about 0.1% of the diet are usually called macro minerals, in distinction to trace minerals that are needed in very small amounts. Macro minerals include calcium, phosphorus, sodium, chlorine, potassium, magnesium, and sulfur. Of those, only calcium, phosphorus, sodium and chlorine are typically limiting in most practical diets. Potassium, magnesium, and sulfur needs are usually covered by contributions from natural ingredients (NRC, 1998; BSAS, 2003). Recommended macro-mineral specifications for piglet diets are in Table 5.9.

Table 5.9. Recommended macro-mineral specifications for piglet diets. (Based on recommendations of NRC, 1998; ITP, 2002; BSAS, 2003.)

Body weight (kg)	Ca[a] (%)	P (%)	Digestible P (%)	Na (%)	Cl[b] (%)	K[b] (%)	Mg[b] (%)	dEB (mEq/kg)
4–6	0.90	0.80	0.38	0.45	0.45	0.35	0.10	250
6–8	0.85	0.75	0.36	0.40	0.40	0.35	0.10	250
8–12	0.80	0.70	0.34	0.35	0.35	0.35	0.10	200
12–20	0.75	0.65	0.32	0.30	0.30	0.35	0.10	200
20–30	0.70	0.60	0.30	0.25	0.25	0.35	0.10	200

dEB, dietary electrolyte balance.

[a] Calcium to total phosphorus should not exceed 1.2:1 in piglet diets to avoid buffering stomach acidity.

[b] Most practical diets contain levels in excess of these amounts.

Ash

The sum of macro and trace minerals comprises ash, which is determined easily by burning a sample of material at 600°C for 4–6 h. A high concentration of ash in nursery diets is considered undesirable, because it may have a laxative effect that is often mistaken for diarrhea. Formulas based on ingredients of animal origin are usually high in ash, although certain vegetable ingredients can be quite rich as well. Such ingredients include fishmeal, meat-and-bone meal, poultry meal, and peanut meal. For such ingredients, ash concentration is usually taken into account in quality assurance schemes.

Calcium

Calcium is the least expensive nutrient because its main sources, calcium carbonate and limestone, are relatively inexpensive. Thus, many commercial products contain excess calcium because calcium carbonate is a common carrier. However, calcium carbonate has a strong buffering capacity that markedly lowers the acidity of the gastrointestinal contents (Peddireddi *et al.*, 2004), thus interfering with protein digestion. It is strongly recommended that dietary calcium specifications do not exceed actual requirements by more than 0.1% Ca (i.e. a small margin of error). For the same reason, the calcium to phosphorus ratio should be no more than 1.2:1. A wide calcium to phosphorus ratio also reduces the absorption of phosphorus, especially in diets supplemented with phytase (Cromwell *et al.*, 1995), and depresses growth, especially in diets marginal in phosphorus (NRC, 1998).

Phosphorus

Phosphorus is the third most expensive nutrient in a pig diet, following energy and lysine. Major sources include phosphate salts of calcium and natural rock phosphates. Of those, dicalcium and monocalcium phosphates are the most commonly used in the feed industry.

Phosphorus bioavailability is high in animal ingredients but it is remarkably low in vegetable ingredients. In plants, around 75% of total phosphorus is bound to phytate, a compound poorly utilized by monogastric animals. In maize and soybean meal, for example, phosphorus bioavailability is only 15 and 30%, respectively (NRC, 1998). In certain vegetable ingredients, however, such as wheat and its by-products, high-moisture maize and sorghum, and low-phytate maize, phosphorus bioavailability may exceed 50% (NRC, 1998). Nevertheless, a considerably large fraction of dietary phosphorus is usually excreted in feces, contributing to eutrophication of surface waters (Lenis and Jongbloed, 1999). It is therefore strongly advised that dietary specifications do not exceed requirements by more than 0.05 percentage units.

Commercial preparations of phytase can be quite useful in controlling phosphorus excretion. Up to 60% less phosphorus in excreta may be anticipated from the use of 500–700 units phytase/kg feed (Pallauf and Rimbach, 1997). In diets supplemented with phytase, digestible phosphorus and calcium specifications must be lowered by 0.1% and 0.08%, respectively (Jongbloed *et al.*, 1995; Radcliffe *et al.*, 1995). Formulation on digestible rather than total phosphorus basis also minimizes dietary phosphorus excesses.

For maximal bone strength and ash content, desirable characteristics for future breeding animals, dietary specifications for both calcium and phosphorus must be increased by at least 0.1% to improve structural soundness (NRC, 1998).

Sodium and chlorine

The main source of sodium and chlorine is common salt (NaCl), which is relatively inexpensive. Most ingredients of animal origin also contain ample quantities of sodium; often enough to meet dietary specifications. Fishmeal is especially rich in salt and is usually marketed with an upper guarantee on salt content. Whey, blood products, and bakery by-products are also good sources of sodium.

Recent research from the University of Ohio (Mahan *et al.*, 1996, 1999) revealed that weaned pigs clearly benefit from concentrations of sodium and chlorine that exceed established requirements. Sodium was partially responsible for the positive responses, but the greater response was attributed to chlorine. Currently, NRC (1998) requirement estimates for sodium and chlorine in piglet diets are around 0.20% for both minerals, but it is strongly recommended that at least twice as much be used. Lower levels may be more satisfactory when fecal looseness is a problem (BSAS, 2003).

Excess salt (up to 2%) does not cause toxicosis as long as pigs have free access to non-saline water (NRC, 1998). But, newly weaned pigs offered diets rich in sodium and chlorine may be at risk of salt toxicosis if they do not know how to operate drinkers. To this end, cup drinkers usually offer an advantage over nipple-type drinkers. When water contains appreciable concentrations of sodium and chlorine (e.g. coastal water may contain up to 200 mg Na/l; Kornegay *et al.*, 1991), dietary salt additions should be reduced accordingly to avoid toxicosis. Apart from toxicosis due to water deprivation, excess salt may also disturb anion–cation electrolyte balance and lead to diarrhea (NRC, 1998).

Magnesium

The magnesium requirements of pigs have not been studied extensively, perhaps because enough magnesium is supplemented via natural ingredients.

Piglets fed liquid milk-based diets require no more than 0.03–0.05% magnesium (Miller *et al.*, 1965). A typical piglet diet contains about 0.15% magnesium, which is 50% bioavailable (Nuoranne *et al.*, 1980). Sow's milk contains 0.045% magnesium on a dry matter basis (Darragh and Moughan, 1998), which is equivalent to 0.05% on a 90% dry matter basis. It is recommended that piglet diets contain at least 0.1% magnesium for safety reasons.

Potassium

Potassium is often ignored in diet formulation because it abounds in most typical ingredients. Minimal requirements are set at 0.26% (NRC, 1998), with most commercial diets containing clearly at least twice this concentration.

A high concentration of potassium may cause diarrhea as it can disrupt osmotic pressure and anion–cation balance, causing excessive water secretion in the gastrointestinal tract. Molasses is especially rich in potassium, and this is believed to cause diarrhea in young pigs, but this has not been proven. Ly (1996) fed pigs with diets containing potassium levels matching those found in diets based on molasses but pigs did not develop diarrhea, indicating that potassium alone is not responsible for digestive upsets.

Sulfur

Sulfur is another essential nutrient that abounds in natural ingredients, and thus no requirement has been established. It is actually excess sulfur that often draws attention, as it may be responsible for secretory diarrhea due to osmotic effects in the gastrointestinal tract, but research on this topic is limited.

Researchers from Germany (Kamphues *et al.*, 2002) investigated the effect of high sulfate concentration in 29 samples of whey on fecal consistency in preruminant calves. Sulfur content in whey ranged from 0.03 to 4.3% per kg dry matter. A high concentration of sulfate in the liquid milk replacer diet (>0.6 g/l) resulted in marked increases in incidents of diarrhea. This concentration would be equivalent to about 0.3% sulfate per kg dry matter. If we assume that results obtained with milk-fed calves are acceptable for piglets, it can be deducted that a safe level of sulfate in most piglet diets should be below 0.25% on an as-fed basis.

Vitamins

The importance of fat- (A, D, E, and K) and water-soluble vitamins (B-vitamins) in pig nutrition is unequivocal (NRC, 1998). Scientific groups frequently publish estimates of requirements and allowances. The latest estimates (BSAS, 2003) are based on an international survey and include considerable safety margins.

Natural ingredients contain highly variable and largely unpredictable vitamin concentrations. It is, thus, common industry practice to supplement piglet feeds with all essential vitamins (usually in the form of a vitamin premix), without taking into account naturally occurring vitamins. In most practical diets, however, not all naturally occurring vitamins are likely to be deficient. Thus, amounts of thiamin, pyridoxine, folic acid, biotin, and choline provided by most common cereals and protein sources are usually more than enough to cover animal needs without fortification (NRC, 1998). Yet, it remains common industry practice to provide a complement of all vitamins, mostly for safety reasons (Fraga and Villamide, 2000). Practical recommendations regarding vitamin additions for piglet diets are presented in Table 5.10.

The exact level of vitamin fortification remains equivocal as academic and industry professionals strongly disagree on optimal levels. Largely unpredictable vitamin losses during manufacturing and storage of complete feeds and premixes only add to this confusion. With vitamins accounting for less than 2–5% of total feed cost, it is considered by many nutritionists safe to err

Table 5.10. Recommended vitamin and trace mineral additions for piglet diets. (Based on recommendations of NRC, 1998; ITP, 2002; BSAS, 2003.)

Vitamin	Unit	Amount	Trace mineral	Unit	Amount
A	IU	10,000	Iron	mg/kg	100
D	IU	1,000	Zinc[b]	mg/kg	100
E	IU	50	Copper[c]	mg/kg	25
K	IU or mg/kg	1	Manganese	mg/kg	25
Niacin	mg/kg	20	Iodine	mg/kg	0.5
Pantothenic acid	mg/kg	15	Selenium[d]	mg/kg	0.3
Riboflavin	mg/kg	5			
B_{12}	mg/kg	0.05			
Biotin[a]	mg/kg	0.15			
Choline[a]	mg/kg	200			
Folacin[a]	mg/kg	1.5			
Thiamin[a]	mg/kg	2			
Pyridoxine[a]	mg/kg	3			

[a] These vitamins are often provided in excess of requirements by natural ingredients.

[b] Pharmacological doses of Zn (1500–3000 mg/kg) from zinc oxide are often used to enhance performance.

[c] Pharmacological doses of Cu (100–250 mg/kg) from copper sulfate are often used to enhance performance.

[d] Maximum Se concentrations permitted by law in the EU and the USA are 0.5 and 0.3 mg/kg, respectively.

on the side of overfortification, especially after several earlier studies suggested that overfortification might actually enhance early growth (Wilson *et al.*, 1991). Thus, many vitamins are often added at ten- or even 100-fold times compared to their established requirements for maximal growth (BSAS, 2003).

Universities rebuke overfortification

In a joint effort by eight US universities (Cline *et al.*, 2002), an extensive study was conducted on the effects of B vitamin overfortification on piglet growth performance. A total of 760 pigs in 35 replicates per treatment in eight different experimental stations were offered a basal diet based on maize, soybean meal, whey, and animal plasma for 2 weeks post-weaning. To this diet, a premix of eight B vitamins (niacin, riboflavin, pantothenic acid, B_{12}, thiamin, biotin, folic acid, and pyridoxine) was added at levels equal to NRC (1998) recommendations or greater (200 and 400%). Results demonstrated that maximal performance was achieved at levels of supplementation no higher than those proposed by NRC (1998). It should be noted, however, that: (i) the diets were in meal form; (ii) feed storage was minimal; and (iii) animal health was satisfactory. Nevertheless, this research is an indication that overfortification is not always warranted in commercial diets.

L-Carnitine

Carnitine is a vitamin-like compound involved in the metabolism of lipids. Previous research reports on the effects of dietary additions of up to 1000 mg carnitine/kg in diets for young pigs are largely inconclusive (for a review, refer to Mavromichalis and Baker, 2000). In a more recent study from the USA (Rincker *et al.*, 2003), dietary L-carnitine additions of up to 100 mg/kg were tested in diets with and without soybean oil. In five trials, graded levels of carnitine (0, 25, 50, 75, and 100 mg/kg) were tested in diets containing varying levels of soybean oil (from 0 to 6%). Carnitine additions did not affect growth performance in phase 1 and 3 of the trials (trials lasted from 34 to 38 days). In phase 2, however, carnitine slightly increased weight gain and feed intake, with a trend toward improved performance for the overall period. In only one trial, the effects of carnitine were pronounced in diets with soybean oil, but this did not approach statistical significance.

Vitamin C and immunity

Pigs, unlike humans and other primates, are able to synthesize vitamin C, and, thus, dietary fortification is not considered essential. Despite this, the issue of supplemental vitamin C in diets for weaned pigs has seen considerable debate during the last 25 years (for a review, refer to Mavromichalis and Baker, 1999). Earlier trials suggested enhanced growth performance in response to vitamin C supplementation, but subsequent studies yielded rather inconsistent results.

Another report from China (Zhao *et al.*, 2002) recently added to this debate. In two experiments, pigs weaned between 20 and 30 days of age were offered diets supplemented with 0, 75, or 300 mg vitamin C/kg for 21 days post-weaning, but growth performance was not affected by supplemental vitamin C. It should be noted, however, that pigs were penned in groups of two and, therefore, the level of stress to which they were exposed was rather limited compared to stress encountered in most commercial facilities. On a positive note, plasma levels of γ-immunoglobulins and antibody titers to bovine serum tended to be higher in pigs fed diets with supplemental vitamin C. This could be an indication of enhanced immunity status that could potentially help pigs cope better in the face of a disease challenge, but this requires further investigation.

Trace Minerals

Today, established requirements for trace minerals exist only for iron, zinc, copper, manganese, iodine, and selenium (NRC, 1998). In accord with commercial vitamin supplementation practices, trace mineral supplementation also ignores amounts furnished by natural ingredients.

Overfortification of trace minerals is usually practiced for manganese, copper, and iodine as dose-titration response trials for these nutrients are several decades old. Iron, zinc, and selenium are often supplied at levels near their established requirements, but when contributions from natural ingredients are taken into account, final levels are many-fold over requirements. Recommended levels presented in Table 5.10 are based on published estimates and commercial practice.

The use of zinc oxide and copper sulfate as antimicrobial and growth-promoting agents is discussed in Chapter 7, as it is the salts and not the individual minerals that exert these beneficial effects. Nevertheless, it should be noted that the use of these additives is declining rapidly in certain parts of the world as trace mineral fortification becomes subject to legislation.

Rare-earth elements

In a German study (He and Rambeck, 2000), young pigs were offered diets that were free of antimicrobial agents but supplemented with chloride salts of rare-earth elements. This was done to verify Chinese reports indicating positive results from the use of lanthanum, cerium, and praseodymium on piglet growth performance.

In the first trial, 72 piglets (7 kg) were offered for 5 weeks two dietary concentrations (75 or 150 mg/kg) of rare-earth elements that were provided via a pure source of lanthanum chloride (98%) or a mixture of rare-earth elements. Growth performance of pigs offered diets with rare-earth elements was numerically increased by up to 5%, but this improvement was not statistically significant. In the second study, however, 14 heavier pigs (17 kg) were offered rare-earth mixture (0 or 150 mg/kg) for 8 weeks. Weight gain was improved by 19% and feed efficiency by 10%, with both figures being significantly different from control. This is the first report indicating potential benefits from rare-earth elements under 'Western' conditions.

Chromium for weaners

Organic chromium is sporadically used in diets for young pigs because it allegedly alleviates post-weaning trauma by enhancing immune system functions. This theory is based on observations with mice and calves. A US research team (van de Ligt *et al.*, 2002) recently evaluated the effects of chromium tripicolinate on immune response and growth performance in weaned pigs. Pigs from 15 litters were used in two experiments. Pigs were born to gilts that were raised on diets with 0 or 200 ppb chromium. After weaning (at 23 days of age) piglets received the same dietary chromium treatments as their dams for 42 days post-weaning. Chromium supplementation did not affect immune system response in terms of serum immunoglobulin production. Similarly, weight gain (511 versus 531 g/day for pigs receiving 0 and 200 ppb chromium, respectively), feed intake (827 versus 851 g/day), and efficiency of feed utilization (1.61 for both groups) were not affected by dietary chromium addition. It appears that the basal diet, which was based on maize, soybean meal, whey, blood products, and fishmeal, contained enough chromium to meet any chromium requirements.

Cobalt

Although there is no scientific evidence that pigs have a dietary requirement for cobalt, other than as a constituent of vitamin B_{12} (NRC, 1998), many commercial trace mineral premixes contain substantial amounts of cobalt. This can only be justified in terms of marketing, as vitamin B_{12} is routinely supplemented in all commercial formulas. Although supplemental cobalt is readily absorbed by enterocytes, almost all of it is rapidly excreted in urine as tissue retention is nearly zero. Currently, BSAS (2003) recommends cobalt be added at 0.2 mg/kg feed.

Boron

Boron is another trace mineral not routinely added in pig diets as naturally occurring forms are considered enough to cover any needs (NRC, 1998). Nevertheless, recent trials (Armstrong and Spears, 2001) indicated that supplementation of 5 mg boron (from sodium borate) per kg feed can elicit a positive growth response in young pigs. As these studies were conducted in only one facility, it merits further investigation to verify the results under more diverse conditions.

Chemical Properties

Little attention is paid to the physicochemical properties of complete feeds. Yet, based on these properties, the organism is called upon to buffer undesirable characteristics or cope with offensive traits.

Acid-binding capacity

Hydrochloric acid is a strong acid secreted by stomach glands to initiate protein digestion. Production of hydrochloric acid is, however, suppressed in suckling pigs (see Chapter 2) and, thus, weaned pigs have limited capacity to digest animal and vegetable protein. In contrast, most piglet diets usually contain ingredients like limestone, calcium salts, soybean meal, and cereals that actually buffer gastric acidity.

It is therefore important to consider the acid-binding or buffering capacity of a piglet formula. British researchers (Pickard *et al.*, 2001) evaluated the effects of dietary acid-binding capacity on gastrointestinal architecture and acidity (pH). A total of 20 pigs weaned at 25 days were offered *ad libitum* access to one of two diets with markedly different concentrations of limestone, and, thus, acid-binding capacity. Two pigs from each treatment were killed on days 2, 4, 6, and 14 and villus height and digesta pH were determined. As expected, villus height (an indicator of gut health) was markedly reduced after weaning in all pigs. However, there was a significant diet × time interaction, such that piglets fed the diet with low acid-binding capacity recovered faster than piglets on the diet with high acid-binding capacity.

It appears that diets with low acid-binding capacity improve gut health, and, thus, such diets may be valuable for pigs recovering from nutritional or pathological digestive upsets that damage the gastrointestinal epithelium. The acid-binding capacities of several common ingredients are listed in Table 5.11. At the moment, there are no recommendations regarding an optimal buffering capacity level other than it should be as low as possible (Gadd, 1989).

Table 5.11. Buffering capacity of selected ingredients used in piglet diets. (Adapted from Gadd, 1989.)

Ingredient	mEq/kg
Maize	160–200
Barley	200–300
Soybean meal	950–1200
Fishmeal	1500–1900
Skim milk	1200–1500
Limestone	20,000
Dicalcium phosphate	1500–1900

Dietary electrolyte balance

The balance of dietary cations (positively charged ions) and anions (negatively charged ions) is in close relationship with pig performance (Patience and Chaplin, 1997) and affects metabolism quite differently than individual ions. Dietary electrolyte balance (dEB), also known as cation–anion difference, is generally calculated using monovalent ions (i.e. sodium, potassium, and chlorine) only:

$$\text{dEB (mEq/kg)} = 1000 \times \{[\text{Na (g/kg)}/23] + [\text{K (g/kg)}/39] - [\text{Cl (g/kg)}/35.5]\}. \quad (5.5)$$

There is a more comprehensive estimate, taking into account also the contribution of divalent ions (i.e. calcium, magnesium, sulfur, and phosphorus), but it is used less often because it requires more chemical analyses.

Dietary electrolyte balance is an indication of the metabolizable ions that can generate or consume acid during metabolism. Diets with negative dEB are more likely to cause metabolic acidosis than diets with positive dEB. Metabolic acidosis has been implicated with reduced feed intake (Yen *et al.*, 1981). Dietary electrolyte balance may also affect energy, amino acid, vitamin, and mineral metabolism. For example, excess dietary alkalinity (positive dEB) may increase lysine oxidation and, thus, increase the requirement for lysine (Scott and Austic, 1978).

It is widely accepted that dEB below 0 mEq/kg is associated with depressed performance in pigs, whereas values between 0 and 300 mEq/kg are considered more appropriate, albeit research results have been variable (Quiniou, 2002). Dietary ingredient selection strongly interacts with dEB. For example (Dersjant-Li *et al.*, 2001), piglets fed a diet high in non-starch polysaccharides (15%), an unusual diet for young pigs, benefited from low dEB (–100 mEq/kg), whereas pigs fed a diet lower in non-starch polysaccharides (10%) benefited from higher dEB (200 mEq/kg). Nutrient digestibility, particularly dry matter, energy, protein, and chlorine, were also affected in a similar fashion by dietary electrolyte balance.

Until more research is conducted, dEB around 250 mEq/kg feed should be satisfactory in most commercial diets (Quiniou, 2002).

Dietary pH

Acidity is measured in units of pH, which indicates the concentration of positively charged protons. A pH below 7 indicates acidity, whereas above 7 indicates alkalinity. Stomach pH is about 2–3 in growing pigs, whereas it is 3–4 in recently weaned piglets (Kidder and Manners, 1978). In contrast, the pH of the small intestine is more alkaline, usually above 7.

To measure dietary pH, a finely ground 10-g sample of feed is mixed with 90 g distilled water (pH 7) for 10 min at room temperature, and then a reading is taken using an inexpensive pH strip that gives a rough estimate based on color change. It is generally advised, although not exactly based on scientific evidence, that a dietary pH between 3 and 4 should be used as a target for piglet diets. To this end, inorganic and organic acids are quite effective in reducing dietary pH, although their effects on stomach acidity are more obscure (Roth and Kirchgessner, 1998).

References

Annison G and Topping DL (1994) Nutritional role of resistant starch: chemical structure vs physiology function. *Annual Reviews of Nutrition* 14:297–320.

ARC (1981) *The Nutrient Requirements of Pigs*. Agricultural Research Council, Commonwealth Agricultural Bureaux, Farnham Royal, UK.

Armstrong TA and Spears JW (2001) Effect of dietary boron on growth performance, calcium and phosphorus metabolism, and bone mechanical properties in growing barrows. *Journal of Animal Science* 79:3120–3127.

Auldist DE, Stevenson FL, Kerr MG, Eason P, and King RH (1997) Lysine requirements of pigs from 2 to 7 kg live weight. *Animal Science* 65:501–507.

Baker DH (1997) *Ideal Amino Acid Profiles for Swine and Poultry and their Applications in Feed Formulation*. Nutri-Quest, Inc., Chesterfield, MO.

Baker DH and Mavromichalis I (2000) *The Role of Branched-Chain Amino Acids in Swine and Poultry Nutrition*. Nutri-Quest, Inc., Chesterfield, MO.

Batterham ES (1970) A nutritional evaluation of diets containing meat meal for growing pigs. 6. Amino acid and mineral–vitamin–antibiotic supplements for maize–meat meal diets. *Australian Journal of Experiments in Agriculture and Animal Husbandry* 10:534.

Beattie VE, Weatherup RN, McCracken KJ, McIlroy SG, and Henry RW (1998) Comparison of a range of NE systems with data obtained from slaughter balance studies on 8–12 week old pigs. *Proceedings of the British Society of Animal Science Annual Meeting*, 154. Midlothian, UK.

Bertol TM, Santos-Filho JI, and Ludke JV (2000) Dietary lactose levels for weaning pigs. *Revista Brasileira de Zootechnia* 29:1387–1393.

Bikker P, Verstegen MWA, Campbell RG, and Kemp B (1994) Digestible lysine requirement of gilts with high genetic potential for lean gain, in relation to the level of energy intake. *Journal of Animal Science* 72:1744–1753.

Black JL, Campbell RG, Williams IH, James KJ, and Davies GT (1986) Simulation of energy and amino acid utilisation in the pig. *Research and Development in Agriculture* 3:121–146.

Boisen S, Hvelplund T, and Weisbjerg MR (2000) Ideal amino acid profiles as a basis for feed protein evaluation. *Livestock Production Science* 64:239–251.

Bolduan G, Jung H, Schnable E, and Schneider R (1988) Recent advances in the nutrition of weaner piglets. *Pig News and Information* 9:381–385.

Bruininx EMAM, van der Peet-Schwering CMC, Schrama JW, Vereijken PFG, Vesseur PC, Everts H, den Hartog LA, and Beynen AC (2001) Individually measured feed intake characteristics and growth performance of group-housed weanling pigs: effects of sex, initial body weight, and body weight distribution within groups. *Journal of Animal Science* 79:301–308.

BSAS (2003) *Nutrient Requirement Standards for Pigs*. British Society of Animal Science, Penicuik, UK

Burrin D and Stoll B (2003) Intestinal nutrient requirements in weanling pigs. In: *Weaning the Pig – Concepts and Consequences*, by Pluske JR, Le Dividich J, and Verstegen MWA (ed), 301–335. Wageningen Academic Publishers, Wageningen, The Netherlands.

Campbell RG, Taverner MR, and Mullaney PD (1975) The effect of dietary concentration of digestible energy on the performance and carcass characteristics of early-weaned pigs. *Animal Production* 21:285–294.

Carter RR and Leibholz J (1991) Effects of extrusion of wheat on dry matter and starch digestibility in the young pig. In: *Manipulating Pig Production III*, by Batterham ES (ed), 86. Australasian Pig Science Association, Werribee, Australia.

Case GL, Phillips RW, Lewis LD, and Connolly B (1981) Effects of osmolality of liquid nutrient diets on plasma equilibration of water and carbohydrate in Yucatan miniature swine. *American Journal of Clinical Nutrition* 34:1861–1867.

Cera KR, Mahan DC, and Reinhart GA (1988) Weekly digestibilities of diets supplemented with corn oil, lard or tallow by weanling swine. *Journal of Animal Science* 66:1430–1437.

Cera KR, Mahan DC, and Reinhart GA (1989) Postweaning swine performance and serum profile responses to supplemental medium-chain free fatty acids and tallow. *Journal of Animal Science* 67:2048–2055.

Cera KR, Mahan DC, and Reinhart GA (1990) Evaluation of various extracted vegetable oils, roasted soybeans, medium-chain triglyceride and an animal–vegetable fat blend for postweaning swine. *Journal of Animal Science* 68:2756–2765.

Cline T, Carter S, Hill G, Kim S, Lewis A, Mahan D, Stein H, and Veum T (2002) Supplemental B-vitamins in pig nursery diets. *Journal of Animal Science* 80(Supplement 2):68.

Cole DJA and van Lunen TA (1994) Ideal amino acid patterns. In: *Amino Acids in Farm Animal Nutrition*, by D'Mello JPF (ed), 99–112. CAB International, Wallingford, UK.

Cole M and Sprent M (2001) Protein and amino acid requirements of weaner pigs. In: *The Weaner Pig – Nutrition and Management*, by Varley MA and Wiseman J (ed), 45–63. CABI Publishing, Wallingford, UK.

Cromwell GL, Lindemann MD, Parker GR, Coffey RD, Monegue HJ, and Randolph JH (1995) Effects of dietary calcium on the efficacy of phytase and on the utilization of phosphorus in low phosphorus diets for pigs. *Journal of Animal Science* 73(Supplement 1):73.

Cromwell GL, Coffey RD, Aaron DK, Lindemann MD, Pierce JL, Monegue HJ, Rupard VM, Cowen DE, Parido MB, and Clayton TM (1996) Differences in growth rate of weanling barrows and gilts. *Journal of Animal Science* 74(Supplement 1):186.

D'Mello JPF (1994) Amino acid imbalances, antagonisms, and toxicities. In: *Amino Acids in Farm Animal Nutrition*, by D'Mello JPF (ed), 63–97. CAB International, Wallingford, UK.

Darragh AJ and Moughan PJ (1998) The composition of colostrum and milk. In: *The Lactating Sow*, by Verstegen MWA, Moughan PJ, and Schrama JW (ed), 3–21. Wageningen Pers, Wageningen, The Netherlands.

Davis ME, Maxwell CV, Brown DC, de Rodas BZ, Johnson ZB, Kegley EB, Hellwig DH, and Dvorak RA (2002) Effect of dietary mannan oligosaccharides and (or) pharmacological additions of copper sulfate on growth performance and immunocompetence of weanling and growing/finishing pigs. *Journal of Animal Science* 80:2887–2894.

de Blas C, Mateos GG, and Rebollar PG (2003) *Tablas FEDNA de composicion y valor nutritivo de alimentos para la fabricacion de piensos compuestos* (2nd edn). FEDNA, Madrid, Spain.

de Vrese M, Frik R, Roos N, and Hagemeister H (2000) Protein-bound D-amino acids, and to a lesser extent lysinoalanine, decrease true ileal protein digestibility in minipigs as determined with N15-labeling. *Journal of Nutrition* 130:2026–2031.

Dersjant-Li Y, Verstegen MWA, Schulze H, Zandstra T, Boer H, Schrama JW, and Verreth JAJ (2001) Performance, digesta characteristics, nutrient flux, plasma composition, and organ weight in pigs as affected by dietary cation anion difference and nonstarch polysaccharide. *Journal of Animal Science* 79:1840–1848.

Dierick NA, Decuypere JA, Molly K, van Beek E, and Vanderbeke E (2002) The combined use of triacylglycerols containing medium chain fatty acids and exogenous lipolytic enzymes as an alternative for nutritional antibiotics in piglet nutrition. *Livestock Production Science* 75:129–142.

Dritz SS, Tokach MD, Nelssen JL, Goodband RD, and Kats LJ (1993) Optimal dried whey level in starter diets containing spray-dried blood meal and comparison of avian and bovine spray-dried blood meals. *Journal of Animal Science* 71(Supplement 1):57.

Edmonds MS, Gonyou HW, and Baker DH (1987) Effect of excess levels of methionine, tryptophan, arginine, lysine or threonine on growth and dietary choice in the pig. *Journal of Animal Science* 65:179–185.

Fenton JP, Roehrig KL, Mahan DC, and Corley JR (1985) Effect of swine weaning age on body fat and lipogenic activity in liver and adipose tissue. *Journal of Animal Science* 60:190–199.

Fowler VR and Gill BP (1989) Voluntary food intake in the young pig. In: *The Voluntary Food Intake of Pigs*, by Forbes JM, Varley MA, and Lawrence TJ (ed), 51–60. Occasional Publication No. 13. British Society of Animal Production, Edinburgh, UK.

Fraga MJ and Villamide MJ (2000) The composition of vitamin supplements in Spanish pig diets. *Pig News and Information* 21:67N–72N.

Fuller MF, Livingstone RM, Baird BA, and Atkinson T (1979) The optimal amino acid supplementation of barley for the growing pig. 1. Response of nitrogen metabolism to progressive supplementation. *British Journal of Nutrition* 41:321–331.

Fuller MF, McWilliam R, Wang TC, and Giles LR (1989) The optimum dietary amino acid pattern for growing pigs 2. Requirements for maintenance and for tissue protein accretion. *British Journal of Nutrition* 62:255–267.

Gadd J (1989) European update. *National Hog Farmer*, 88–90.

Giesting DW, Easter RA, and Roe BA (1985) A comparison of protein and carbohydrate sources of milk and plant origin for starter pigs. *Journal of Animal Science* 61(Supplement 1):299.

Glaser D, Wanner M, Tinti JM, and Nofre C (2000) Gustatory responses of pigs to various natural and artificial compounds known to be sweet in man. *Food Chemistry* 68:375–385.

Graham PL, Mahan DC, and Shields RG Jr (1981) Effect of starter diet and length of feeding regimen on performance and digestive enzyme activity of 2-week old weaned pigs. *Journal of Animal Science* 53:299–307.

He ML and Rambeck WA (2000) Rare earth elements – a new generation of growth promoters for pigs? *Archives of Animal Nutrition* 53:323–334.

Hernandez J, Borbolla A, Mendoza R, and Garcia G (2000) Glutamine stimulates the synthesis of immunoglobulin IgG in infected early weaned pigs. *Journal of Animal Science* 78(Supplement 1):175.

Hongtrakul K, Goodband RD, Behnke KC, Nelssen JL, Tokach MD, Bergstrom JR, Nessmith WB Jr, and Kim IH (1998) The effects of extrusion processing of carbohydrate sources on weanling pig performance. *Journal of Animal Science* 76:3034–3042.

Hyun Y, Ellis M, Riskowski G, and Johnson RW (1998) Growth performance of pigs subjected to multiple concurrent environmental stressors. *Journal of Animal Science* 76:721–727.

ITP (2002) *Tables d'alimentation pour les porcs*. Institut Technique du Porc, Paris, France.

Jongbloed AW, Kemme PA, Mroz Z, and Makinen M (1995) Apparent total tract digestibility of ash and minerals in pigs as affected by phytate, microbial phytase, and lactic acid. *Journal of Animal Science* 73(Supplement 1):188.

Kamphues J, Stolte M, and Rust P (2002) High sulfate content in whey products and milk replacers – a potential reason for changed faeces composition/watery faeces in calves. *XXII World Buiatrics Congress: Diseases of the Calf*, 522. Hanover, Germany.

Kats LJ, Nelssen JL, Tokach MD, Goodband RD, Hansen JA, and Laurin JL (1994) The effect of spray-dried porcine plasma on growth performance in the early-weaned pig. *Journal of Animal Science* 72:2075–2081.

Kelly D, Smyth JA, and McCracken KJ (1991a) Digestive development of the early-weaned pig. 2. Effect of level of food intake on digestive enzyme activity during the immediate post-weaning period. *British Journal of Nutrition* 65:181–188.

Kelly D, Smyth JA, and McCracken KJ (1991b) Digestive development of the early-weaned pig. 1. Effect of continuous nutrient supply on the development of the digestive tract and on changes in digestive enzyme activity during the first week post-weaning. *British Journal of Nutrition* 65:169–180.

Kerr BJ and Easter RA (1995) Effect of feeding reduced protein, amino acid-supplemented diets on nitrogen and energy balance in grower pigs. *Journal of Animal Science* 73:3000–3008.

Kidder DE and Manners MJ (1978) *Digestion in the Pig*. Scientechnica, Bristol, UK.

Kornegay ET, Lindemann MD, and Bartlett HS (1991) The influence of sodium supplementation of two phosphorus sources on performance and bone mineralization of growing-finishing swine evaluated at two geographical locations. *Canadian Journal of Animal Science* 71:537–547.

Krider JL, Becker DE, Curtin LV, and van Poucke RF (1949) Dried whey products in drylot rations for weanling pigs. *Journal of Animal Science* 8:112–120.

Le Dividich J and Seve B (2001) Energy requirements of the young pig. In: *The Weaner Pig – Nutrition and Management*, by Varley MA and Wiseman J (ed), 17–44. CAB International, Wallingford, UK.

Lee CH, Han YK, Lee KU, Kim JD, Cho WT, Ko TG, and Han IK (2000) Study on the nutritive value of dextrin as a carbohydrate source for pigs weaned at 21 days of age. *Journal of Animal and Feed Sciences* 9:647–663.

Lenis NP, van Diepen HTM, Bikker P, Jongbloed AW, and van der Meulen J (1999) Effect of the ratio between essential and nonessential amino acids in the diet on utilization of nitrogen and amino acids by growing pigs. *Journal of Animal Science* 77:1777–1787.

Lenis NP and Jongbloed AW (1999) New technologies in low pollution swine diets: diet manipulation and use of synthetic amino acids, phytase and phase feeding for reduction of nitrogen and phosphorus excretion and ammonia emission-review. *Asian-Australian Journal of Animal Science* 12:305–327.

Lepine AJ, Mahan DC, and Chung YK (1991) Growth performance of weanling pigs fed corn–soybean meal diets with or without dried whey at various L-lysine HCl levels. *Journal of Animal Science* 69:2026–2032.

Lorschy ML and Patience JF (1999) Defining the tryptophan requirement for pigs based on protein deposition rate: 47 to 75 kg body weight. In: *Manipulating Pig Production VII*, by Cranwell PD (ed), 132. Australasian Pig Science Association, Werribee, Australia.

Ly J (1996) The pattern of digestion and metabolism in high sugar feeds for pigs. *Cuban Journal of Agricultural Science* 30:117–129.

Lynch PB, Van Cauwenberghe S, and Fullarton P (2000) Response of weaned pigs to level of tryptophan in the diet. *Proceedings of the British Society of Animal Science Occasional Meeting 'The Weaner Pig – Nutrition and Management'*, 28. University of Nottingham, Nottingham, UK.

Mahan DC (1992) Efficacy of dried whey and its lactalbumin and lactose components at two dietary lysine levels on postweaning pig performance and nitrogen balance. *Journal of Animal Science* 70:2182–2187.

Mahan DC and Newton EA (1993) Evaluation of feed grains with dried skim milk and added carbohydrate sources on weanling pig performance. *Journal of Animal Science* 71:3376–3382.

Mahan DC, Newton EA, and Cera KR (1996) Effect of supplemental sodium chloride, sodium phosphate, or hydrochloric acid in starter pig diets containing dried whey. *Journal of Animal Science* 74:1217–1222.

Mahan DC, Wiseman TD, Weaver E, and Russell L (1999) Effect of supplemental sodium chloride and hydrochloric acid added to initial starter diets containing spray-dried blood plasma and lactose on resulting performance and nitrogen digestibility of 3-week-old weaned pigs. *Journal of Animal Science* 77:3016–3021.

Mahan DC, Fastinger ND, and Peters JC (2004) Effects of diet complexity and dietary lactose levels during three starter phases on postweaning pig performance. *Journal of Animal Science* 82:2790–2797.

Mavromichalis I, Webel DM, Emmert JL, Moser RL, and Baker DH (1998) Limiting order of amino acids in a low-protein corn–soybean meal–whey-based diet for nursery pigs. *Journal of Animal Science* 76:2833–2837.

Mavromichalis I and Baker DH (1999) Vitamin C sets a nursery puzzle. *Pig International* 29(4):27–28.

Mavromichalis I and Baker DH (2000) Queries about carnitine. *Pig International* 30(2):35–36.

Mavromichalis I (2000a) Lactose equivalents as a cheaper energy source in starter diets. *Pig Progress* 16(7):25–27.

Mavromichalis I (2000b) A close look at fats in nursery pig diets. *Feed International* 21(5):15–16.

Mavromichalis I, Hancock JD, Hines RH, Senne BW, and Cao H (2001) Lactose, sucrose, and molasses in simple and complex diets for nursery pigs. *Animal Feed Science and Technology* 93:127–135.

Mavromichalis I and Varley MA (2003) Transition feeding systems for weaned pigs. In: *Perspectives of Pig Science*, by Wiseman J, Varley MA, and Kemp KBF (ed), 405–456. Nottingham University Press, Nottingham, UK.

Miller ER, Ullrey DE, Zutaut CL, Baltzer BV, Schmidt DA, Hoefer JA, and Luecke RW (1965) Magnesium requirement of the baby pig. *Journal of Nutrition* 85:13–20.

Nessmith WB Jr, Nelssen JL, Tokach MD, Goodband RD, Bergstrom JR, Dritz SS, and Richert BT (1997a) Evaluation of the interrelationships among lactose and protein sources in diets for segregated early-weaned pigs. *Journal of Animal Science* 75:3214–3221.

Nessmith WB Jr, Nelssen JL, Tokach MD, Goodband RD, and Bergstrom JR (1997b) Effects of substituting deproteinized whey and (or) crystalline lactose for dried whey on weanling pig performance. *Journal of Animal Science* 75:3222–3228.

Noblet J and Perez JM (1993) Prediction of digestibility of nutrients and energy values of pig diets from chemical analysis. *Journal of Animal Science* 71:3389–3398.

Noblet J, Fortune H, Shi XS, and Dubois S (1994) Prediction of net energy value of feeds for growing pigs. *Journal of Animal Science* 72:344–354.

NRC (1987) *Predicting Feed Intake of Food-Producing Animals.* National Academy Press, Washington, DC.

NRC (1998) *Nutrient Requirements of Swine* (10th edn). National Academy Press, Washington, DC.

Nuoranne PJ, Raunio RP, Saukko P, and Karppanen H (1980) Metabolic effects of a low-magnesium diet in pigs. *British Journal of Nutrition* 44:53–60.

Pallauf J and Rimbach G (1997) Nutritional significance of phytic acid and phytase. *Archives of Animal Nutrition* 50:301–319.

Patience JF and Chaplin RK (1997) The relationship among dietary undetermined anion, acid–base balance, and nutrient metabolism in swine. *Journal of Animal Science* 75:2445–2452.

Peddireddi L, Yager AL, Saddoris KL, Wilson LM, Walsh MC, Sholly DM, Hinson RB, Richert BT, and Radcliffe JS (2004) The effects of dietary calcium source and level on growth performance, *E. coli* shedding, and gastric pH and buffering capacity in nursery pigs. *Journal of Animal Science* 82(Supplement 2):74.

Pickard JA, Wiseman J, and Varley MA (2001) Influence of diet acid binding capacity on gut morphology and digesta pH in piglets. *Proceedings of the Annual Meeting of the British Society of Animal Science*, 163. York, UK.

Pluske JR, McDonald DE, Pethick DW, Mullan BP, and Hampson DJ (2001) Nutritional management of the gastrointestinal tact to reduce enteric diseases in pigs. *Recent Advances in Animal Nutrition in Australia* 73:127–134.

Prohaszka L and Baron D (1980) The predisposing role of high dietary protein supplies in enteropathogenic *Escherichia coli* infections of weaned pigs. *Zentralblätte für Veterinärmedizin* 27:222–232.

Quiniou N (2002) Le point sur l'equilibre acido-basique chez le porc et le bilan electrolytique des aliments. *Techni Pork* 25(3):19–24.

Radcliffe JS, Kornegay ET, and Conner DE Jr (1995) The effect of phytase on calcium release in weanling pigs fed corn–soybean meal diets. *Journal of Animal Science* 73(Supplement 1):173.

Rincker MJ, Carter SD, Real DE, Nelssen JL, Tokach MD, Goodband RD, Dritz SS, Senne BW, Fent RW, Pettey LA, and Owen KQ (2003) Effects of increasing dietary L-carnitine on growth performance of weanling pigs. *Journal of Animal Science* 81:2259–2269.

Roth FX and Kirchgessner M (1998) Organic acids as feed additives for young pigs: nutritional and gastrointestinal effects. *Journal of Animal and Feed Sciences* 7:25–33.

Russell LE, Kerr BJ, and Easter RA (1987) Limiting amino acids in an 11% crude protein corn–soybean meal diet for growing pigs. *Journal of Animal Science* 65:1266–1272.

Scott RL and Austic RE (1978) Influence of dietary potassium on lysine metabolism in the chick. *Journal of Nutrition* 108:137–144.

Tokach MD, Nelssen JL, and Allee GL (1989) Effect of protein and (or) carbohydrate fractions of dried whey on performance and nutrient digestibility of early weaned pigs. *Journal of Animal Science* 67:1307–1312.

Touchette KJ, Crow SD, Allee GL, and Newcomb MD (1995a) Lactose response is dependent on plasma in the diet of weaned pigs. *Journal of Animal Science* 73(Supplement 1):171.

Touchette KJ, Crow SD, Allee GL, and Newcomb MD (1995b) Weaned pigs respond to lactose (day 0–14 postweaning). *Journal of Animal Science* 73(Supplement 1):70.

van Barneveld RJ, Batterham ES, and Norton BW (1991) Utilization of ileal digestible lysine from heat-treated field peas by growing pigs. In: *Manipulating Pig Production III*, by Batterham ES (ed), 184. Australasian Pig Science Association, Werribee, Australia.

van de Ligt JLG, Lindemann MD, Harmon RJ, and Cromwell GL (2002) Effect of chromium tripicolinate supplementation on porcine immune response during the postweaning period. *Journal of Animal Science* 80:449–455.

Vargane-Visi E, Meresz P, Terlakyne Balla E, and Csapo J (2004) The effect of the extrusion temperature and the residence time on the D-amino acid content of corn extrudates. *Acta Agraria Kaposvariensis* 8:59–68.

Veum TL and Mateo JP (1981) Utilization of glucose, sucrose or corn starch with casein or isolated soybean protein supplemented with amino acids by 8-day-old pigs reared artificially. *Journal of Animal Science* 53:1027–1038.

Wahlstrom RC and Libal GW (1974) Gain, feed efficiency and carcass characteristics of swine fed supplemental lysine and methionine in corn–soybean meal diets during the growing and finishing periods. *Journal of Animal Science* 38:1261–1266.

Wahlstrom RC, Hauser LA, and Libal GW (1974) Effects of low lactose whey, skim milk and sugar on diet palatability and performance of early weaned pigs. *Journal of Animal Science* 38:1267–1271.

Webel DM, Johnson RW, and Baker DH (1998) Lipopolysaccharide-induced reductions in food intake do not decrease the efficiency of lysine and threonine utilization for protein accretion in chickens. *Journal of Nutrition* 128:1760–1766.

Weber E and Ehrlein HJ (1998) Glucose and maltodextrin in enteral diets have different effects on jejunal absorption of nutrients, sodium, and water and on flow rate in mini pigs. *Deutsche Tierärztliche Wochenschrift* 105:446–449.

Whittemore CT and Fawcett RH (1976) Theoretical aspects of a flexible model to simulate protein and lipid growth in pigs. *Animal Production* 22:87–96.

Whittemore CT, Aumaitre A, and Williams IH (1978) Growth of body components in young weaned pigs. *Journal of Agricultural Science, Cambridge* 91:681–692.

Whittemore CT (1998) *The Science and Practice of Pig Production* (2nd edn). Blackwell Science Ltd, Oxford, UK.

Whittemore CT and Green DM (2001) Growth of the young weaned pig. In: *The Weaner Pig – Nutrition and Management*, by Varley MA and Wiseman J (ed), 1–15. CAB International, Wallingford, UK.

Williams NH, Stahly TS, and Zimmerman DR (1997a) Effect of chronic immune system activation on the rate, efficiency, and composition of growth and lysine needs of pigs fed from 6 to 27 kg. *Journal of Animal Science* 75:2463–2471.

Williams NH, Stahly TS, and Zimmerman DR (1997b) Effect of level of chronic immune system activation on the growth and dietary lysine needs of pigs fed from 6 to 112 kg. *Journal of Animal Science* 75:2481–2496.

Williams NH, Stahly TS, and Zimmerman DR (1997c) Effect of chronic immune system activation on body nitrogen retention, partial efficiency of lysine utilization, and lysine needs of pigs. *Journal of Animal Science* 75:2472–2480.

Wilson ME, Pettigrew JE, Johnston LJ, Hawton JD, Rust JW, and Chester-Jones H (1991) Provision of additional B-vitamins improves growth rate of weanling pigs. *Journal of Animal Science* 69(Supplement 1):106.

Wiseman J, Pickard J, and Zarkadas L (2001) Starch digestion in piglets. In: *The Weaner Pig – Nutrition and Management*, by Varley MA and Wiseman J (ed), 65–80. CAB International, Wallingford, UK.

Wu G, Meier SA, and Knabe DA (1996) Dietary glutamine supplementation prevents jejunal atrophy in weaned pigs. *Journal of Nutrition* 126:2578–2584.

Yen JT, Pond WG, and Prior RL (1981) Calcium chloride as a regulator of feed intake and weight gain in pigs. *Journal of Animal Science* 52:778–782.

Zhao JM, Li DF, Piao XS, Yang WJ, and Wang FL (2002) Effects of vitamin C supplementation on performance, iron status and immune function of weaned piglets. *Archives of Animal Nutrition* 56:33–40.

Feedstuffs

6

Introduction

The study of feed ingredients (bromatology) is a difficult topic to cover in a whole book let alone a couple of chapters. Unfortunately, there is no single title that covers this topic comprehensively, especially in today's fast changing political and economic environment. This chapter and the next one provide enough information to allow the reader to understand the basic functions of most common feed ingredients. They also provide an insight into current advances in research regarding novel and promising ingredients for piglet diets.

Feed ingredients are traditionally classified into feedstuffs and additives. Feedstuffs are usually ingredients with a nutritional role, in that they serve primarily as sources of energy, proteins, lipids, fibers, minerals, and vitamins. Additives are usually ingredients with functional properties that may or may not be connected with the general role of feed as a source of nutrients.

Nutrient Composition Tables

One of the most intriguing questions arising in the study and practice of bromatology is 'Which of the published tables of nutrient analysis are best?' In truth, only actual analysis of a representative sample of the ingredient in question can serve as the best estimate of the nutritive value of the whole lot. However, real-time data are often impractical to acquire as several analyses are expensive (e.g. vitamins and amino acids), time-consuming (e.g. fiber), or just impossible due to the lack of appropriate facilities at hand (e.g. energy and amino acid digestibility values). Thus, nutritionists do need to use 'table' values where actual data are missing. Quite often, these 'table' values are adjusted based on empirical experience to reflect a slightly different profile for a well-known ingredient.

Among the most popular publications providing tables of nutrient analyses for ingredients suitable for piglet feeds are the following:

- INRA (2003) *Tables de composition et de valeur nutritive des matieres premieres destinees aux animaux d'elevage.* http://www.inapg.fr/dsa/afz/tables/index.htm (in French).
- NRC (1998) *Nutrient Requirements of Swine.* http://www.nap.edu/openbook/0309059933/html (in English).
- CVB (2002) *Veevoedertabel.* http://www.cvb.pdv.nl/nederlands/CVB_Produkten/page666.php (in Dutch).
- FEDNA (2003) *Tablas de composition y valor nutritivo des alimentos para la fabrication de piensos compuestos.* http://www.etsia.upm.es/fedna/introtabla.htm (in Spanish).

Variability in nutrient analysis

Analytical variability among chemical laboratories can be as great as between two batches of the same ingredient, according to a recent report (NCR-42 Committee on Swine Nutrition, 1999). In an investigation involving 22 analytical laboratories, 16 sources of maize and soybean meal were analyzed for dry matter, crude protein, calcium, phosphorus, amino acids, and selenium. Nutrient composition varied greatly by source of origin and, with few exceptions (i.e. crude protein), variability was as great between laboratories.

Selenium was found to have the greatest variability, with values ranging from 0.02 to 0.29% (a difference of 1350%) in maize, and from 0.08 to 0.95% (a difference of 1088%) in soybean meal. Calcium concentrations in maize and soybean meal (regular or high-protein) were also quite variable and affected mostly by source and less by analytical laboratory.

The significance of this work is that not only do feed and ingredients need to be assayed frequently for major nutrients, but also a reliable analytical laboratory must be carefully selected. Some laboratories will definitely perform certain analyses with greater accuracy and repeatability than other laboratories.

Recommended Maximum Inclusion Levels

Maximum inclusion levels for feedstuffs are usually needed only for those ingredients that pose a threat to animal health and (or) growth performance when they are used in excessive concentrations. These ingredients are usually relatively inexpensive and, thus, a balance is often sought between feed cost and animal performance. Setting maximum limits for ingredients that are relatively safe (except for unbalancing diets) is redundant, but it is often seen in older publications, and usually represents common practice rather than upper limits of tolerance.

Defining the maximum inclusion level for each possible ingredient is quite a risky task. First, ingredient quality may vary considerably from batch to batch for a great number of reasons that can often be unpredictable or even unknown. Thus, lowering maximum inclusion levels for ingredients of questionable quality is often a good strategy, albeit not always the least-cost one. Second, research is constantly revealing that advances in processing methods and plant genetics result in improved quality of several ingredients previously thought challenging to use (e.g. canola versus rapeseed). Third, tolerance to anti-nutritional factors, usually present in high concentrations in several ingredients, increases with age, maturation of the digestive system, enhanced gut health, and high feed intake.

Basic guidelines for several feedstuffs are proposed in Table 6.1 as a starting point. It should be noted, however, that these values are rather conservative, reflecting concerns stated above. Practical experience, field tests, and new research should form the basis for transforming table values into formulation specifications.

Table 6.1. Suggested maximum inclusion levels (%) for non-traditional feedstuffs.

	Body weight (kg)					Major factors that
Feedstuff	4–6	6–8	8–12	12–20	20–30	limit usage
Bakery/biscuit meal	5	10	15	20	25	Excess sodium and oil rancidity
Barley, raw	5	10	15	20	30	Fiber and NSP
Barley, hulless	10	15	20	25	30	NSP, may be sole cereal with enzymes
Beet pulp	–	5	10	15	20	Fiber and low energy density
Blood meal, flash	–	1	2	3	3	Low amino acid digestibility, low palatability
Blood meal, spray-dried	–	2	3	3	3	Low in isoleucine and palatability
Blood red cells, spray-dried	1	2	3	3	3	Low in isoleucine and palatability
Brewer's grains, barley	–	5	10	15	15	Fiber and variable quality
Canola meal, solvent-extracted	–	5	10	20	30	Glucosinolates and erucic acid
Canola seeds, extruded	5	10	15	20	30	Glucosinolates and erucic acid
Carob meal	–	–	5	5	5	Fiber, low in energy
Maize germ meal	5	5	10	10	10	Oil rancidity and protein quality
Maize gluten feed, 20%	–	–	5	10	15	Low energy density
Maize gluten meal, 60%	5	5	10	10	10	Palatability

Table 6.1. *Continued*

Feedstuff	Body weight (kg)					Major factors that limit usage
	4–6	6–8	8–12	12–20	20–30	
Ethanol DDGS	–	5	10	15	20	Overall quality and low energy
Fishmeal	10	10	10	10	10	Over 1% fish oil may depress feed intake
Lentils	–	10	15	20	25	Protease inhibitors and lectins
Lupines, raw	–	5	10	15	20	Alkaloids and lathyrogens
Lupines, extruded	5	10	15	20	25	Alkaloids and lathyrogens
Meat-and-bone meal	5	10	10	15	15	High ash (calcium)
Meat meal	10	15	20	20	20	Overall quality and processing
Molasses, beet or cane	5	10	10	10	15	Manufacturing capabilities
Oats	–	5	10	15	20	Fiber and low in energy
Peas, raw	–	5	10	15	20	Protease inhibitors, lectins, and tannins
Peas, extruded	5	10	15	20	25	Protease inhibitors, lectins, and tannins
Potato protein	–	1	2	3	4	Glycoalkaloids with bitter taste
Poultry by-product meal	–	5	5	10	10	Ash concentration and lipid rancidity
Rapeseed meal, solvent-extracted	–	5	10	15	20	Glucosinolates and erucic acid
Rye	–	–	5	10	15	NSP, Fiber and low in energy
Sorghum, low-tannin	25	50	50	NL	NL	Tannins otherwise it may be sole cereal
Soybean meal, 44–48%	5	10	15	20	25	TIA and lectins
Soybeans, extruded	10	15	20	25	30	TIA must be below 5 mg/g
Soybeans, roasted	–	5	10	15	20	Low protein quality, TIA and lectins
Sunflower meal, 45%	–	5	10	15	20	Fiber
Tapioca, 72%	–	5	10	15	20	Cyanides
Triticale	5	10	20	NL	NL	Fiber and NSP
Wheat, raw	20	40	NL	NL	NL	NSP but it may be sole cereal
Wheat bran	–	–	–	5	5	Fiber and low energy density
Wheat middlings	–	5	5	10	10	Fiber and NSP

DDGS, distiller's dried grains with solubles; NL, no limit; NSP, non-starch polysaccharides; TIA, trypsin inhibitor activity.

Advances in Non-traditional Feedstuffs

The search for new feedstuffs or new uses for existing ingredients is driven mostly by the need to reduce feed cost, as it is now well established that maximal growth performance can be easily achieved by typical feedstuffs of high quality. Below are research summaries from scientific reports that merit consideration. This is not an inclusive review of all recent research. Instead, reports were selected critically based on their relevance and importance to field practices, adherence to proper statistical analyses and experimental design, and applicability.

Less common cereals

Low-phytate maize

The most common ways of reducing phosphorus excretion in the environment are by means of reduced dietary phosphorus concentration and (or) added phytase. Both approaches are based on the fact that phosphorus bioavailability in most cereals is extremely low, usually below 15%. The development of a new maize line with the same concentration of total phosphorus but only half the amount of phytate-bound phosphorus as that found in normal maize offers a new possibility in controlling the amount of phosphorus excreted. Research at the University of Missouri (Spencer *et al.*, 2000) demonstrated that the bioavailability of phosphorus in low-phytate maize was 62% compared to only 9% in normal maize using a slope-ratio assay with young pigs, in which monosodium phosphate was the standard. These values agreed well with an *in vitro* test that yielded values of 57 and 11% phosphorus bioavailability for low-phytate and normal maize, respectively. Phosphorus excretion was reduced by about 30% when low-phytate maize was fed. In addition, the nitrogen to phosphorus ratio in the manure was also more favorable for land application, whereas even calcium digestibility was improved when pigs were offered diets based on low-phytate maize. Although promising from nutritional and environmental points of view, such genetically modified hybrids may not be suitable for all parts of the world due to regulation restrictions.

Light wheat

Although wheat is a most common feedstuff in many parts of the world, wheat of light bushel weight is often bypassed as it is traditionally considered of inferior quality for both human and animal diets. However, bushel weight does not always reflect accurately the nutritive value of wheat for pigs. Previous research (Pearce *et al.*, 1997) indicated that wheat variety is actually the single most important characteristic that determines nutritive value. British researchers (Miller *et al.*, 2000) evaluated two wheat varieties (feed and food grade) at two different bushel weights (low = 66 or high = 72.5 kg/hl) in diets for piglets (24 days of age and 7 kg body weight). Ground raw wheat was included in diets at 500 g/kg to amplify response in terms of growth performance. All diets were made iso-nutrient and were fed for 20 days post-weaning. Results indicated that bushel weight did not influence growth performance during the entire grow-out period (Table 6.2). Surprisingly, wheat variety also did not influence performance as feed-grade wheat supported performance comparable to that from feeding food-grade wheat. This indicates that, with proper diet balancing, even low-quality wheat can be used effectively in pig diets. To this end, wheat-specific enzymes have been most successful (Cadogan *et al.*, 2000; see also Chapter 7). In conclusion, bushel weight should not be used as an indicator of wheat quality for feed applications.

Table 6.2. Wheat variety and bushel weight (low or high) does not affect piglet performance. (Adapted from Miller *et al.*, 2000.)

	Feed-grade (Buster)		Food-grade (Riband)	
	Low	High	Low	High
Initial weight (kg)	6.9	6.9	6.9	6.9
Final weight (kg)	13.9	13.8	14.0	13.6
Weight gain (g/day)	341	341	342	321
Feed/gain	1.10	1.17	1.14	1.14

Sorghum

Although in sorghum-producing areas (e.g. Kansas) sorghum (milo) is used freely in piglet diets, in other parts of the world there is still considerable concern regarding its suitability and safety. A Brazilian research group (Fialho *et al.*, 2004) conducted a metabolism assay and a growth trial to evaluate the effects of low-tannin sorghum on piglet performance. Sorghum replaced 0, 33, 66, and 100% of maize in experimental diets. Results indicated that nitrogen retention was not different among pigs fed any of the experimental diets. Crude protein digestibility (85% for the diet with 100% maize versus 85.8% for the diet with 100% sorghum) was also not affected by cereal source. Digestible energy (3821 versus 3793 kcal/kg) and metabolizable energy (3619 versus 3670 kcal/kg) were also comparable between the two cereals. Feed intake, weight gain, and feed efficiency were also not affected by cereal source, indicating that low-tannin sorghum can readily replace maize in piglet diets.

Hulless barley

Hulless barley varieties are considered a premium ingredient for piglet diets because they provide protein and energy without the excessive fiber found in regular barley. Both barley types, however, contain β-glucans, which resist digestion and increase intestinal viscosity. Researchers from the University of Minnesota (Yin *et al.*, 2001a,b) evaluated two varieties of hulless barley, having low and high concentrations of β-glucans and xylose, with or without an enzyme preparation of β-glucanase and xylanase in diets for weaned piglets (21 days old). As expected, in pigs fed barley with a high concentration of non-starch polysaccharides, digesta viscosity was increased, whereas enzyme addition decreased viscosity only at the distal part of the small intestine. Apparent ileal digestibility of dry matter, energy, amino acids, and non-starch polysaccharides was also increased by dietary enzyme addition, but this effect was greater in hulless barley with the higher concentration of non-starch polysaccharides. In conclusion, it appears that an appropriate enzyme preparation should be used in diets based on hulless barley, but its inclusion rate should be determined according to barley quality.

Triticale

Triticale is a cross between wheat and rye. Arabinoxylans are the main anti-nutritional factor in triticale, and their concentration is intermediate between that found in wheat and rye. Therefore, there is often considerable skepticism regarding the use of triticale in diets for young pigs. Myer (2001) evaluated triticale as a replacement for maize in three trials with a total of 324 weaned pigs (6.7 kg) in 22 replicates. Pigs were weaned at 3 weeks of age and fed the experimental diets for 5 weeks post-weaning. Triticale and maize were ground to similar particle size and incorporated into iso-lysine diets as the only cereal source. Triticale had 12% crude protein, 13.4% neutral detergent fiber, and 0.4% total lysine. Surprisingly, the substitution of triticale for maize yielded slightly better growth performance. Pigs fed triticale-based diets grew at 510 g/day, compared with 490 g/day for pigs fed maize-based diet, but feed efficiency was not affected by cereal substitution. Interestingly, pigs fed triticale-based diets exhibited superior growth rate only during the second phase of the experiment (days 12 to 35 post-weaning), which may imply a nutrient imbalance in the maize diet during this period. In conclusion, it appears that the nutritive value of good-quality triticale is at least comparable to that of maize in well-balanced diets. Triticale may thus be used as the sole cereal in diets for weaned pigs.

Cooked cereals

Maize versus barley

Cooked cereals are often considered a must in high-quality piglet diets, although research results are often conflicting. A report from Spain (Medel *et al.*, 1999) indicated that piglets offered diets based on processed (extruded or micronized) maize or barley had significantly improved growth rates (+7%) and feed efficiency (+6%) compared to pigs that were fed raw cereal-based diets. There was no difference between the two processing methods. The greatest response in terms of growth performance was observed with barley (+14%), whereas there was a negative response to processed maize (–4%)

during the first two weeks post-weaning, perhaps due to overprocessing of maize.

A further growth trial from the same group (Medel *et al.*, 2003) was conducted to evaluate the effects of feeding maize versus barley, in raw or cooked-flaked form, as pellets or meal in a $2 \times 2 \times 2$ factorial arrangement, using weaned piglets (22 days of age). At 42 days of age, piglets fed diets based on maize had improved feed efficiency compared to piglets fed diets based on barley (1.2 versus 1.4%, respectively). Cooked cereals increased growth rate at 32 days of age (135 versus 114 g/day for cooked and raw cereals, respectively). Finally, pelleting improved feed conversion but it did not affect weight gain. At 52 days of age, considerable differences existed between maize and barley treatments for weight gain, and between pellets and meal treatments for feed efficiency. Maize-based diets and heat-treated cereals resulted in improved total tract apparent nutrient digestibility. In conclusion, the best performance in piglets is achieved with cooked maize-based diets in pellet form (Fig. 6.1).

Barley

Accumulating data from Europe indicate that cooked barley is beneficial for weaned pigs in terms of growth performance, especially during the period following weaning. To these data, a further Spanish trial (Medel *et al.*, 2000) is offering confirming evidence on the use of raw barley versus barley

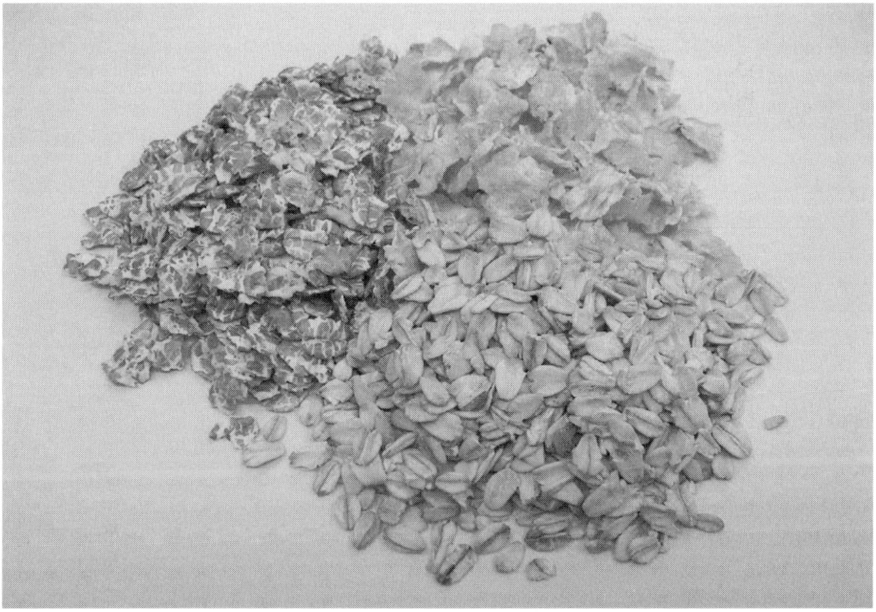

Fig. 6.1. Common cooked cereals include maize, wheat, and oats.

processed via extrusion or micronization. A single batch of winter barley, with 10% protein, 3.5% β-glucans, and 6.0% xylans, was divided in equal fractions and was then either ground (2.5 mm screen), micronized and flaked, or extruded in a single-screw extruder. Thermal processing increased starch gelatinization from about 19% in raw barley to 30% in cooked barley (Table 6.3). In a 28-day growth experiment, weaned pigs (20 days and 5.7 kg) were offered a complex diet, without antimicrobial agents, that contained 50% of each barley sample. Cereal cooking enhanced growth rates by about 13.5% during the first 2 weeks post-weaning. However, feed intake was not affected by any dietary treatment. There was no difference between micronized and extruded barley. The benefits of barley processing diminished during the following 2 weeks, resulting in no significant differences for the entire 4-week period. Diets based on processed barley had increased dry matter digestibility, but this was not reflected in the digestibility of energy or protein.

Rice

Australian researchers (Montagne *et al.*, 2003; Pluske *et al.*, 2003) investigated the use of cooked white rice as a means of reducing dietary fiber that is considered detrimental for achieving high growth rates in piglets. A total of 30 piglets in six replicates were assigned to the following dietary treatments for 14 days post-weaning:

1. Cooked white rice plus animal protein (very low in dietary fiber).
2. Cooked white rice plus high-amylose maize starch.
3. Cooked white rice plus lupine isolate (very high in dietary fiber).
4. Cooked white rice plus high-amylose maize starch plus lupine isolate.
5. Commercial weaner diet.

Table 6.3. Effect of cooked barley-based diets on piglet performance. (Adapted from Medel *et al.*, 2000.)

	Raw	Extruded	Micronized
Starch gelatinization (%)	19	30	31
Day 0 to 14			
Weight gain (g/day)	204[a]	225[b]	238[b]
Feed intake (g/day)	210	224	232
Day 0 to 28			
Weight gain (g/day)	337	353	370
Feed intake (g/day)	440	463	473
Total tract apparent digestibility (%)			
Dry matter	78[a]	81[b]	83[b]
Energy	77	79	80
Protein	75	77	77

[a,b] Means within a row with unlike superscript letters are different ($P < 0.05$).

Total dietary fiber ranged from 2.7 to 30% in diets 1 and 3, respectively. Pigs fed diet 1 consumed more feed than pigs fed diets 4 and 5. They also tended to grow faster than pigs fed diets with higher levels of dietary fiber. Pigs receiving diet 1 did not break out with scours nor did they receive any antibiotic injections, even though this diet contained 5% soybean meal. In contrast, pigs offered all other diets suffered from diarrhea and received numerous injections per treatment (as needed). In conclusion, it appears that a highly digestible diet is extremely effective against the development of diarrhea in young pigs, possibly through the absence of sufficient substrate to support proliferation of gut microflora. To this end, cooked rice and maize can play a significant role.

Rice versus maize

A more practical study (Vicente *et al.*, 2004) evaluated the effects of replacing cooked maize with raw or cooked rice using 25-day-old piglets in eight replicates per treatment. Treatments included a positive control with 50% cooked maize or the same diet with maize replaced with raw or cooked rice. During the 2 week trial, piglets fed rice-based diets grew faster (+29%), ate more (+23%), and had better feed conversion (–6%) than piglets fed maize-based diets. Piglets fed cooked rice grew faster (+6%) and with a better feed efficiency (–6%) than piglets fed raw rice. Total tract digestibility values for organic matter, energy, and dry matter were lower for maize-fed piglets than rice-fed piglets at 27 days of age, but differences diminished with age. This study is a clear indication that rice is a choice ingredient for piglet diets.

Agro-industrial products

Molasses

Molasses is often used in piglet diets in relatively small concentrations (1–2%) as a pelleting agent and appetizer. Higher concentrations of molasses are generally avoided mainly due to feed manufacturing issues, but also due to a misconception that high-molasses diets may cause diarrhea. At Kansas State University (Mavromichalis *et al.*, 2001), cane molasses was tested as a replacement for lactose in simple and complex diets using 210 piglets (19 days of age and 4.6 kg body weight) in two experiments. Molasses replaced crystalline lactose at 50 or 100%, and was thus included at 10 and 20% of the final diet; much above current recommended levels. All diets were fed in a pellet form and contained antimicrobial agents. Results indicated that piglets utilized molasses with the same efficiency as they did food-grade crystalline lactose. Growth performance was not affected by even 20% dietary molasses. Despite expectations, the health of the pigs was exceptional and there were no incidences of diarrhea due to dietary treatments. Nevertheless, fecal color was considerably darker in pigs fed molasses-based diets compared with pigs fed lactose-based diets. Not surprisingly, molasses enhanced feed intake as was expected based on the popular belief that young pigs favor sweet diets, but this was a transient effect. It should be noted, though, that the basal diet contained antimicrobial agents and zinc oxide, which certainly influenced the behavior of gut microflora.

Sugarbeet pulp

Another co-product of the sugar industry, dried sugarbeet pulp has too much fiber (20%), and traditionally has been considered a second-class ingredient for piglet diets. However, it is now believed that the easily fermented non-starch polysaccharide fraction of sugarbeet pulp may be of benefit to piglets susceptible to diarrhea. Therefore, a joint study between British and French researchers (Gill *et al.*, 2000) was undertaken to investigate partial replacement of wheat with relatively high levels of sugarbeet pulp (18.5%) in simple piglet diets. Pigs were weaned at 28 days of age and offered dietary treatments for a period of 4 weeks. Results indicated that, apart from the first week post-weaning, growth performance was not affected by the addition of sugarbeet pulp (Table 6.4). Previous research has already demonstrated the ability of young pigs to utilize high levels of sugarbeet pulp (15%) in complex starter diets (Edwards *et al.*, 1991). It is speculated that the transient depression of growth performance during the first week post-weaning was a reflection of the lower density of the high-fiber diet. In conclusion, unmolassed dried sugarbeet pulp can support acceptable performance in piglets and, thus, it can be used in levels of 10 to 20% in second-stage diets to reduce cost. However, its high fiber content may prevent pigs from achieving acceptable levels of feed intake immediately after weaning and, therefore, it should not be used in first-stage diets.

Maize syrup

Liquid milk replacers for young pigs are usually based on lactose to simulate sow's milk that contains about 30% lactose on a dry matter basis. But, as prices for dairy products continue to be at a premium throughout the world, ingredients that can replace lactose are always in high demand. A research team from the USA (Oliver *et al.*, 2001) recently evaluated maize syrup, an ingredient used in beverages, to replace 40% crystalline lactose in a liquid diet offered *ad libitum* to 1-day-old pigs until weaning at 20 days of age. Maize syrup (of either 20 or 42 dextrose equivalent grade) did not affect growth performance or digestive development and architecture compared to lactose. Piglets grew at an astonishing rate of about 380 g/day, reaching almost 10 kg body weight at only 20 days of age. This study demonstrated

Table 6.4. Sugarbeet pulp as a partial replacement of cereals in piglet diets. (Adapted from Gill *et al.*, 2000.)

Growth performance	Control	18.5% sugarbeet pulp
Weight gain (g/day)		
Week 1	191[a]	126[b]
Week 2	329	296
Week 3	419	483
Week 4	459	513
Overall	349	354
Feed intake (g/day)		
Week 1	245[a]	219[b]
Week 2	479	469
Week 3	642	651
Week 4	713	795
Overall	519	534

[a,b] Means within a row with unlike superscript letters are different ($P < 0.05$).

not only the ability of very young pigs to utilize alternative sources of simple sugars, but also the impediment imposed to piglet growth when reared only on sow's milk before weaning.

Dry distiller's grains with solubles

Increasing production of ethanol from maize in Midwest USA yields substantial amounts of distiller's dried grains with solubles (DDGS; so-called 'ethanol' or 'new generation' DDGS), which are readily available for feeding to all classes of livestock. Pig producers and nutritionists are especially interested in the potential cost savings from feeding this new raw material, as 100 kg 'ethanol' DDGS per tonne feed can replace 88 kg maize, 9 kg soybean meal, and about 3 kg dicalcium phosphate. 'New generation' DDGS produced by wet milling ethanol plants have about the same energy density as maize (3350 kcal/kg) and contain about 0.91% lysine and 0.78% phosphorus. Lysine digestibility is about 54% and phosphorus bioavailability around 90% (more information can be obtained at www.ddgs.umn.edu). In a recent study (Witney and Shurson, 2003), a total of 196 pigs in two trials were offered diets with 0, 5, 10, 15, 20, and 25% DDGS to determine the maximum dietary concentration of 'ethanol' DDGS tolerable by young pigs. Pigs (6–7 kg body weight) were weaned on a common starter diet (without DDGS) for 4 days post-weaning, followed by trial diets for 5 weeks. All test diets had similar nutrient and energy density. Overall weight gain, feed intake and feed efficiency were not affected by level of 'ethanol' DDGS even when added up to 25% of the diet. In one of the two trials, feed intake (but not growth) was linearly depressed during the first two weeks, indicating a possible quality problem in the source of DDGS. This only emphasizes the importance of selecting reliable sources of 'ethanol' DDGS.

Novel lipids

Encapsulated fat

It is well documented that weaned piglets cannot utilize fats of animal origin very efficiently. Such fats, however, are attractive as energy sources because they are generally less expensive than oils. A recent study from North Carolina State University (Xing *et al.*, 2004) investigated the effects of using encapsulated fat in piglet diets. A total of 144 piglets (6 kg) were allotted in a 3×2 factorial design, with factors being: (i) source and level of fat; and (ii) diet form (pelleted or meal). The basal diet contained 1% lard, whereas test diets contained 5% additional lard in natural or encapsulated spray-dried form. Lard decreased growth performance, but improved feed efficiency. Pelleting improved both growth performance and feed efficiency. Fat encapsulation significantly increased weight gain and improved feed efficiency during the second phase post-weaning (days 15 to 28), but not during the first two weeks post-weaning. In conclusion, encapsulated fat is a valid source of lipids suitable for piglets past the weaning phase. It should not be used to replace oils in the first 2 weeks post-weaning.

Fish oil

Fish oil is a rich source of long-chain *n*-3 polyunsaturated fatty acids (*n*-3 PUFA) that allegedly prevent the growth-depressing effects of a disease challenge by altering the cascade of events leading to pro-inflammatory cytokine production (Carroll *et al.*, 2001). However, the use of fish oil under practical conditions without clinical disease challenges has not been evaluated. A US research group (Meyer *et al.*, 2001) recently evaluated the effects of different levels of *n*-3 PUFA from fish oil in diets for pigs weaned at 21 days of age (6.8 kg). Complex diets with 5% added oil were formulated to *n*-6/*n*-3 ratios of 0.7, 1.9, 6.9, 35.5, and 70 by altering fish and maize oil additions. At the end of 28-day growth assay, pig performance in terms of weight gain, feed intake, and efficiency of feed utilization were not affected by dietary treatment. Assessment of cell-mediated immunity by intradermal injection of phytohemaglutenin solution in the ear did not reveal any dietary treatment effects. Furthermore, villi height at duodenum and jejunum was not affected by fish oil additions, although crypt depth at jejunum was increased in a quadratic form, indicating minimal deterioration of gut health at intermediate levels of fish oil additions. In conclusion, fish oil addition up to 5% in complex diets does not confer any beneficial effects on piglets reared under practical conditions with minimal health challenges.

Milk products

Casein

Xiao *et al.* (2000) evaluated the response of macrophages (cells of the immune system in the first line of defense against invading pathogens) to an antigen (lipopolysaccharide, LPS; a component of bacterial cell wall) in the presence of milk-derived oligopeptides. As expected, macrophages quickly released large amounts of cytokines when triggered by LPS, but they did not respond to casein peptides alone in the absence of the antigen. When macrophages were incubated with a combination of casein-derived peptides and LPS, their response was greatly enhanced compared to LPS alone. These results indicate that casein-based diets for piglets may exert a prophylactic effect against the establishment of disease by amplifying the immune system reaction in the presence of pathogenic microorganisms.

Milk immunoglobulins

Whey protein is a rich source of immunoglobulins, which also abound in animal plasma. This high concentration of immunoglobulins (mainly IgG) in animal plasma is believed to be responsible for enhancing piglet performance (Stahly *et al.*, 1995b). Due to its relatively high price or unavailability in certain parts of the world, replacements for animal plasma are always in strong demand. A Kansas State University team (Grinstead *et al.*, 2000) used a total of 1750 weaned pigs (12 to 19 days of age) in five trials and two types of facilities (university and commercial) to evaluate the effects of replacing animal plasma with other sources of immunoglobulins. Results indicated that in complex diets based on skim milk, plasma or whey proteins exerted minimal effects on growth performance. When pigs were offered simple diets based on dried whey, a minimal concentration of animal plasma (2.5%) was needed to stimulate feed intake during the first seven days post-weaning. It appears that skim milk is reducing the need for animal plasma in formulas for early-weaned pigs.

Liquid skim milk

Undoubtedly, there is enormous growth potential in suckling piglets, which is not easily realized because of inadequate intake of sow's milk and creep feed. Provision of a milk replacer in the form of a liquid diet before and just after weaning has been extensively tested in Europe and the USA with more than encouraging results (Azain *et al.*, 1996). A new study from Australia (Dunshea *et al.*, 1999) focused on the feasibility of feeding liquid skim milk before and shortly after weaning to enhance weaning weights and assist in the transition to dry feed. From day 10 after birth and until weaning on day 20, pigs that were offered supplemental liquid skim milk grew significantly faster (291 versus 223 g/day) than pigs with access only to sow's milk. Sow live weight change and backfat loss were not affected by dietary treatments, which indicates the potential for piglets to grow beyond the milking capacities of their dams. After weaning, pigs on the skim milk regimen were allowed a 2-day period of adjustment, in which time they were fed only skim milk. Consumption of dry matter (257 versus 30 g/day) and growth rates (213 versus –30 g/day) were greater when compared to pigs that received no liquid skim milk before weaning and only dry pellets after weaning. Thereafter, pellets were gradually introduced into skim milk over a period of 5 days to ensure a smooth transition from the liquid to an all-dry diet. Piglets on the skim milk regimen were 33% and 10% heavier at 41 and 120 days of age, respectively, compared with pigs that had access only to sow's milk during suckling and dry pellets after weaning. The researchers indicated that some feed refusal was observed when pellets were first introduced into the skim milk but all piglets consumed solid feed after 7 days post-weaning. It appears that skim milk is a viable option to commercial milk replacers when cost permits it.

Animal plasma

Mechanism of action

That spray-dried animal plasma enhances feed intake and overall growth performance in the first couple of weeks post-weaning is well documented (see a review by van Dijk *et al.*, 2001). It is also known that animal plasma exerts its effect mostly in pigs of average-to-low health status (Stahly *et al.*, 1995a). In a study to identify the mechanism of action of animal plasma, researchers at the University of Missouri and the Agricultural Research Service of the US Department of Agriculture (Touchette *et al.*, 2000) used a total of 20 pigs (5 kg and 14 days of age) allotted in a 2×2 factorial design, in an isolated nursery facility. Dietary treatments included two levels of animal plasma (0 versus 7%) and two intraperitoneal injections (saline or LPS antigen). The latter was used to simulate pathogenic activation of the immune system by causing a mild inflammation and fever. Pigs that were challenged with LPS had increased levels of cytokines, which are responsible for the loss of appetite in disease, compared to pigs injected with saline (placebo). Other elements of the innate immunity system, such as TNF-α and interferon-γ, were also elevated in LPS-challenged pigs. These indicators of immune system function appeared even more elevated in LPS-injected pigs that received 7% animal plasma in their diets compared to challenged pigs that were not fed animal plasma. In conclusion, it appears that animal plasma provides significant immunological protection in weaned pigs.

Animal plasma in antibiotic-free diets

Although animal plasma has been recently re-allowed in the EU (2005), the ban on all feed-grade antimicrobial agents in piglet feeds (2006) encourages research on the effects of plasma on animal health as a potential antibiotic replacement. Recent research from Spain (Torrallardona *et al.*, 2003) indicated that animal plasma confers protection against experimental infection by *E. coli* similar to that bestowed by an antibiotic (colistin sulfate). Forty-eight piglets at 24 days of age were allotted in a 2×2 factorial trial with two levels of animal plasma (0 or 7%) and colistin (0 or 300 mg/kg). All piglets were infected at the beginning of the trial with *E. coli* strain K99. Animal plasma (+54 g) and colistin (+75 g) markedly improved weight gain during the first 2 weeks post-weaning, whereas feed efficiency was improved by 35 and 32%, respectively. These effects were not additive. Examination of gastrointestinal health parameters revealed that colistin supported better mucosa integrity (longer villi) and reduced pathogenic bacteria. Animal plasma favored growth of beneficial lactobacilli, but had no effect on gastrointestinal architecture. Clearly, more research is needed to further elucidate the beneficial effects of animal plasma in the absence of antibiotics.

Plasma and antimicrobials

Another two trials were conducted in The Netherlands (Bikker *et al.*, 2004) to investigate the interactive effects of diet composition and an antimicrobial growth promoter with animal plasma on piglet growth. In the first trial, piglets were offered a simple or complex diet, with (4%) or without animal plasma, in a 2×2 factorial arrangement of treatments. In the second trial, piglets were offered diets with (4%) or without animal plasma, and an antimicrobial growth promoter (avilamycin) at 0 or 40 ppm, again in a 2×2 factorial. As expected, during the first week post-weaning, animal plasma improved growth performance by approximately 20% in both trials. This effect was more pronounced when plasma was combined with the complex diet in trial 1 and without avilamycin in trial 2. In conclusion, it appears that animal plasma is more effective in diets that enable rapid growth in piglets and when antibiotics are not included in the first diet post-weaning.

Salt and plasma

Although whey-based diets contain ample quantities of sodium and chlorine, previous research from Ohio State University demonstrated beneficial effects from supplementing starter diets with salt (NaCl) beyond established requirements during the first two weeks post-weaning (Mahan *et al.*, 1996). Sodium was partially responsible for the positive response to salt additions, but the greater response was attributed to chlorine supplementation. Today, starter diets with 4 to 8% animal plasma protein may contain more than enough Na and Cl, as this specialty ingredient is rich in both Na (0.58%) and Cl (1.4%). However, recent reports from the same research group (Mahan *et al.*, 1999) revealed that diets that contain animal plasma protein require additional salt to reach a total dietary Cl concentration of at least 0.40%. Currently, NRC requirement estimates for Cl in post-weaning diets call for only 0.20% Cl for pigs weighing 5 to 10 kg. Care should be exercised when diets rich in whey, animal plasma, and fishmeal are fed to newly weaned pigs to ensure that they have free access to non-saline water and that they know how to use the drinkers, to avoid salt toxicosis.

Soybeans

Soybean meal source

It is often assumed that soybean meals from different sources can be used interchangeably on a protein basis. Yet, not all soybeans are created equal and not all soybean-processing methods are the same. A research team from Korea (Kim *et al.*, 2002) evaluated three sources of soybeans (Korean, Brazilian, and Indian) in diets for young pigs to investigate potential differences in soybean meal quality due to source. In the first experiment, 180 weaned pigs (21 days) were assigned to receive a typical complex diet for 7 days followed by a second-stage diet for another 21 days. The second experiment was conducted with growing pigs (38 kg). The only difference between treatments in these trials was the source of soybean meal. Pigs receiving diets with Korean or Brazilian had statistically similar growth performance, although there were numerical differences (Table 6.5). Nevertheless, their performance was far superior to the performance of pigs receiving Indian soybean meal. In the first experiment, growth rate and feed intake were reduced by 10 and 8%, respectively, in pigs offered soybean meal from India. Similarly, in the experiment with growing pigs, growth rate was depressed by 19% and feed intake by 5% in pigs fed diets based on Indian soybean meal. Numerical differences among treatments existed for feed efficiency in both trials. Quality within a country of origin may be as variable as quality among countries. Quality control programs should therefore be designed to monitor quality in incoming soybean meal loads. This study should be used only as an example of potential differences among different sources of soybean meal.

Expelled soybean meal

Conventional soybean meal is produced by dehulling, solvent extraction of oil, and partial addition of hulls to toasted meal. With solvent extraction being a very effective method, the meal is left with less than 1% oil, whereas

Table 6.5. Effect of soybean meal origin on piglet performance. (Adapted from Kim *et al.*, 2002.)

	Korean	Brazilian	Indian
Trial 1			
Weight gain (g/day)	450[a]	420[a]	390[b]
Feed intake (g/day)	770	760	710
Feed/gain	1.71	1.81	1.82
Trial 2			
Weight gain (g/day)	640[a]	650[a]	540[b]
Feed intake (g/day)	1670	1640	1580
Feed/gain	2.61	2.52	2.93

[a,b] Means within a row with unlike superscript letters are different ($P < 0.05$).

soybeans contain around 18% oil. Dry extrusion-expelling of whole soybeans is a novel method of oil extraction that produces a drier soybean meal with more oil (5%) and protein (50%), but with anti-nutritional properties similar to conventional soybean meal. A US research group (Woodworth *et al.*, 2001) evaluated dry extruded-expelled soybean meal in diets for young pigs in a series of growth trials, amino acid digestibility assays, and energy balance experiments. Expelled soybean meal with or without hulls was compared against conventional soybean meal without hulls, which is the most common soybean meal used in piglet diets. The growth assay, which involved 216 pigs (10.6 kg and 35 days of age), indicated that there were no adverse effects of replacing conventional soybean meal with expelled soybean meal during a 21-day grow-out period. Apparent ileal digestibility of amino acids and digestible or metabolizable energy concentrations were not affected by hull inclusion in the expelled soybean meal. Digestibility of lysine, isoleucine, and valine was slightly increased (+2.5%) in expelled soybean meal, but digestibility of sulfur amino acids, threonine, and tryptophan was comparable to conventional soybean meal. As expected based on its higher oil content, expelled soybean meal had about 15% more digestible and metabolizable energy than conventional soybean meal. In conclusion, properly processed expelled soybean meal has nutritive value superior to high-protein, solvent-extracted soybean meal. Expelled soybean meal may be valuable in high-nutrient density diets for young pigs, depending on cost relative to other fat and protein sources.

Dry roasting

Dry roasting is a common on-farm heat treatment of whole (full-fat) soybeans. In general, heating soybeans destroys protease inhibitors that reduce protein digestibility in pigs. Overheating, however, markedly affects protein quality by rendering amino acids unavailable for metabolism. On the other hand, of course, underprocessing is equally detrimental to animal performance. Therefore, applying optimal roasting conditions in terms of temperature, time, and moisture are of paramount importance in the final quality of the product. In a recent study, US researchers (White *et al.*, 2000) determined the optimum roasting conditions for full-fat soybeans destined to be used in piglet diets. The beans were brought to a dry matter content of 80 or 90% and then roasted at 110°C (60 s) or 125°C (90 s). Diets based on heat-treated solvent-extracted soybean meal (25%), raw soybeans (40%), and heat-treated soybeans (40%) were then fed to 5-kg pigs for 35 days. As expected, raw soybeans contained excessive amounts of trypsin inhibitor and drastically depressed growth performance compared with control pigs that received the soybean-meal based diet. Heating 90% DM soybeans at 110°C was not effective in restoring growth performance of pigs because of residual high levels of trypsin inhibitor activity. However, heating 90% DM soybeans to 125°C partially restored performance. Soybeans of reduced moisture required lower temperatures to inactivate trypsin inhibitor, but performance was improved with increasing processing temperatures. Apparently, temperatures higher than 125°C would be needed to fully inactivate anti-nutritional factors in 90% DM soybeans, whereas even higher temperatures would be needed for 80% DM soybeans. The latter would probably result in significant protein deterioration. In conclusion, dry roasted soybeans should be reserved for older pigs.

Micronized/extruded soybeans

Researchers from the UK (Zarkadas and Wiseman, 2000) determined the optimal processing conditions for micronized or extruded soybeans. In the first trial, micronized soybeans were cooked with low or full steam for a short (10 s) or long period of time (40 s). In the second trial, extruded soybeans were cooked for 30 s at 70, 90, 110, and 150°C in a twin-screw extruder. The soybeans were included at 30% in simple diets and were fed to young pigs from 10 to 27 kg body weight. Thermal processing reduced considerably the trypsin inhibitor activity, an indicator of the anti-nutritional properties in soybean seeds irrespective of processing method. As expected, this reduction in trypsin inhibitor activity had a marked effect on animal growth and feed efficiency (Fig. 6.2). The best performance was achieved in pigs offered the micronized soybean seeds that were cooked for a longer time and in pigs offered extruded soybean seeds cooked at 150°C. In conclusion, the optimum trypsin inhibitor activity in processed soybean should be below 5 mg/g for maximal animal performance (soybean meal has around 34 mg trypsin inhibitor activity/g). In absolute terms, performance was optimized when trypsin inhibitor activity intake was below 1.5 g/day.

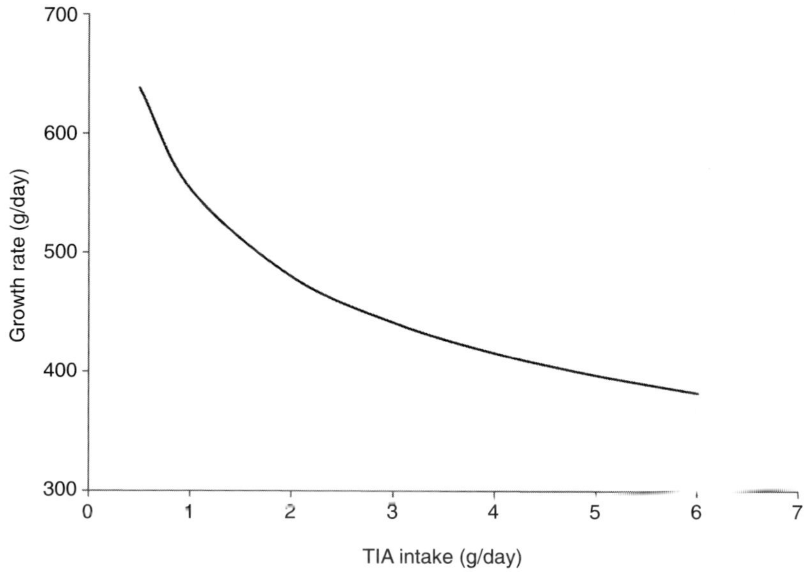

Fig. 6.2. Trypsin inhibitor activity (TIA) below 5 mg/g is recommended for soybeans in piglet diets. (From Zarkadas and Wiseman, 2000.)

Minor legumes

Lentils and peas

The increasing demand for plant-derived protein sources has rekindled interest in several non-traditional legume crops such as lentils and peas, especially in areas where soybeans are not readily available. Currently, raw lentils and peas are used effectively up to 10% in piglet diets to replace soybean meal. Higher inclusion levels usually depress growth performance because lentils and peas contain anti-nutritional factors such as protease inhibitors and lectins. Canadian research (Jaikaran, 2001) evaluated the use of lentils and peas at increased concentrations in diets for piglets. A total of 120 pigs (28 days of age) were allotted to five treatments (four pens per treatment) in two 4-week growth assays. Dietary treatments included:

1. Positive control (soybean meal);
2. Raw lentils or peas (15%);
3. Raw lentils or peas (30%);
4. Extruded lentils or peas (15%); and
5. Extruded lentils or peas (30%).

Results indicated that raw lentils did not depress growth performance compared to soybean meal even at 30%, whereas extruded lentils did not improve performance (Table 6.6). Raw peas, however, negatively affected weight gain and feed efficiency at 30% but not at 15%. Extrusion of peas

Table 6.6. Lentils and peas in piglet diets. (Adapted from Jaikaran, 2001.)

Treatment	Lentils: Weight gain (g/day)	Lentils: Feed/gain	Peas: Weight gain (g/day)	Peas: Feed/gain
1. Positive control (soybean meal)	590	1.35	520^{x}	1.32^{x}
2. Raw lentils or peas (15%)	607	1.42	573^{x}	1.33^{x}
3. Raw lentils or peas (30%)	551	1.38	466^{y}	1.49^{y}
4. Extruded lentils or peas (15%)	609	1.35	539^{x}	1.33^{x}
5. Extruded lentils or peas (30%)	605	1.33	540^{x}	1.29^{x}

^{x,y} Means within a column with unlike superscript letters are different ($P < 0.05$).

restored growth performance to control levels. In conclusion, it appears lentils may be used in diets for piglets at relatively high concentrations (30%) without negatively impacting performance. Peas, however, must be thermally processed when used at high levels in piglet diets.

Peas

A Canadian research group (Owusu-Asiedu *et al.*, 2002) conducted two trials to investigate the effects of heat treatment and enzyme supplementation in pea-based diets for young pigs. In the first experiment, 16-day-old cannulated pigs were fed diets with raw, extruded, or micronized peas and supplemented with amylase and xylanase. Heat processing improved apparent and true ileal digestibility of most amino acids, including the limiting amino acids lysine, methionine, and threonine. Micronization improved collective digestibility of essential amino acids from 79 to 88%. Enzyme supplementation further improved digestibility of amino acids in heat-treated peas. In a second growth trial, 16-day-old piglets were fed diets based on raw, extruded, or micronized peas with or without enzyme supplementation from 4.5 to 20 kg body weight. Enzyme supplementation improved feed efficiency from 1.4 to 1.2 (kg feed/kg gain) in pigs that were fed diets with raw peas. Similar results were observed with heat processing of peas.

Yellow lupines

Considerable debate exists regarding the maximum inclusion level of lupines in pig diets. Levels as high as 40% have been suggested for finishing pigs, whereas recommendations for piglets are usually lower. It is argued that the alkaloid content of lupines is the most important factor in determining maximal inclusion level. It is suggested, thus, that pig diets fed *ad libitum* should contain no more than 200 ppm alkaloids. However, the source of alkaloids must not be overlooked. White lupines contain lupanine and sparteine that are more toxic than lupinine, the predominant alkaloid in yellow lupines. Polish researchers (Bugnacka *et al.*, 2001) used raw yellow lupines (variety Juno) in two assays to evaluate feed preference and animal growth. The control diet was based on soybean meal, barley, and wheat. Lupines replaced 75 and 100% of soybean meal protein, with additions of crystalline methionine and lysine. Soybean meal concentration in the control diet was 21% and alkaloid concentration in lupine seeds was 390 ppm. In a feed preference test, 12 pigs (22.5 kg) were placed in individual pens and they were given free access, successively for 4 h, to each of the three diets. In the growth assay, 36 pigs (18.8 kg) were allotted in six replicates per treatment to receive one of the three experimental diets for 28 days. When pigs were given a choice between the three diets, they clearly preferred the soybean meal-based diet over lupine-based diets. Feed intake was reduced linearly as alkaloid content increased (Table 6.7). In the second experiment, however, when pigs were not allowed to select among diets, feed intake was not affected by lupine additions. Weight gain and feed intake were not affected as well by replacing soybean with lupines. In conclusion, yellow lupine seeds appear to support performance comparable to soybean meal in grower diets. Although pigs are able to detect even low concentrations of alkaloids (less than 100 ppm) in complete diets, such levels are not sufficient to affect growth performance under practical feeding conditions.

Animal proteins

Low-temperature fishmeal

Fishmeal is one of the choice animal proteins available for young pigs. It is rich in protein (amino acids), readily available throughout most of the world, and competitively priced against other animal proteins (milk and blood). Species selection and drying conditions are the major factors affecting

Table 6.7. Yellow lupines in diets for young pigs. (Adapted from Bugnacka *et al.*, 2001.)

	Soybean meal	Lupines (75%)	Lupines (100%)
Preference assay			
Feed intake of each diet (g/day)[a]	760	736	700
Growth assay			
Feed intake (g/day)	1520	1490	1580
Weight gain (g/day)	676	706	693
Feed/gain	2.25	2.11	2.28

[a] Linear effect ($P < 0.01$).

amino acid concentration and digestibility in fishmeal, which in turn determine its quality and price. US researchers (Kim and Easter, 2001) evaluated four fishmeal sources in diets for young pigs:

1. Menhaden (dried at 70°C).
2. Mackerel (dried at 85°C).
3. Mackerel (dried at 70°C).
4. Herring (dried at 70°C).

Amino acid digestibility was estimated weekly in eight cannulated pigs for 4 weeks post-weaning (at 3 weeks of age). The basal diet contained 16% fishmeal, a blend of maize starch and lactose, amino acids, vitamins, and minerals. Overall, amino acid digestibility was about 15% greater in low-temperature (LT) mackerel (70°C) and herring fishmeal than in menhaden or higher-temperature mackerel (85°C) fishmeal. In a second experiment, 120 weaned pigs (20 days of age), in six replicates, were offered four diets based on the same sources of fishmeal for 4 weeks post-weaning. Fishmeal was added on a protein basis and, thus, its concentration ranged from 9.5 to 11%. Overall, weight gain and feed intake were not affected by fishmeal source. Feed efficiency was improved, however, by about 10% in pigs offered mackerel or herring fishmeal. In a third experiment, 160 weaned pigs (14 days of age), in eight replicates, were fed diets with LT mackerel fishmeal included at 0, 2.5, and 5%, or diets with animal plasma added at 2.5 and 5%, for 15 days post-weaning. Weight gain and feed intake were not affected by inclusion of either fishmeal or plasma, although they were numerically higher compared with control. Feed efficiency, however, was improved in a linear fashion as fishmeal and plasma levels increased. In conclusion, selection of fishmeal for piglet diets must be based not only on chemical composition, but also on processing conditions that affect amino acid digestibility.

Inedible egg product

Although spray-dried egg powder (i.e. egg contents without shells) is a prized, albeit expensive, ingredient for piglet diets, other egg-based products are frequently made available at competitive prices. These products are usually derived from off-quality eggs that are unfit for human consumption. Such an inedible egg product, derived from a 50:50 mixture of whole eggs and whites, was tested as a source of protein in piglet diets (Zimmerman, 2000). The dried egg product contained 55.2% protein and 28.6% fat. A total of 124 weaned pigs (6.4 kg body weight and 18 days of age) were offered a complex diet that contained 5% animal plasma for 2 weeks post-weaning, followed by a less complex diet for another 2 weeks. The egg product was added at 0, 3, 6, and 9% of each diet to replace soybean meal and soy oil on an equal lysine and energy basis. Increasing concentrations of egg product linearly decreased weight gain and efficiency of feed utilization,

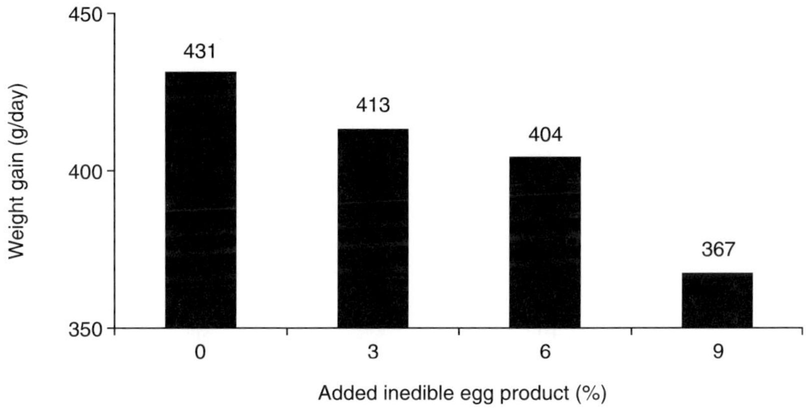

Fig. 6.3. Inedible egg products are not suitable for piglet diets. (From Zimmerman, 2000.)

but feed intake was not affected (Fig. 6.3). In a second experiment (James *et al.*, 2000), 144 weaned pigs (6.7 kg body weight and 18 days of age) were fed a maize–whey soybean meal diet that was supplemented with animal plasma (4%), egg product (6.3%), or a mixture of plasma (3.15%) and egg product (2%) on an equal nutrient basis for 2 weeks post-weaning. Animal plasma increased weight gain by 24% over control, but egg product did not improve growth performance. In conclusion, inedible egg product is not a suitable protein source for piglet diets.

References

Azain MJ, Tomkins T, Sowinski JS, Arentson RA, and Jewell DE (1996) Effect of supplemental pig milk replacer on litter performance: seasonal variation in response. *Journal of Animal Science* 74:2195–2202.

Bikker P, van Dijk AJ, Dirkzwager A, Fledderus J, Ubbink-Blanksma M, and Beynen AC (2004) The influence of diet composition and an anti-microbial growth promoter on the growth response of weaned piglets to spray dried animal plasma. *Livestock Production Science* 86:201–208.

Bugnacka D and Falkowski J (2001) The effect of dietary levels of yellow lupine seeds (*Lupinus luteus* L.) on feed preferences and growth performance of young pigs. *Journal of Animal and Feed Sciences* 10:133–142.

Cadogan DJ, Partridge GG, and Simmins PH (2000) Effect of xylanase addition in feed containing either pre-characterised wheat or wheat by-products on the performance of growing pigs. *Proceedings of the Annual Meeting of the British Society of Animal Science*, 21. York, UK.

Carroll JA, Fritsche KL, Spencer JD, Gaines AM, Allee GL, Matteri RL, Kattesh HG, Roberts MP, Beausang LA, and Zannelli ME (2001) Effect of fish oil supplementation on the young pig's immunological response to an endotoxic challenge. *Journal of Animal Science* 79(Supplement 2):34.

Dunshea FR, Kerton DJ, Eason PJ, and King RH (1999) Supplemental skim milk before and after weaning improves growth performance of pigs. *Australian Journal of Agricultural Research* 50:1165–1170.

Edwards SA, Taylor AG, and Harland JI (1991) The inclusion of sugar beet pulp in diets for early weaned piglets. *Animal Production* 52:599–600.

Fialho ET, Rodrigues PB, Lima JAF, Silva HO, and Oliveira V (2004) Performance and nutrient digestibility of low-tannin sorghum fed to pigs from 10 to 30 kg. *Journal of Animal Science* 82(Supplement 1):22.

Gill BP, Mellange J, and Rooke JA (2000) Growth performance and apparent nutrient digestibility in weaned piglets offered wheat-, barley- or sugar-beet pulp-based diets supplemented with food enzymes. *Animal Science* 70:107–118.

Grinstead GS, Goodband RD, Dritz SS, Tokach MD, Nelssen JL, Woodworth JC, and Molitor M (2000) Effects of a whey protein product and spray-dried animal plasma on growth performance of weanling pigs. *Journal of Animal Science* 78:647–657.

Jaikaran S (2001) Using ground and extruded lentils and peas in weaner diets. http://www.albertapork.com.

James BW, Sparks JC, Jurgens MH, and Zimmerman DR (2000) Comparison of inedible egg product and spray-dried plasma as sources of protein for weanling pigs. *Annual Swine Research Report No. ASL-1659*. Iowa State University, Ames, IA,

Kim JG, Shin YM, Park YH, Kim HS, and Whang K-Y (2002) Effect of soybean meal origin on the growth performance in broilers and pigs. *Journal of Animal Science* 80(Supplement 1):160.

Kim SW and Easter RA (2001) Nutritional value of fish meals in diets for young pigs. *Journal of Animal Science* 79:1829–1839.

Mahan DC, Newton EA, and Cera KR (1996) Effect of supplemental sodium chloride, sodium phosphate, or hydrochloric acid in starter pig diets containing dried whey. *Journal of Animal Science* 74:1217–1222.

Mahan DC, Wiseman TD, Weaver E, and Russell L (1999) Effect of supplemental sodium chloride and hydrochloric acid added to initial starter diets containing spray-dried blood plasma and lactose on resulting performance and nitrogen digestibility of 3-week-old weaned pigs. *Journal of Animal Science* 77:3016–3021.

Mavromichalis I, Hancock JD, Hines RH, Senne BW, and Cao H (2001) Lactose, sucrose, and molasses in simple and complex diets for nursery pigs. *Animal Feed Science and Technology* 93:127–135.

Medel P, Salado S, de Blas JC, and Mateos GG (1999) Processed cereals in diets for early-weaned piglets. *Animal Feed Science and Technology* 82:145–156.

Medel P, Garcia MC, Lazaro R, de Blas JC, and Mateos GG (2000) Particle size and heat treatment of barley in diets for early-weaned piglets. *Animal Feed Science and Technology* 84:13–21.

Medel P, Latorre MA, de Blas C, Lazaro R, and Mateos GG (2003) Heat processing of cereals in mash or pellet diets for young pigs. *Animal Feed Science and Technology* 113:127–140.

Meyer TA, Lindemann MD, Cromwell GL, and Monegue HJ (2001) Use of menhaden oil to alter *n*-6:*n*-3 fatty acid ratios in nursery pig diets. *Journal of Animal Science* 79(Supplement 1):21.

Miller HM, Toplis P, Arnold S, Cook DR, and Marshall C (2000) A comparison of two wheat varieties at two different bushel weights had no effect on weaner pig performance. *Proceedings of the British Society of Animal Science Occasional Meeting 'The Weaner Pig – Nutrition and Management'*, 34. University of Nottingham, Nottingham, UK.

Montagne L, Pluske JR, and Hampson DJ (2003) A review of interactions between dietary fibre and the intestinal mucosa, and their consequences on digestive health in young non-ruminant animals. *Animal Feed Science and Technology* 108:95–117.

Myer RO (2001) Evaluation of triticale and soft red wheat in nursery diets for pigs weaned at three weeks of age. *Proceedings of the Annual Midwestern Meeting of the American Society of Animal Science*, 55. Des Moines, IA.

NCR-42 Committee on Swine Nutrition (1999) Variability among sources and laboratories in nutrient analyses of maize and soybean meal. *Journal of Animal Science* 77:3262–3273.

Oliver WT, Mathews SA, Phillips O, Jones EE, Odle J, and Harrell RJ (2001) Efficacy of partially hydrolyzed maize syrup solids as a replacement for lactose in manufactured liquid diets for neonatal pigs. *Journal of Animal Science* 80:143–153.

Owusu-Asiedu A, Baidoo SK, and Nyachoti CM (2002) Effect of heat processing on nutrient digestibility in pea and supplementing amylase and xylanase to raw, extruded or micronized pea-based diets on performance of early-weaned pigs. *Canadian Journal of Animal Science* 82:367–374.

Pearce AN, Rose SP, Kettlewell PS, and Schulze H (1997) A comparison in growth performance of young pigs fed six different cultivars of wheat. *Proceedings of the Annual Meeting of the British Society of Animal Science*, 64. York, UK.

Pluske JR, Black B, Pethick DW, Mullan BP, and Hampson DJ (2003) Effects of different sources and levels of dietary fiber in diets on performance, digesta characteristics and antibiotic treatment of pigs after weaning. *Animal Feed Science and Technology* 107:129–142.

Spencer JD, Allee GL, and Sauber TE (2000) Phosphorus bioavailability and digestibility of normal and genetically modified low-phytate corn for pigs. *Journal of Animal Science* 78:675–681.

Stahly TS, Cook DR, and Zimmerman DR (1995a) The effect of dietary level and source of plasma proteins on rate and efficiency of gain in pigs postweaning fed from 13 to 37 pounds body weight. *Swine Research Report No. ASL-R1158*:6–10. Iowa State University, Ames, IA.

Stahly TS, Swenson SG, Zimmerman DR, and Williams NH (1995b) Impact of porcine plasma proteins on postweaning growth of pigs with a low and high level of antigen exposure. *Swine Research Report No. ASL-R1157*:3–6. Iowa State University, Ames, IA.

Torrallardona D, Conde MR, Badiola I, Polo FJ, and Brufau J (2003) Effect of fishmeal replacement with spray-dried animal plasma and colistin on intestinal structure, intestinal microbiology, and performance of weanling pigs challenged with *Escherichia coli* K99. *Journal of Animal Science* 81:1220–1226.

Touchette KJ, Carroll JA, Allee GL, Matteri RL, Dyer CJ, Beausang LA, and Zannelli ME (2000) Feeding spray-dried plasma alters the immunological response of the weaned pig to a lipopolysaccharide challenge. *Journal of Animal Science* 78(Supplement 1):43.

van Dijk AJ, Everts H, Nabuurs MJA, Margry RJCF, and Beynen AC (2001) Growth performance of weanling pigs fed spray-dried animal plasma: a review. *Livestock Production Science* 68:263–274.

Vicente B, Valencia DG, Lazaro R, Latorre MA, and Mateos GG (2004) Use of rice in substitution of corn in diets for young pigs. *Journal of Animal Science* 82(Supplement 1):456.

White CE, Campbell DR, and McDowell LR (2000) Effects of dry matter content on trypsin inhibitors and urease activity in heat treated soya beans fed to weaned piglets. *Animal Feed Science and Technology* 87:105–115.

Witney MH and Shurson GC (2003) Growth performance of nursery pigs fed diets containing increasing levels of maize distiller's dried grains with solubles. *Journal of Animal Science* 81(Supplement 2):80.

Woodworth JC, Tokach MD, Goodband RD, Nelssen JL, O'Quinn PR, Knabe DA, and Said NW (2001) Apparent ileal digestibility of amino acids and the digestible and metabolizable energy content of dry extruded-expelled soybean meal and its effects on growth performance of pigs. *Journal of Animal Science* 79:1280–1287.

Xiao C, Jin LZ, and Zhao X (2000) Bovine casein peptides co-stimulate naive macrophages with lipopolysaccharide for proinflammatory cytokine production and nitric oxide release. *Journal of the Science of Food and Agriculture* 81:300–304.

Xing JJ, van Heugten E, Li DF, Touchette KJ, Coalson JA, Odgaard RL, and Odle J (2004) Effects of emulsification, fat encapsulation, and pelleting on weanling pig performance and nutrient digestibility. *Journal of Animal Science* 82:2601–2609.

Yin YL, Baidoo SK, Schulze H, and Simmins PH (2001a) Effects of supplementing diets containing hulless barley varieties having different levels of non-starch polysaccharides with β-glucanase and xylanase on the physiological status of the gastrointestinal tract and nutrient digestibility of weaned pigs. *Livestock Production Science* 71:97–107.

Yin YL, Baidoo SK, Jin LZ, Liu YG, Schulze H, and Simmins PH (2001b) The effect of different carbohydrase and protease supplementation on apparent (ileal and overall) digestibility of nutrients of five hulless barley varieties on young pigs. *Livestock Production Science* 71:109–120.

Zarkadas LN and Wiseman J (2000) Inclusion of differently processed full-fat soya bean in diets for piglets. *Proceedings of the British Society of Animal Science Occasional Meeting 'The Weaner Pig – Nutrition and Management'*, 45–46. University of Nottingham, Nottingham, UK.

Zimmerman DR (2000) Effect of inedible egg product on growth performance of weanling pigs. *Annual Swine Research Report No. ASL 1659*. Iowa State University, Ames, IA.

Feed Additives

7

Introduction

Additives may be defined as ingredients used for purposes other than directly supplying essential nutrients and energy. Additives are used to enhance performance or prevent loss of performance. Additives may be classified as 'zootechnical', in that they interact with the animal, or 'technical', in that they interact mainly with feed quality. The former are the focus of this chapter, whilst the latter – having no nutritional value – are described briefly at the end.

Most countries have their own definitions and classifications of additives and often regulate their application to some extent. Users are advised to consult with authorities and suppliers before employing additives of unknown status.

Evaluating Research on Additives

Additives are the focus of modern research worldwide as their trade plays a major part in the international animal nutrition business. For most products, results from their use under most practical conditions remain largely inconclusive and quite often difficult to evaluate, perhaps because the conditions under which they might be beneficial are difficult to understand without proper research efforts.

Common pitfalls in the experimental design of trials often used to promote commercial additives include (but are not limited to) the following.

No negative control

It is often assumed that a long-established additive (e.g. antibiotics) is always effective when used under standard conditions. Thus, when such a product is replaced by a novel additive (e.g. organic acids) without any loss in performance, it is often claimed that the two additives are of equal potency in enhancing animal performance or health. However, there is no value in comparing the two additives without a negative control (a diet without any of the two additives) to guard against the event of no response to the standard additive that would render the whole trial ineffectual.

No positive control

Without a positive control, on the other hand, it is quite difficult to evaluate the return on investment from the use of a novel additive that may or may not support performance equal to the standard additive.

Arbitrary dosage

Without proper dose–response trials, dosages often recommended by some manufacturers are educated guesses, based on theoretical calculations, at best. It is equally likely for a smaller or larger dose to elicit a similar or even greater response, respectively.

No statistical analysis

Numerical differences without statistical analysis are never a sufficient basis for a decision on replacing or using a novel additive.

Inappropriate statistics

It is widely accepted that a probability value of 5% ($P < 0.05$) is sufficient to discern experimental data. Under commercial conditions, a stretched value of 10% ($P < 0.10$) is acceptable, especially in large-scale experiments, but even then it should be used as an indication (trend) and not as a definite result. Conclusions based on greater values are meaningless.

Insufficient replicates

Quite often, experiments are conducted with limited replicates. In such cases, it is extremely difficult to detect small differences in response as such differences are likely to be due to biological variation or random effects. Trials with less than six to ten replicates per treatment (e.g. ten pens for each treatment) are usually of limited value.

Experimental conditions

Practical trials conducted under non-commercial conditions should be interpreted with care for application under commercial practices. For example, results obtained with one or two piglets per pen are not likely to be repeated in larger pens holding ten or 20 pigs, as feeding behavior is quite different in large groups. The same logic applies in diets used for experimental purposes.

Applied versus basic research

Data generated *in vitro* or in basic research programs do not always result in improved performance or profitability under commercial conditions. For example, additives that improve indices of digestive tract health do not always improve growth performance. In such cases, it is best to establish under which conditions these additives are most effective.

Gut Conditioners

Feed-grade 'antibiotics'

Feed-grade antimicrobial agents are well-established additives that control the gastrointestinal microflora and enhance feed efficiency, resulting in improved growth performance (Cromwell, 2002). In young pigs, the magnitude of response depends on the level of hygiene in facilities and the health status of pigs. Under most commercial conditions, it is expected that antimicrobial agents increase growth performance by 5–15% over non-supplemented controls. Nevertheless, the use of feed-grade antimicrobial agents is declining worldwide due to concerns regarding increasing bacterial resistance to these compounds (Goransson, 2001). Effective alternatives are currently in great demand.

Zinc oxide

The beneficial effects of zinc oxide supplementation are well documented (reduces scouring and improves growth performance) and its use is widespread (where still allowed by law), but its mode of action remains elusive (Hill *et al.*, 2001). Current speculation leans toward the theory of modification and control of the gastrointestinal microflora as its main mechanism of improving animal performance (Katouli *et al.*, 1999). On average, 3000 ppm Zn from zinc oxide are sufficient to elicit the above responses in the first couple of weeks post-weaning, followed by diminishing concentrations in the following weeks until exit from the nursery. Unfortunately, the use of zinc oxide is viewed negatively from the environmental perspective and in many countries it is prohibited or strictly controlled by law. Effective alternatives are not available at the moment.

Zinc oxide and antimicrobials

Considerable confusion exists concerning the addition of zinc oxide, a potent growth promoter, in the presence of antimicrobials, especially in the USA. Although both agents improve post-weaning performance and prevent or alleviate symptoms of diarrhea, their interactive effects are still perplexing. A regional study (Mahan *et al.*, 2000) conducted in seven US states investigated the effects of 0, 1500, and 3000 ppm Zn from zinc oxide with or without an antimicrobial agent (carbadox). During a 4-week study, which involved 918 pigs (14 to 21 days of age) in 20 replicates, a complex diet (1.5% lysine) was offered during the first week, followed by a less complex diet (1.3% lysine) during the remaining period. Results from this project indicated that during the first week post-weaning, carbadox did not enhance growth performance. However, there was a trend for improved growth in pigs offered diets fortified with zinc oxide. During weeks 2 to 4, both carbadox and zinc oxide increased gain and feed intake, with the effects being additive. Additionally, the response to zinc oxide was maximized at 1500 ppm Zn, which is in agreement with most recent data suggesting a plateau around 2000 ppm Zn from zinc oxide. It is therefore concluded that when growth-promoting antimicrobials are used, they should be reserved for the late nursery period, whereas zinc oxide should be fed from the beginning.

Copper sulfate

The use of copper sulfate dates before the advent of zinc oxide (Cromwell *et al.*, 1978). This salt elicits responses similar to those elicited by zinc oxide, but the latter is more effective in the post-weaning period. As their actions are not additive, it is often suggested that zinc oxide is used in the first couple of weeks post-weaning followed by copper sulfate until exit from the nursery. The maximum tolerable dose is 250 ppm Cu from copper sulfate, although satisfactory results are often obtained with smaller doses (125–175 ppm). Copper sulfate is another salt under restrictions imposed by law in several countries. Effective alternatives are not available at the moment.

Copper sulfate and zinc oxide

Today, many piglet formulas still include both additives, disregarding preliminary research indicating that the actions of zinc oxide and copper sulfate are not additive. To provide a clear-cut answer to this issue, two regional committees representing 12 university experimental stations in the

USA (NCR-42 and S-145, 2000) employed 1356 weaned pigs that averaged 6.6 kg and 22 days of age in a 28-day growth assay with 55 replicates per treatment. Experimental diets contained antimicrobial agents and the four dietary treatments were:

1. The basal diet;
2. The basal diet supplemented with 3000 ppm Zn from zinc oxide;
3. The basal diet supplemented with 250 ppm Cu from copper sulfate; and
4. The basal diet supplemented with Zn and Cu (as in 2+3).

Average daily gain, feed intake, and efficiency of feed utilization improved by the addition of zinc, copper, and their combination, but the responses were independent and not additive (Table 7.1). Pigs fed zinc oxide outperformed pigs fed copper sulfate only during the second week post-weaning but not during the entire experimental period. Fecal color was darker in Cu-fed pigs and fecal consistency was improved by zinc and copper alike. In conclusion, zinc oxide is more efficacious than copper sulfate during the first couple of weeks post-weaning and there is no need for both additives to be used together.

Organic acids

The advent of organic acids was the outcome of the ban on most antimicrobial agents in the EU (Mroz, 2003). Organic acids are considered today the closest replacements for antibiotics, in the absence of zinc oxide and copper sulfate. Earlier research indicated that rather high concentrations of organic acids (1–2%) are needed to effectively enhance performance in young pigs (Roth and Kirchgessner, 1998). Recent practice, however, limits use to less than 1%. It is currently accepted that blends of organic acids are usually more potent than single organic acids (Namkung *et al.*, 2004).

Table 7.1. Zinc and copper in piglet diets[a]. (Adapted from NCR-42 and S-145, 2000.)

	Control	3000 ppm Zn	250 ppm Cu	Zn+Cu
Weight gain (g/day)	375	422	409	415
Feed intake (g/day)	637	690	671	681
Feed/gain	1.70	1.64	1.64	1.64
Fecal color	3.2	3.2	4.3	3.6
Fecal consistency	2.4	2.1	2.1	2.1

[a] A total 1356 pigs (6.6 kg and 22 days of age) in a 28-day growth assay with 55 replicates per treatment.

The mode of action of organic acids is believed to be: (i) through lowering of stomach pH, which creates an unfavorable environment for pathogens to proliferate; and (ii) through directly killing pathogenic bacteria at the small intestinal level (Roth and Kirchgessner, 1998). The first concept is not well documented, but it is a logical one, at least if organic acids remain undissociated at the stomach level. For this, their pK_a should be lower than stomach pH or else they dissociate and are absorbed by the stomach epithelium. The second concept assumes that undissociated organic acids are absorbed by pathogens and then dissociate inside the cell, disrupting normal functions and resulting in cell death.

The most common organic acids used in piglet feeds with their main effects in enhancing piglet performance are presented in Table 7.2 from a comprehensive literature review (Freitag *et al.*, 1998; as cited by Koch, 2005). Several organic acids are not permitted in certain countries and, thus, local laws must be consulted before using them. Also, dosage remains an art rather than a science, with most common levels being 0.5–1% for the first diet post-weaning followed by decreasing levels in subsequent diets.

Most acids are liquid and corrosive, and pose a health hazard during handling at the feed mixing point. Thus, buffered salts on a solid carrier are frequently preferred, but their efficacy is obviously diminished unless their dietary concentration is adjusted accordingly.

Citric and acetic acids

Citric and acetic acids are relatively inexpensive and readily available, but data are limited on their antimicrobial properties. A recent report (Lee *et al.*, 2002) indicated that although both acids have strong antimicrobial properties, they are effective against different pathogens. Citric acid is most effective against Gram-positive bacteria, like *Clostridium perfringens*, whereas acetic acid is more effective against Gram-negative bacteria, like

Table 7.2. Relative performance enhancement from organic acids in piglet diets compared to diets without growth-promoting agents. (Adapted from Freitag *et al.*, 1998; as cited by Koch, 2005.)

Ingredient[a]	Trials	Weight gain (%)	Feed intake (%)
Avilamycin	6	12	5
Formic acid	9	15	7
Sorbic acid	5	20	9
Fumaric acid	14	6	3
Other acids	12	3	1
Formates	11	4	1
Acid blends	20	10	6

[a] Consult manufacturer's directions before using any specific product.

Salmonella choleraesuis and *E. coli*. Their combination did not show synergism or antagonism. This study demonstrated that organic acids cannot be used interchangeably. Additionally, it appears that the commercial practice of using blends of organic acids may be most appropriate for combating the plethora of bacteria hosted in the pig's gastrointestinal system.

Sorbic acid

Sorbic acid has wide applications in the human food industry as a preservative, but it appears also to have great potential for inclusion in piglet diets. Maribo (2000) evaluated sorbic acid in post-weaning diets using 444 pigs in 19 replicates per treatment. Pigs were weaned at 24 days of age at an average body weight of 6.8 kg. During the first 2 weeks post-weaning, pigs were offered a weaner diet, followed by a starter diet for another 4 weeks. Dietary treatments were: (i) control without organic acids; (ii) control with 1.25% calcium formate; and (iii) control with 0.2% sorbic acid. As expected, calcium formate improved growth performance over control diets, mainly via an improvement in feed efficiency (–10%) during the first 2 weeks post-weaning. Weight gain was also improved by 7% during the same period. These effects practically disappeared during the subsequent 4 weeks. Sorbic acid, added only in the weaner diet, dramatically increased weight gain (+37%) and improved feed efficiency (+22%) during the first 2 weeks post-weaning. Overall, calcium formate and sorbic acid applications increased profitability by 6% and 11%, respectively. In conclusion, organic acids appear to be most effective during the period immediately after weaning. Calcium formate continues to yield consistent results under field conditions, whereas sorbic acid merits further investigation to substantiate these results.

Digestive Enhancers

Enzymes

Enzymes are used to enhance digestion of specific nutrients (starch, proteins, and lipids) or enable, at least partially, digestion of otherwise indigestible compounds (mainly non-starch polysaccharides and phytate). In Table 7.3, several enzyme preparations are presented along with their target compounds and relative efficacy. In young pigs, the ability to digest starch, proteins, and lipids is not enhanced by dietary supplementation of corresponding enzymes, at least to the point to justify their cost. Research has been rather inadequate and confusing at best. Most authorities agree that young pigs fed high-quality diets are not likely to benefit markedly from such enzymes (Partridge, 2001).

Table 7.3. Description of enzymes available for piglet feeds[a].

Enzyme	Main target	Ingredients	Effectiveness in piglets
Amylase	Starch	All cereals	Small
β-Glucanase	NSP[b]	Barley, wheat, rye, triticale	Medium
Lipase	Lipids	Lipids and oil seeds	Trivial
Phytase	Phytate	All plant-based ingredients	High for P/Ca
Protease	Proteins	Plant-derived ingredients	Unclear
Xylanase	NSP[b]	Wheat, triticale, barley, rye	Depends on cereal quality

[a] Consult manufacturer's directions before using any specific product.
[b] Non-starch polysaccharides (NSP) like β-glucans and arabinoxylans.

Carbohydrases

Carbohydrases specific for non-starch polysaccharides can be rather effective if used appropriately. Not all cereals benefit from such enzymes, however, as research has revealed. When the concentration of non-starch polysaccharides is below average (good-quality cereals), enzymes are more often than not ineffective (Mavromichalis *et al.*, 2000). But, with low-quality cereals (i.e. high in non-starch polysaccharides) enzyme supplementation usually confers benefits in terms of enhanced growth performance (Partridge, 2001).

Enzymes and poor wheat quality

Australian and British teams (Cadogan *et al.*, 2000) established the quality of three wheat batches in a pilot growth experiment and classified them as poor, medium, and high. Three diets containing each of the three wheat classes were then formulated with or without a carbohydrase (xylanase from *Trichoderma longibrachiatum* at 4000 units/g product) and fed to growing-finishing pigs. Growth performance linearly decreased with decreasing quality of wheat. Pigs fed low-quality wheat had the poorest growth rates compared to pigs offered high-quality wheat, whereas pigs offered medium-quality wheat had intermediate growth rates (see Fig. 7.1). Feed efficiency was not significantly affected by wheat quality. Enzyme supplementation restored growth rates in pigs fed low- or medium-quality wheat to the levels achieved by pigs fed high-quality wheat. These effects are expected to be more pronounced in young pigs. In conclusion, wheat quality can significantly affect animal performance but carbohydrases can reduce the negative impact of low-quality wheat.

Enzymes and good wheat quality

It is a common belief that young pigs fed diets based on wheat would benefit constantly from enzyme supplementation. A Canadian team (Zijlstra

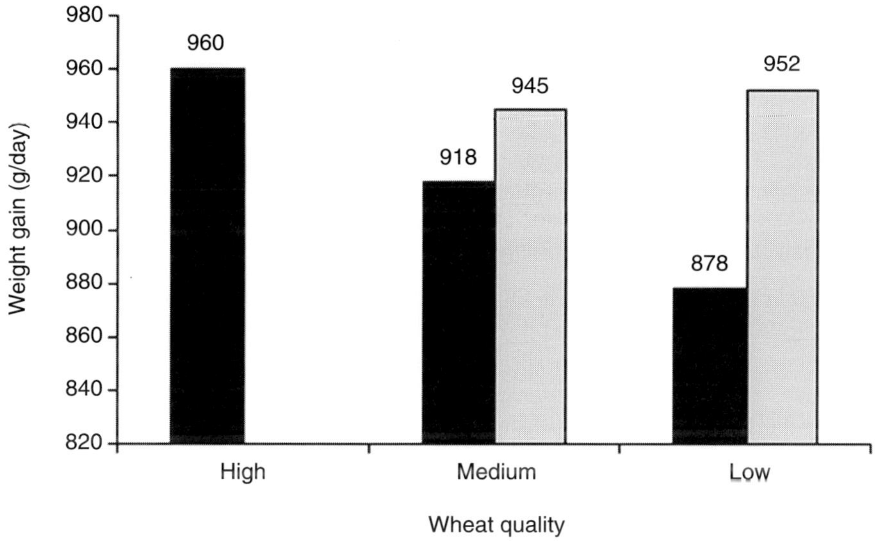

Fig. 7.1. Enzyme supplementation (▒, enzyme; ■, control) restored growth rate in pigs fed medium- and low-quality wheat. (From Cadogan *et al.*, 2000.)

et al., 2004) recently evaluated the effects of enzyme supplementation (xylanase) in diets for young pigs (12 kg) using six samples of wheat varying considerably in neutral detergent fiber concentration (20 to 36%). In the first 7 days post-weaning, enzyme supplementation improved pig performance in five samples of wheat (+0.26 kg at day 7), whereas it actually decreased growth performance in the sixth sample (–0.30 kg at day 7). Growth performance was also affected by wheat source. For the overall period of the trial (21 days), enzyme supplementation or wheat source did not affect weight gain, but enzyme supplementation marginally improved feed efficiency by 2%. In conclusion, the source of wheat appears to affect growth performance during the first week post-weaning and enzyme supplementation appears to improve performance when used in conjunction with some but not all sources of wheat. During the whole nursery period, enzyme supplementation offered negligible benefits in terms of improved feed efficiency. More work is needed to properly classify wheat quality before feeding to animals.

Phytase

The most frequently used enzyme is phytase, an enzyme that enhances phosphorus utilization from plant-derived feedstuffs (Jongbloed *et al.*, 1995). On average, 500 units of phytase (or the dose recommended by the manufacturer) can replace about 0.08% digestible/available phosphorus and 0.05% digestible calcium from inorganic salts (e.g. dicalcium phosphate and calcium carbonate). Quite often, though, the only reason that justifies the use of phytase is legislation that aims to protect the environment from phosphorus pollution, as any savings are often negated by the cost of phytase.

Phytase and protein digestibility

Several research reports indicate that phytase improves protein and amino acid digestibility when added in diets containing phytate-bound phosphorus. However, there has been a dispute whether these findings are meaningful because other reports revealed that phytase does not increase the bioavailability of any released protein and amino acids. In a joint study conducted at Texas A&M University and the University of Kentucky (Traylor *et al.*, 2000), researchers fed a soybean meal-based diet to cannulated pigs (25 kg body weight). The soybean meal contained 0.4% Ca, 0.7% P, 49% crude protein, and 0.32% lysine. The diet was completed with starch, vitamins and minerals, and four levels of phytase were fed: 0, 500, 1000, and 1500 units per kg of complete diet. True digestibility of Ca in soybean meal tended to increase with increasing doses of phytase but the effect was not significant. As expected, phosphorus true digestibility was significantly improved by phytase addition in a quadratic fashion, with most of the improvement at 500 units/kg (see Fig. 7.2). True digestibility of crude protein was not affected by phytase addition except for a slight non-significant improvement (0.8%) at the 500 units phytase/kg level. In conclusion,

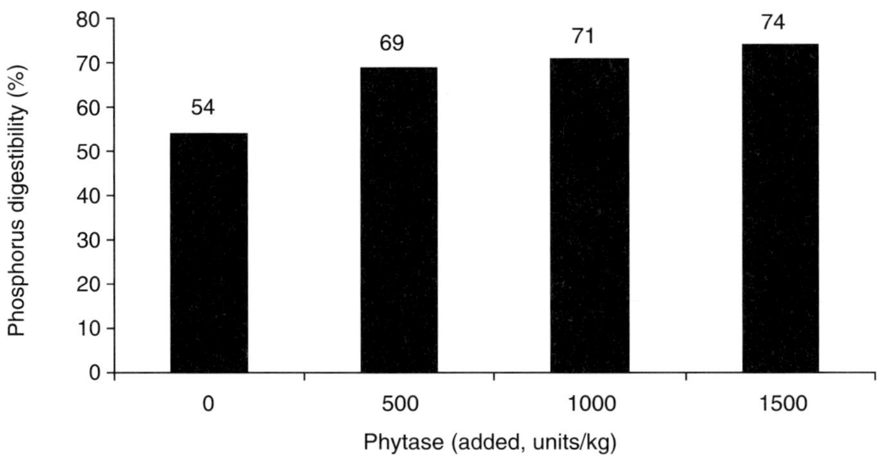

Fig. 7.2. Supplemental phytase improved phytic phosphorus digestibility in piglets. (From Traylor *et al.*, 2000.)

phytase is a potent additive to improve phosphorus digestibility in high-phytate diets, but it offers little if any advantages in terms of protein and amino acid digestibility.

Plant extracts

Plant extracts from herbs and spices have a long history in human traditional medicine, and they have emerged recently as novel additives for antibiotic-free diets (Kamel, 2000). Their mode of action is largely unknown, but claims exist for enhanced appetite and digestion, along with stimulation of the immune system and control of the gastrointestinal microflora (Gill, 1999). Table 7.4 presents the major extracts used today in most commercial preparations. Research on the efficacy of plant extracts in young pigs is rather limited and largely undocumented.

Chinese herbs

In the search for antibiotic replacements, scientists often refer to Chinese ancient medicine for possible solutions. Dried roots of Chinese rhubarb contain anthraquinones that affect large intestine functions and have antibacterial, antifungal, and antiviral properties, all well documented in international journals. A research team from Switzerland (Gebert *et al.*, 2003) fed incremental dietary doses of Chinese rhubarb (0, 0.25, 0.5, and 1%) to 8-kg weaned pigs for 31 days post-weaning. At 0.25% concentration, rhubarb supplementation improved feed intake (+32%) and weight gain (+17%), especially during the first couple of weeks post-weaning. Pigs also had improved energy and nitrogen metabolism. At 0.5%, the beneficial effects of rhubarb were not detectable, whereas at 1%, growth performance (–35%) and feed intake (–15%) were severely depressed. Animals fed 1% rhubarb also suffered from diarrhea due to the strong laxative effect of this

Table 7.4. Common plant extracts used in diets for piglets[a]. (Adapted from Kamel, 2000.)

Source	Active compound(s)	Properties
Cinnamon	Cinnamaldehyde	Appetite and digestion stimulant, antiseptic
Oregano	Carvacrol	Appetite stimulant, antiseptic
Clove	Eugenol	Appetite and digestion stimulant, antiseptic
Garlic	Allicin	Digestion stimulant, antiseptic
Capsicum	Capsaicin	Anti-diarrheic, anti-inflammatory
Thyme	Thymol	Appetite stimulant, antiseptic, antioxidant

[a] Consult manufacturer's directions before using any specific product.

herb. In an earlier trial, growth performance was enhanced with 0.1% dietary rhubarb, but the concentration of anthraquinones was higher (1.53%) than in the current experiment (1.02%). In conclusion, it appears that Chinese rhubarb may enhance animal performance post-weaning, but the concentration of anthraquinones, which is variable, should be carefully controlled to avoid diarrhea and associated growth depression. A dose-titration trial with purified anthraquinones would be interesting.

Immunoglobulins

Animal plasma

Although animal plasma is an excellent source of amino acids for young pigs, its extremely high price prohibits its use as such an ingredient. Animal plasma has been shown to greatly (25–50%) increase feed intake and growth performance during the first two weeks post-weaning (Gatnau *et al.*, 1991; van Dijk *et al.*, 2001). This effect is more pronounced in pigs of average health (Stahly *et al.*, 1995) and it is believed that the high concentration of immunoglobulins in plasma is mainly responsible for its beneficial effects (Owen *et al.*, 1995). Animal plasma has been recently re-allowed in the EU.

Egg protein

Egg powder from hens hyperimmunized against specific pathogens (usually *E. coli* strains) is a rich source of immunoglobulins. Its use in piglet diets has been shown to improve growth performance and reduce scouring (see also Table 9.5), but, in general, the effect is not as great as that obtained with plasma, perhaps because the response is more pathogen-specific.

A British research group (Rizvi *et al.*, 2001) recently evaluated the use of hyperimmunized eggs in a liquid milk replacer for neonatal pigs. The spray-dried eggs contained antibodies against *E. coli* and rotavirus and were added at 5% on a dry matter basis. A regular spray-dried egg was also added as a positive control treatment. At birth, 15 piglets were allowed to consume colostrum for 24 h, whereas another 15 littermates were deprived of colostrum. Following a 3-day adaptation period with a regular milk replacer, piglets were offered the experimental diets for another 3-day period, at the end of which they were infected with rotavirus and *E. coli* (K88) pathogens. Piglets were euthanized after 0, 1, 2, 3, and 4 days for bacteriological examination of the gastrointestinal tract. The experiment was repeated three times. Feeding hyperimmunized eggs prevented *E. coli* infection, regardless of colostrum treatment, as evidenced by markedly reduced colony counts in the lumen of the gastrointestinal tract. Regular egg powder was not effective in preventing infection. Weight gain was 0.27, 0.08, and 0.03 kg/day post-infection for piglets receiving diets with hyperimmunized eggs, normal eggs, or plain milk replacer, respectively. Rotavirus infection, however, was not deterred by dietary treatment. In conclusion, it appears that hyperimmunized eggs may have a place in milk replacers for neonatal pigs that are susceptible to colibacillosis infection. The optimum inclusion level, though, remains to be determined.

Top-dressed immunoglobulins

Researchers from the UK (Miller and Toplis, 2000) used 64 crossbred piglets that were weaned at 23 days of age (5.3 kg), without prior access to creep feed, to evaluate a top-dressed supplement rich in immunoglobulins for 4 days post-weaning. The supplement was based on a whey globulin concentrate containing 4% immunoglobulins and it was offered at 60 g/day per piglet. All piglets were offered high-quality starter pellets for the duration of the experiment.

Overall, supplemented piglets were 4% heavier at the end of the 20-day grow-out period compared to their counterparts that had access only to pellets. The difference in growth performance was evident during the second week post-weaning, during which time supplementation had ceased, suggesting an enduring beneficial effect of immunoglobulins ingested early in the post-weaning period.

Novel Applications for Minerals

Organic zinc versus zinc oxide

Preliminary research reports indicated that organic zinc may promote performance with the same efficacy as high doses of zinc oxide (Schell and Kornegay, 1996). The significance of organic zinc is certainly increasing in certain areas of the world where zinc oxide additions are under legislative pressure.

A regional study (Hollis *et al.*, 2001) conducted in seven experimental stations in the USA evaluated the efficacy of zinc methionine at 125, 250, and 500 mg Zn/kg versus 2500 mg Zn/kg from zinc oxide and a negative control with no extra zinc added (basal diet contained 124 mg Zn/kg). A total of 616 weaned pigs (21 days of age and 6.3 kg) were assigned to 26 replicates per treatment. During the first 7 days post-weaning, zinc additions did not improve growth performance compared with the negative control. This is a common observation in most trials with pharmacological doses of zinc. Although overall growth performance (days 0 to 28 post-weaning) was improved by zinc methionine, zinc oxide offered the greatest improvements

(Table 7.5). In conclusion, it appears that up to 500 mg Zn/kg from zinc methionine may improve growth performance in weaned pigs, but not as effectively as zinc oxide. Organic forms of zinc, however, may be the only alternative to zinc oxide where its use is restricted.

Organic trace minerals

The effect of dietary trace mineral concentration and source on performance and fecal mineral excretion from weaning until market age was recently evaluated (Creech *et al.*, 2004) in 216 weaned pigs (6.7 kg). Pigs were offered a positive control diet containing the following levels of trace minerals: 25 ppm Cu, 150 ppm Zn, 180 ppm, Fe, and 60 ppm Mn during the nursery phase; and 15 ppm Cu, 100 ppm Zn, 100 ppm Fe, and 40 ppm Mn during the remaining period until market age. Trace minerals were supplied through sulfate salts. A second treatment included the same basal diet supplemented with reduced levels of trace minerals in all phases: 5 ppm Cu, 25 ppm Zn, 25 ppm Fe, and 10 ppm Mn; whereas in a third treatment only half of these levels were supplied by sulfate salts, the other half being supplied by organic trace minerals. Results indicated that trace mineral concentrations did not affect performance from weaning until slaughter, although during the nursery period pigs offered the diet with reduced inorganic minerals had higher feed/gain ratio compared to piglets offered the diet with the inorganic/organic combination. Fecal excretion of all trace minerals studied was substantially lower when pigs were offered diets with reduced dietary trace mineral levels regardless of source.

From this trial and in agreement with numerous other studies, the following conclusions may be drawn:

- Compared to inorganic trace minerals, organic forms offer no significant growth performance benefits, at least at tested concentrations.
- Current trace mineral specifications overestimate true requirements and result in increased feed cost and unnecessary environmental burden.

Table 7.5. The replacement of zinc oxide by zinc methionine (ZnMet)[a]. (Adapted from Hollis *et al.*, 2001.)

Zn (mg/kg)	Source	Weight gain (g/day)	Feed/gain
0	–	371	1.71
125	ZnMet	391	1.62
250	ZnMet	389	1.65
500	ZnMet	396	1.62
2500	ZnO	415	1.56

[a] A total of 616 weaned pigs (21 days of age and 6.3 kg) in 26 replicates per treatment.

Chromium

Quite often, chromium is recommended as an alternative feed additive for alleviating post-weaning growth depression. Indeed, a higher expenditure of chromium during periods of stress (i.e. weaning, moving, mixing, disease) demonstrated by elevated urinary excretion has been suggested as an indication of higher dietary requirements (Anderson, 1998).

Researchers in Italy (Baldi *et al*., 1999) demonstrated no beneficial effects in terms of growth performance and immune system activity from dietary supplementation of chromium-yeast (330 ppb Cr) in pigs from 10 days after birth until 7 days after weaning. Not only was chromium supplementation uneventful in the case of weaning stress, but it also did not help pigs overcome severe high-stress conditions imposed by injected cortisol. These results are not surprising. Accumulating evidence from several US research institutions indicates that chromium supplementation via chromium tripicolinate, chromium nicotinate, or chromium-yeast alone cannot reduce the negative effects of weaning nor can it enhance immune status or resistance to diseases (for a review, see Mavromichalis and Baker, 1999a). Today, there is no established dietary requirement for chromium in pigs because there is no accurate assessment of chromium status, although its metabolic significance has been clearly demonstrated. Apparently, natural ingredients supply enough chromium to negate dietary supplementation even in times of higher requirements.

Rare-earth elements

Chinese reports indicated that such rare-earth elements as lanthanum, cerium, and praseodymium can improve growth performance of young pigs by as much as 20%. To validate these claims under Western conditions, German researchers (He and Rambek, 2000) prepared diets free of antimicrobial agents but supplemented with chloride salts of these rare-earth elements.

In the first trial, 72 pigs (7.3 kg) were offered two dietary concentrations (75 or 150 mg/kg) of rare-earth elements that were provided via a pure source of lanthanum chloride (98%) or a mixture of rare-earth elements. Although growth performance of pigs offered diets supplemented with rare-earth elements was numerically increased by up to 5% compared to control during the 5-week trial, these improvements were not statistically different. In a second study, however, 14 pigs (17 kg) were offered 0 or 150 mg rare-earth mixture/kg for 8 weeks. Weight gain was improved by 19% and feed efficiency by 10%, both figures significantly different from control. This is the first report indicating potential benefits from rare-earth elements under Western conditions. These pilot studies merit further investigation under more practical conditions and more replications.

Special Roles for Vitamins

Vitamin C and immunity

The issue of supplemental vitamin C in diets for weaned pigs has seen considerable debate during the last 20 years. Earlier trials suggested enhanced growth performance in response to vitamin C supplementation, but subsequent studies yielded rather inconsistent results (see Mavromichalis and Baker, 1999b for a review).

A report from China (Zhao *et al.*, 2002) recently added to this debate. In two experiments, pigs weaned between 20 and 30 days of age were offered diets supplemented with 0, 75, or 300 mg vitamin C/kg for 21 days post-weaning. Growth performance was not affected by supplemental vitamin C. It should be noted, however, that pigs were penned in groups of two and, therefore, the level of stress to which they were exposed was rather limited compared to the stress encountered in most commercial facilities. On a positive note, plasma levels of γ-immunoglobulins and antibody titers to bovine serum tended to be higher in pigs fed diets with supplemental vitamin C. This may be an indication of enhanced immunity status that could potentially help pigs cope better in the face of a disease challenge. But, this requires further investigation.

L-Carnitine

Previous research reports on the effects of dietary additions of up to 1000 ppm carnitine in diets for young pigs are largely inconclusive (Hoffman *et al.*, 1993; Owen *et al.*, 1996). A review was presented by Mavromichalis and Baker (2000).

In a more recent study (Rincker *et al.*, 2003), dietary L-carnitine additions of up to 100 ppm were tested in diets with and without soybean oil (carnitine is involved in lipid metabolism). In five trials, graded levels of carnitine (0, 25, 50, 75, and 100 ppm) were tested in diets containing varying levels of soybean oil (from 0 to 6%). There were between five and eight replicates per treatment and each pen had four to six piglets. Carnitine additions did not affect growth performance in phase 1 and 3 of the trials (trials lasted from 34 to 38 days). In phase 2, however, carnitine slightly increased weight gain and feed intake, with a trend toward improved performance for the overall period. In the last trial, the effects of carnitine were more pronounced in diets with soybean oil, but did not approach statistical significance. In conclusion, research regarding carnitine in diets for young pigs remains equivocal. More research is needed to clarify whether the effects during the second phase are reproducible under commercial conditions, and why similar effects were not observed in other periods of growth.

Luminal Nutrition

This is an emerging area of scientific research that is becoming increasingly important as nutrition now depends less on well-established antimicrobial agents to control the gastrointestinal microflora. In these early stages of research, it is not always possible to establish a positive relationship between indices of increased luminal health and growth performance. Certainly, more research is expected on this area.

Glutamine against *Escherichia coli*

Glutamine plays a major role in gastrointestinal metabolism as a fuel source for enterocytes, including cells of the immune system. It has been demonstrated that enterocytes consume most dietary glutamine, mainly for energy production (Wu, 1996; Watford, 1999).

In a Spanish study (Hernandez *et al*., 2000), piglets weaned at 14 days of age were offered a diet supplemented with 0, 0.50, 0.77, and 1.50% glutamine. After 1 week, they were infected with *E. coli* serotype 66. Glutamine supplementation significantly increased serum levels of IgG against antigen infection in a linear pattern (Fig. 7.3). Infection symptoms in the abdominal cavity were also reduced in pigs fed glutamine at the 0.77 and 1.50% level. In conclusion, it appears that glutamine deserves closer attention in production systems with a high risk of *E. coli* infection, especially with the advent of antimicrobial-free diets. An excellent source of glutamine is wheat gluten.

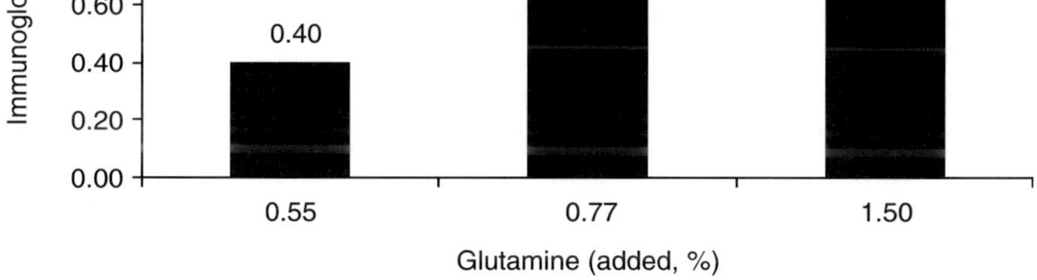

Fig. 7.3. Glutamine increased serum immunoglobulin G (IgG) levels in infected pigs. (From Hernandez *et al*., 2000.)

Ornithine and creatine

Ornithine α-ketoglutarate, an amino acid derivative of intermediate metabolism, has been demonstrated to benefit human trauma patients and rats under severe immunological stress. Ornithine, thus, could help weaned pigs to overcome the stress of weaning at an early age. Likewise, creatine, an energy-dense source, could provide an extra source of calories in piglets experiencing low feed intakes during the early post-weaning period.

In four experiments, American researchers (Guzik *et al.*, 2000) evaluated graded doses of dietary ornithine, ranging from 0 to 0.75%, and creatine, ranging from 0 to 0.5%, in pigs weaned between 15 and 23 days of age. Oral supplements (capsules) of ornithine and creatine were also tested during the last four days before weaning. Overall, results were disappointing in that ornithine slightly increased weight gain in one experiment and decreased the efficiency of feed utilization in another. Creatine supplementation linearly decreased growth performance and plasma albumin and urea nitrogen. Oral supplements were equally ineffective in enhancing growth performance. It appears that the beneficial responses to ornithine and creatine supplementation that are observed in other species cannot be associated with post-weaning stress in pigs.

Miscellaneous Additives

Yucca extract

Feeding high-protein diets usually results in excessive nitrogen excretion in absolute terms, which is a rather common phenomenon during the nursery phase where diets may contain as much as 25% crude protein. Nitrogen in manure is rapidly converted to volatile ammonia that can become problematic in facilities with solid floors or deep pits because ammonia is detrimental to animal health and production. Ammonia emission depends on dry matter and nitrogen concentration in manure, temperature and acidity, and air velocity.

Researchers from Nebraska (Colina *et al.*, 2000) investigated the addition of *Yucca shidigera* extract and calcium chloride in diets for early-weaned pigs. Yucca is a tree native to South America and its extract is known to inhibit urease and thus reduce ammonia emission from manure. Calcium chloride is a relatively inexpensive salt that binds ammonia. A total of 390 weaned pigs (3–5 kg) were employed in three experiments to test the two dietary intervention strategies to lower ammonia emission in a 3-week growth period. Each treatment/group was housed in separate, yet comparable, rooms. Temperature, ventilation, and humidity were kept constant across rooms. Treatments were:

1. Negative control;
2. *Y. shidigera* extract; and
3. Calcium chloride.

As expected, ammonia emission was significantly reduced by the addition of *Y. shidigera* extract despite the fact that control ammonia emission levels were deemed relatively low. Calcium chloride also reduced aerial ammonia levels but it additionally reduced growth rate. Calcium chloride is known to be an appetite depressant because it disrupts electrolyte balance. Pigs that were fed the *Y. shidigera* extract-supplemented diet had growth performance comparable with pigs fed the control diet.

Lecithin

Lecithin is a natural lipid emulsifier usually extracted from soybeans. It is widely used in milk replacers that are high in lipids and require reconstitution in water.

Spanish researchers (Soares and Lopez-Bote, 2002) conducted a 2×3 factorial digestibility experiment with weaned pigs to investigate lecithin supplementation (0 or 1%) in diets with soybean oil, lard, or a soy–lard (80:20) blend. Lecithin was added at the expense of the respective lipid source, which was included at 5% in the control diet. Contrary to expectations, lecithin addition did not improve lipid digestibility in lard-based diets, which was clearly inferior compared to lipid digestibility in diets based on soybean oil and (or) fat–oil blend. As expected, lipid digestibility was lower during the first 2 weeks post-weaning compared to the following 2 weeks. In conclusion, soybean oil remains a choice source of lipids for piglet diets, whereas lard appears to be equally effective at least past the critical post-weaning period. Lecithin supplementation does not improve lipid digestibility in diets based on soybean oil or lard.

Oligosaccharides

Oligosaccharides are believed to exert a tropic effect on the gut microflora, favoring the development and establishment of beneficial bacterial species (Patterson and Burkholder, 2003).

A Danish research team (Mikkelsen *et al.*, 2003) evaluated the effects of feeding fructose- or galacto-oligosaccharides to 4-week weaned piglets. Piglets were fed identical diets with 4% oligosaccharides replacing maize starch and cellulose. Measurements included determination of pH, organic acid concentration, microbial population distribution, and identity of dominant bacterial species in fecal samples collected on days 0, 3, 7, 14, and 28 after weaning. Results indicated that dietary supplementation with oligosaccharides had no effect on growth performance. Also, dietary oligosaccharides did not affect fecal physicochemical and bacterial characteristics. Only in piglets fed fructo-oligosaccharides was fecal concentration of yeast elevated. In conclusion, the effect of oligosaccharides remains controversial, and, thus, no firm recommendations can be made regarding practical application of such technology.

Technical Additives

It is the absence rather than the presence of technical additives that creates potential problems in manufacturing, storing, distributing, and handling animal feed products. In general, good-quality feed that is based on a well-designed formula and prepared under appropriate manufacturing conditions requires little or nothing at all in terms of agents preserving or enhancing its physicochemical characteristics. But, under most commercial practices, certain technical additives are deemed essential. Below is a non-exclusive list of the most common technical additives.

Flavoring agents

Although piglets do not respond to feed flavors when they are given a fresh diet of good quality (Wahlstrom *et al.*, 1974), flavoring agents and aromas are frequently used based on the marketing appeal of a flavored diet to the person buying or handling such feed. Common flavors (in order of preference by humans based on non-scientific evidence) are coconut, milk/vanilla, and strawberry.

Colorants

Colorants (yellow and orange) may be used to mask changes in ingredient composition that significantly alter the color of the finished product. Flavors may be used to the same effect.

Insecticides

Insecticides are used only when certain raw materials or products may become susceptible to insect infestation due to prolonged storage under unfavorable conditions. Diatomaceous earth is a natural insecticide (Mewis and Ulrichs, 2001).

Antioxidants

Antioxidants are strongly recommended for diets containing high concentrations of lipids. Common examples include ethoxyquin, butylated hydroxytoluene, citric acid, and vitamin C. The last two antioxidants are usually too expensive to be used as antioxidants in most piglet diets.

Mold inhibitors

These products prevent growth of molds already present in raw materials and feed. The most common mold inhibitor is propionic acid in various commercial preparations (Mellor, 2001). Mold inhibitors do not bind mycotoxins.

Mycotoxin binders

These compounds inactivate mycotoxins produced by molds present in raw materials and finished feed. Common mycotoxin binders include bentonite, zeolite, yeast cell derivatives, activated charcoal, and aluminosilicate preparations (Hohler, 2000). Mycotoxin binders do not inhibit growth of molds.

Pellet binders

Pellet binders markedly improve pellet durability, but very hard pellets reduce feed intake in the early post-weaning period (see Chapter 8). The most common pellet binders include molasses, clays, starches, and various lignin and hemicellulose products.

Flow enhancers

These additives are used in meal-type products to improve flowability, especially with high inclusion rates of hydroscopic dairy ingredients. Common examples include sepiolite, zeolite, and flaked oats. Flow agents usually dilute the nutrient density of the finished product.

References

Anderson RA (1998) Recent advances in the clinical and biochemical manifestation of chromium deficiency in human and animal nutrition. *Journal of Trace Elements in Experimental Medicine* 11:241–250.

Baldi A, Bomtempo V, Dell'Orto V, Cheli F, Fantuz F, and Savoini G (1999) Effects of dietary chromium-yeast in weaning-stressed piglets. *Canadian Journal of Animal Science* 79:369–374.

Cadogan DJ, Partridge GG, and Simmins PH (2000) Effect of xylanase addition in feed containing either pre-characterised wheat or wheat by-products on the performance of growing pigs. *Proceedings of the Annual Meeting of the British Society of Animal Science*, 21. York, UK.

Colina JJ, Lewis AJ, Miller PS, and Fischer RL (2000) Effects of the addition of *Yucca shidigera* extract and an acidified diet on reducing ammonia emission in nursery pig facilities. *Journal of Animal Science* 78(Supplement 1):186.

Creech BL, Spears JW, Flowers WL, Hill GM, Lloyd KE, Armstrong TA, and Engle TE (2004) Effect of dietary trace mineral concentration and source (inorganic vs. chelated) on performance, mineral status and fecal mineral excretion in pigs from weaning through finishing. *Animal Production* 82:2140–2147.

Cromwell GL, Hays VW, and Clark TL (1978) Effects of copper sulfate, copper sulfide and sodium sulfide on performance and copper stores of pigs. *Journal of Animal Science* 46:692–698.

Cromwell GL (2002) Why and how antibiotics are used in swine production. *Animal Biotechnology* 13:7–27.

Gatnau R, Zimmerman DR, Diaz T, and Johns J (1991) Determination of optimum levels of spray dried porcine plasma (SDPP) in diets for weanling pigs. *Journal of Animal Science* 69(Supplement 1):369.

Gebert S, Straub R, Wanner M, and Wenk C (2003) Growth performance, energy and nitrogen balance of weanling pigs fed cereal based diets supplemented with Chinese rhubarb. *54th Annual Meeting of the European Association for Animal Production*, 167–170. Wageningen Academic Publishers, Wageningen, The Netherlands.

Gill C (1999) Herbs and plant extracts as growth enhancers. *Feed International*: 20–24.

Goransson L (2001) Alternatives to antibiotics-the influence of new feeding strategies for pigs on biology and performance. In: *Recent Developments in Pig Nutrition 3*, by Wiseman J and Garnsworthy PC (ed), 39–50. Nottingham University Press, Nottingham, UK.

Guzik AC, Southern LL, Matthews JO, Bidner TD, and Ladner JP (2000) Ornithine α-ketoglutarate and creatine effects on growth and plasma metabolites of nursery pigs. *Journal of Animal Science* 78:1022–1028.

He ML and Rambeck WA (2000) Rare earth elements – a new generation of growth promoters for pigs? *Archives of Animal Nutrition* 53:323–334.

Hernandez J, Borbolla A, Mendoza R, and Garcia G (2000) Glutamine stimulates the synthesis of immunoglobulin IgG in infected early weaned pigs. *Journal of Animal Science* 78(Supplement 1):175.

Hill GM, Mahan DC, Carter SD, Cromwell GL, Ewan RC, Harrold RL, Lewis AJ, Miller PS, Shurson GC, and Veum TL (2001) Effect of pharmacological concentrations of zinc oxide with or without the inclusion of an antibacterial agent on nursery pig performance. *Journal of Animal Science* 79:934–941.

Hoffman LA, Ivers DJ, Ellersieck MR, and Veum TL (1993) The effect of L-carnitine and soybean oil on performance and nitrogen and energy utilization by neonatal and young pigs. *Journal of Animal Science* 71:132–138.

Hohler D (2000) A brief survey on important mycotoxins and possible detoxification methods. *Feed Tech* 4(5/6):44–46.

Hollis GA, Mahan DC, Carter SD, Crenshaw TD, Cromwell GL, Hill GM, Lewis AJ, and Veum TL (2001) The efficacy of zinc methionine and zinc oxide in promoting nursery pig performance. *Journal of Animal Science* 79(Supplement 1):149.

Jongbloed AW, Kemme PA, Mroz Z, and Makinen M (1995) Apparent total tract digestibility of ash and minerals in pigs as affected by phytate, microbial phytase, and lactic acid. *Journal of Animal Science* 73(Supplement 1):188.

Kamel C (2000) A novel look at a classic approach of plant extracts. *Feed Mix* 8(3):16–18.

Katouli M, Melin L, Jensen-Waern M, Wallgren P, and Mollby R (1999) The effect of zinc oxide supplementation on the stability of the intestinal flora with special reference to composition of coliforms in weaned pigs. *Journal of Applied Microbiology* 87:564–573.

Koch F (2005) Organic acids in animal nutrition. *AminoNews* 6(1):11–18.

Lee YL, Cesario T, Owens J, Shanbrom E, and Thrupp LD (2002) Antibacterial activity of citrate and acetate. *Nutrition* 18:665–666.

Mahan DC, Carter SD, Cromwell GL, Hill GM, Harrold RL, Lewis AJ, and Veum TL (2000) Efficacy of added zinc oxide levels with or without an antibacterial agent in the postweaning diets of pigs. *Journal of Animal Science* 78(Supplement 1):41.

Maribo H (2000) Effect of calcium formate and sorbic acid in feed for weaners 7–30 kg. *Proceedings of the British Society of Animal Science Occasional Meeting 'The Weaner Pig – Nutrition and Management'*, 31. University of Nottingham, Nottingham, UK.

Mavromichalis I and Baker DH (1999a) A chromium supplement after weaning? *Pig International* 29(3):23–24.

Mavromichalis I and Baker DH (1999b) Vitamin C in nursery diets. *Pig International* 29(4):27–28.

Mavromichalis I and Baker DH (2000) Queries about carnitine. *Pig International* 30(2):35–36.

Mavromichalis I, Hancock JD, Senne BW, Gugle TL, Kennedy GA, Hines RH, and Wyatt CL (2000) Enzyme supplementation and particle size of wheat in diets for nursery and finishing pigs. *Journal of Animal Science* 78:3086–3095.

Mellor S (2001) Mycotoxins in feed: a global challenge. *Feed Mix* 9(3):26–28.

Mewis I and Ulrichs C (2001) Red flour beetle bites the dust in diatomaceous earth-insecticides. *Feed Tech* 5(5):35–37.

Mikkelsen LL, Jakobsen M, and Jensen BB (2003) Effects of dietary oligosaccharides on microbial diversity and fructo-oligosaccharide degrading bacteria in faeces of piglets post-weaning. *Animal Feed Science and Technology* 109:133–150.

Miller HM and Toplis P (2000) Supplement containing immunoglobulins fed post-weaning promotes nursery pig performance. *Proceedings of the Annual Meeting of the British Society of Animal Science*, 106. York, UK.

Mroz Z (2003) Organic acids of various origins and physico-chemical forms as potential alternatives to antibiotic growth promoters for pigs. *Proceedings of the 9th International Symposium on Digestive Physiology in Pigs (Volume 1)*, 267–293. University of Alberta, Canada.

Namkung H, Li M, Gong J, Yu H, Cottyill M, and de Lange CFM (2004) Impact of feeding blends of organic acids and herbal extracts on growth performance, gut microbiota and digestive function in newly weaned pigs. *Canadian Journal of Animal Science* 84:697–704.

NCR-42 and S-145 (2000) Growth promotion effects and plasma changes from feeding high dietary concentrations of zinc and copper to weanling pigs (regional study). *Journal of Animal Science* 78:1010–1016.

Owen KQ, Nelssen JL, Goodband RD, Tokach MD, Friesen KG, Richert BT, Smith JW, and Russell LE (1995) Effects of various fractions of spray-dried porcine plasma on performance of early weaned pigs. *Journal of Animal Science* 73(Supplement 1):81.

Owen KQ, Nelssen JL, Goodband RD, Weeden TL, and Blum SA (1996) Effect of L-carnitine and soybean oil on growth performance and body composition of early-weaned pigs. *Journal of Animal Science* 74:1612–1619.

Partridge GG (2001) The role and efficacy of carbohydrase enzymes in pig nutrition. In: *Enzymes in Farm Animal Nutrition*, by Bedford MR and Partridge GG (ed), 161–198. CABI Publishing, Wallingford, UK.

Patterson JA and Burkholder KM (2003) Prebiotic feed additives: rationale and use in pigs. *Proceedings of the 9th International Symposium on Digestive Physiology in Pigs (Volume 1)*, 319–331. University of Alberta, Canada.

Rincker MJ, Carter SD, Real DE, Nelssen JL, Tokach MD, Goodband RD, Dritz SS, Senne BW, Fent RW, Pettey LA, and Owen KQ (2003) Effects of increasing dietary L-carnitine on growth performance of weanling pigs. *Journal of Animal Science* 81:2259–2269.

Rizvi S, Harbour DA, Pearson GR, Patel D, Stokes CR, and Miller BG (2001) The use of hyper-immunized egg as a source of prophylactic antibodies in the neonatal piglet. *Proceedings of the Annual Meeting of the British Society of Animal Science*, 23. York, UK.

Roth FX and Kirchgessner M (1998) Organic acids as feed additives for young pigs: nutritional and gastrointestinal effects. *Journal of Animal and Feed Sciences* 7:25–33.

Schell TC and Kornegay ET (1996) Zinc concentration in tissues and performance of weanling pigs fed pharmacological level of zinc from ZnO, Zn-methionine, Zn-lysine, or $ZnSO_4$. *Journal of Animal Science* 74:1584–1593.

Soares M and Lopez-Bote CJ (2002) Effects of dietary lecithin and fat unsaturation on nutrient utilization in weaned piglets. *Animal Feed Science and Technology* 95:169–177.

Stahly TS, Cook DR, Swenson SG, Williams NH, and Zimmerman DR (1995) Growth responses of pigs to dietary plasma protein (PP) additions as influenced by pig antigen exposure and PP source. *Journal of Animal Science* 73(Supplement 1):81.

Traylor SL, Cromwell GL, Plunkett MS, Lindemann MD, and Knabe DA (2000) Effects of level of phytase on ileal digestibility of calcium, phosphorus, crude protein, and amino acids in dehulled soybean meal. *Journal of Animal Science* 78(Supplement 1):169.

van Dijk AJ, Everts H, Nabuurs MJA, Margry RJCF, and Beynen AC (2001) Growth performance of weanling pigs fed spray-dried animal plasma: a review. *Livestock Production Science* 68:263–274.

Wahlstrom RC, Hauser LA, and Libal GW (1974) Effects of low lactose whey, skim milk and sugar on diet palatability and performance of early weaned pigs. *Journal of Animal Science* 38:1267–1271.

Watford M (1999) Is there a requirement for glutamine catabolism in the small intestine? *British Journal of Nutrition* 81:261–262.

Wu G, Meier SA, and Knabe DA (1996) Dietary glutamine supplementation prevents jejunal atrophy in weaned pigs. *Journal of Nutrition* 126:2578–2584.

Zhao JM, Li DF, Piao XS, Yang WJ, and Wang FL (2002) Effects of vitamin C supplementation on performance, iron status and immune function of weaned piglets. *Archives of Animal Nutrition* 56:33–40.

Zijlstra RT, Overend D, Schalm M, Owusu-Asiedu A, Simmins PH, and Patience JF (2004) Effect of wheat quality and xylanase supplementation on performance of weaned pigs fed pelleted diets. *Journal of Animal Science* 82(Supplement 2):71.

Feed Manufacturing

8

Introduction

Feed manufacturing is the bridge between the science of animal nutrition and the practice of feeding. In the preparation of feed, selection of raw materials and processes determines the quality of the finished products. Quality may be defined in terms of feed safety, preservation or even enhancement of nutritive value, and changes in form and texture. This chapter deals with aspects of feed manufacturing that affect growth performance in young pigs. Technical aspects of feed manufacturing may be found in McEllhiney (1994).

The Maillard Reaction

The Maillard reaction, also known as non-enzymatic browning, is an integral part of feed and food manufacturing. It is a natural phenomenon that involves the binding of amino groups, such as those found in amino acids and several vitamins, to the carbonyl groups of reducing sugars such as glucose and lactose (Maillard, 1912, 1916). Although sugar losses are greater and more intense than losses of amino acids and certain vitamins (Adrian *et al.*, 1962), it is the deterioration of protein quality that is of most concern (Adrian, 1974). Under controlled conditions, the Maillard reaction enhances the flavor and palatability of certain foods (e.g. crusted bread, grilled meat, cooked cereals). Without proper control, however, the Maillard reaction damages the nutritive value of ingredients (e.g. burned milk products, overprocessed soybean meal). Feed manufacturers are concerned more about the negative effects of the Maillard reaction rather than its largely unexplored beneficial effects.

Browning is often confused with the intensity of the Maillard reaction (Fig. 8.1). However, coloration and nutrient destruction are two independent phenomena of the Maillard reaction that differ radically (Lea and Hannan, 1950). During the initial stages of the Maillard reaction, products remain colorless but, nevertheless, nutrients become unavailable although they are still detectable by chemical analysis (Lewis and Lea, 1950). It is the formation of late-Maillard reaction products, such as melanoides, that reduces the amount of chemically analyzed nutrients (Zhang and Parsons, 1994, 1996) and causes changes in color. Therefore, chemical analyses and color changes are not adequate indicators of protein quality damage, which begins rather early in the process.

The adverse effects of the Maillard reaction are experienced via reduced nutrient availability due to excess thermal processing and (or) prolonged storage of raw materials and finished products. The Maillard reaction takes place even at room temperature, but its intensity increases as time, temperature, moisture (maximum at 40 to 70%), and alkalinity (linear between pH 3 and 8) increase (Lea and Hannan, 1949). Under conditions of elevated temperature and humidity, any compound with a free amino group is vulnerable to the Maillard reaction, and this includes free amino acids (Johnson *et al.*, 1977; Robbins and Baker, 1980), ε-amino groups of protein-bound lysine, and free amino groups of thiamin, folacin, and gossypol (Baker, 1995). Lysine is the most susceptible amino acid in intact

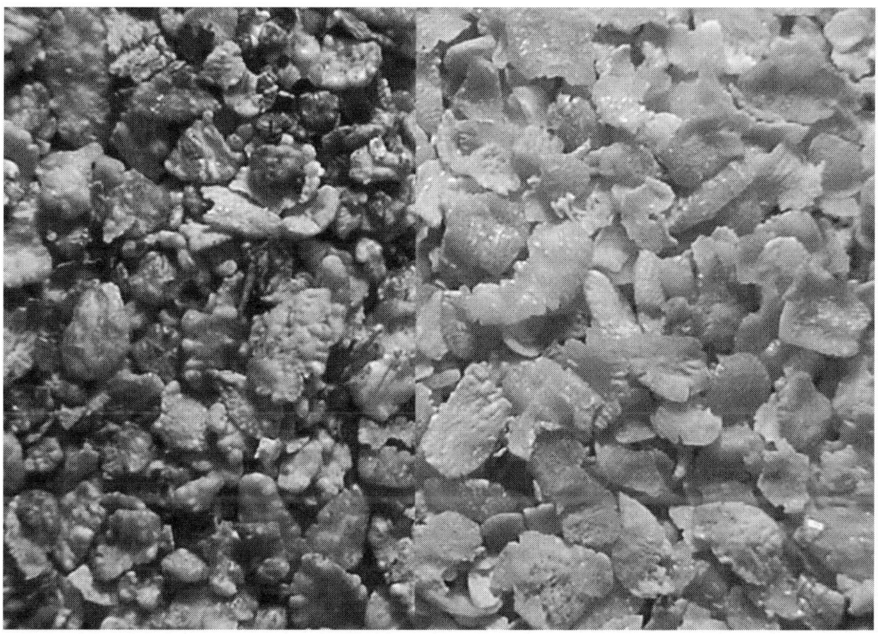

Fig. 8.1. Cooked maize showing different degrees of browning.

proteins because it has a free amino group at the ε-carbon unit that is readily available to react with reducing sugars. Free lysine is even more reactive because it has two free amino groups. Early Maillard reaction derivatives of lysine include *N*-(1-deoxy-D-fructosyl) lysine and *N*-(1-deoxy-D-lactulosyl) lysine (Finot and Mauron, 1972). These compounds are deaminated only by the intestinal microflora and thus are not available to mammals and birds (Bleyl *et al.*, 1980). Because destruction of lysine is often five to 15 times greater than that occurring with other amino acids (e.g. methionine, cystine, tryptophan, leucine), changes in its bioavailability indicate both the occurrence and the intensity of the Maillard reaction (Adrian, 1967).

The adverse effects of the Maillard reaction on lysine bioavailability have been extensively demonstrated in feed ingredients such as fishmeal (Kim and Easter, 2001), field peas (van Barneveld *et al.*, 1994), soybean meal (Hancock *et al.*, 1990; Fernandez and Parsons, 1996), fish protein isolate (Plakas *et al.*, 1988), milk products (Mahan and Newton, 1993; Moughan *et al.*, 1996), egg products (Sgarbieri *et al.*, 1973), canola meal (Anderson-Hafermann *et al.*, 1993), peanut meal (Zhang and Parsons, 1996), and sunflower meal (Zhang and Parsons, 1994). It has been repeatedly demonstrated that thermal overprocessing of high-protein feedstuffs reduces lysine bioavailability, depending on temperature levels and the duration of heat application. In some instances (Table 8.1), changes in nutrient availability are not represented accurately by digestibility assays (Batterham *et al.*, 1990; van Barneveld *et al.*, 1991). It appears that there is an inverse relationship between temperature and time such that, as temperature declines, more time is needed for the same loss of lysine bioavailability, and vice versa (Adrian, 1974).

Most diets for young pigs are rich in milk products, which contain relatively high amounts of lactose and lysine. Moreover, such diets usually contain a plethora of equally sensitive ingredients such as blood products, egg products, refined plant proteins, and fishmeal, which readily contribute to the Maillard reaction problem. Before pelleting, 2 to 6% moisture is usually added to the mash during conditioning at temperatures that can range from 50 to 90°C for several seconds to over 20 min (Fairfield, 1994). Extremely high temperatures also develop during the formation of pellets from friction between the die walls and the conditioned mash (Fairfield,

Table 8.1. Effect of overheating peas on lysine digestibility and availability[a]. (Adapted from van Barneveld *et al.*, 1991.)

Item (%)	Raw	110°C	135°C	150°C	165°C
Ileal digestibility	75	82	78	75	62
Availability[b]	72	65	64	58	42

[a] Trial lasted 29 days post-weaning.

[b] Estimated ratio of deposited lysine/ileal digestible lysine intake.

1994). Thus, pelleting and other aggressive feed processing methods, such as expansion, extrusion, double pelleting, and prolonged mash conditioning, all increase the risk of nutrient destruction via the Maillard reaction.

Prolonged storage of heat-sensitive material can also initiate a second cycle of Maillard reactions, because the initial Maillard products have autocatalytic properties that further intensify the effects of heat treatment and storage (Henry *et al.*, 1946; Bensabat *et al.*, 1958). For example (Table 8.2), exposure of a pig starter diet for 1 week in a hot nursery environment reduced lysine bioavailability by about 9% (Mavromichalis and Baker, 2000). Also, storage of a milk powder with 10% residual moisture for 10 weeks at 30°C destroyed 20% of bioavailable lysine (Erbersdobler, 1970). Nutrient losses from exposure of ingredients and finished diets to adverse environmental conditions may also occur during storage in silos and warehouses, especially during summer months.

Gelatinization and Retrogradation

Starch in its natural form exists in granules as a polymer of D-glucose units, which form essentially linear (amylose) or highly branched (amylopectin) chains. Amylose is amorphous and rather soluble in water, whereas amylopectin is partially crystalline and much less soluble in water. The ratio of amylopectin to amylose in most cereals is relatively constant at about 4:1 (Hoseney, 1994). Mutant lines for several cereals exist with almost 100% amylopectin (waxy cereals), whereas certain maize mutants have up to 70% amylase (Collins *et al.*, 1999). Under polarized light, starch granules show birefringence, which appears as a 'Maltese cross' over a round black background, due to the high degree of crystallinity in amylopectin. The starch granule as a whole is about 30% crystalline and absorbs about 30% water under room temperature.

When starch is heated with water (e.g. extrusion), the granule absorbs water and swells slightly. When temperature exceeds a certain value (around 60°C), amylose starts to solubilize and leak out of the granule, whereas the granule starts to lose its birefringence properties because amylopectin is distorted. When 98% of birefringence is lost, starch reaches complete gelatinization (Wiseman *et al.*, 2001). Continued heating with excess water

Table 8.2. Effect of storing feed inside a hot nursery facility on relative lysine bioavailability[a]. (Adapted from Mavromichalis and Baker, 2000.)

Diet form	Sample from freezer	Sample from barn	Difference (%)
Meal	97	88	–9
Pellets	100	92	–8

[a]Samples from a self-feeder after 1 week in a hot nursery facility.

causes more amylose, and even amylopectin, to leach, and increases the viscosity of the solubilized starch until the whole granule is completely soluble at 120°C. The degree of solubilization and gelatinization depends on the final temperature to which the starch is exposed and not on the time of holding at a specific temperature. When starch is heated with limited water (e.g. pelleting), swelling and distortion of starch granules is limited. The amount of available water affects the degree of completion of the gelatinization process at a given temperature, but it does not affect the temperature at which starch starts to gelatinize (McWilliams, 1997). Excessive heating causes amylopectin to leach. When starch is heated without water (e.g. roasting), starch quickly reacts with water naturally present in ingredients. Hydrolysis of starch produces dextrins, which are shorter chains of glucose readily digestible by digestive enzymes (isomaltases).

Starch from different cereals starts to gelatinize at different temperatures (Table 8.3), with granule size having a partial effect; small granules generally require less heating to solubilize. Starch from wheat, barley, rye, and triticale loses 50% of birefringence at about 53°C, whereas starch from maize and sorghum loses 50% of birefringence at about 67°C. Oat starch requires the lowest temperature (55°C) among common cereals to reach 50% gelatinization, and rice starch the highest (70°C), although both rice and oats have rather small starch granules (Hoseney, 1994). To achieve complete loss of birefringence, starch must be heated to the upper temperature of the gelatinization range, which is rather impractical under most commercial conditions as it may decrease protein quality.

Loss of crystallinity and other changes in starch characteristics above the point of gelatinization are not reversible. As gelatinized starch begins cooling, solubilized starch chains become less energetic and start to interact with each other, forming hydrogen bonds by expelling water (McWilliams, 1997). As gelatinized starch ages, chains (and especially amylose) continue to interact to form stronger bonds that eventually lead to the formation of crystals (retrogradation). Retrograded starch is less soluble in water and, thus, less digestible (resistant starch) even than raw starch (Wiseman *et al.*, 2001). Amylopectin is more resistant to retrogradation but forms stronger bonds than

Table 8.3. Average starting gelatinization temperature and starch granule size. (Adapted from Hoseney, 1994.)

Cereal	Temperature (°C)	Size (μm)
Barley	55	22
Oats	56	6
Wheat	60	27
Maize	67	15
Sorghum	73	25
Rice	73	5

amylose. Thus, retrogradation is more prominent in high-amylose starches, during prolonged storage, and in starches heated beyond gelatinization. In contrast, in thermally processed waxy cereals retrogradation is extremely low (Berry, 1986). The distribution of resistant versus digestible starch for several cereals is given in Table 8.4 (Patil *et al.*, 1998).

Gelatinization is usually determined with an enzymatic hydrolysis test measuring release of glucose using α-amylase *in vitro*. Because of the nature of this test, fine grinding that disrupts starch granules and increases solubility appears to increase 'gelatinization'. Indeed, finely ground raw cereals are more digestible than coarsely ground raw cereals (Wondra *et al.*, 1995a). Thus, more sophisticated methods are used to accurately assess the effects of thermal processing on starch quality. For example, X-ray diffraction measures crystallinity by distinguishing between ordered and disordered states (Wiseman *et al.*, 2001).

Lipid Oxidation

Oxidation of lipids, also called oxidative rancidity, is a natural reaction between unsaturated fatty acids and free oxygen. Such fatty acids exist in all fats and oils, but certain vegetable oils such as soybean and maize oil are especially rich in them. For example, the ratio between saturated and unsaturated fatty acids in coconut oil is over 11, whereas in maize oil it is only 0.15, indicating the richness of maize oil in unsaturated, and thus vulnerable to oxidation, fatty acids (Table 8.5). Lipid oxidation is enhanced by exposure to air (open bags), light, high temperatures, and certain inorganic minerals such as iron and copper. The reaction is autocatalytic; once started, oxidized fatty acids continue to form and peroxides, the end product of oxidation, accumulate.

Antioxidants are frequently added to most diets for young pigs that tend to contain rather elevated levels of lipids. Antioxidants can only delay the process by stabilizing reactive fatty acids; given enough time, fatty acids will eventually react with available oxygen.

Table 8.4. Starch fractions in selected cooked cereals. (Adapted from Patil *et al.*, 1998.)

Cereal	Total (% in dry matter)	Rapidly digested (% of total)	Slowly digested (% of total)	Resistant (% of total)
Maize	78	47	21	32
Sorghum	79	37	18	46
Barley	55	45	22	33
Wheat	50	60	14	26
Brewer's rice	88	45	22	33

Table 8.5. Saturated to unsaturated fatty acids (S/U) ratio in selected lipid sources. (Adapted from McWilliams, 1997.)

Lipids	Saturated (%)	Unsaturated (%)	S/U ratio
Tallow	49.8	45.8	1.09
Lard	39.2	56.3	0.70
Soybean oil	14.4	81.2	0.18
Maize oil	12.7	82.9	0.15
Coconut oil	86.5	7.6	11.38

Oxidized fatty acids, which contain free radicals, react not only with other fatty acids but also with amino acids, rendering them unavailable to the animal (Nielsen *et al.*, 1985). Methionine and tryptophan are particularly susceptible to oxidation by free radicals. Methionine and tryptophan are second-limiting amino acids in starter diets and they are often added in the form of crystalline amino acids to supplement natural ingredients. In a controlled study (Horvatic and Vedrina-Dragojevic, 2000), lipid oxidation caused by flaking reduced the bioavailability of methionine and tryptophan in wheat, rye, barley and oats by as much as 26%.

Other side-effects of rancidity include the creation of objectionable flavors such as 'fishy' or 'beany' flavor in oils rich in linoleic and linolenic fatty acids (e.g. soybean, rapeseed and fish oils). This process, called reversion, can take place even under anaerobic conditions and currently there is no way to prevent it (McWilliams, 1997).

It is evident that, with most starter diets being enhanced with fats and oils to increase energy intake in pigs and facilitate the pelleting process, lipid oxidation can easily become problematic. Increased rancidity in choice white grease (lard), added at 6% of the diet, linearly depressed growth rates and feed intake in weaned pigs that were fed complex starter diets (DeRouchey *et al.*, 1999). From the same study (Fig. 8.2), it was demonstrated that dietary concentrations of peroxides should not exceed 240 mEq to prevent depression of growth performance.

Vitamin Stability

Vitamins are organic compounds sensitive to a myriad of physical and chemical reactions that affect their potency (Adams, 1972). For example, vitamin A has five double bonds highly susceptible to oxidation, whereas vitamin E is a natural antioxidant that is rapidly oxidized without protection. During feed manufacturing and storage, oxidative conditions often arise that may reduce vitamin stability (Scott, 1972). Unless vitamin destruction is prevented or compensated, animal performance may be reduced depending on the severity and duration of the imposed vitamin deficiency.

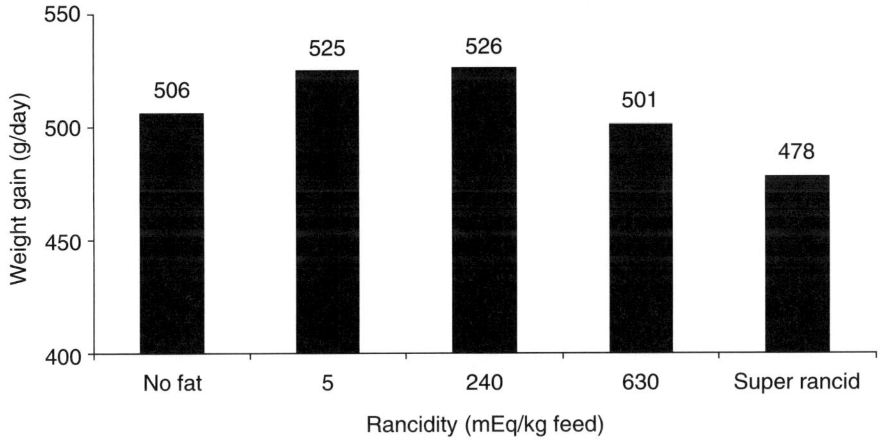

Fig. 8.2. Effects of fat rancidity on piglet performance post-weaning. (From DeRouchey *et al.*, 1999.)

The chemical form of vitamins affects their stability and resistance to oxidation (BASF, 2000). For example, pure vitamin A (retinol) is more susceptible than its ester (retinyl acetate), which in turn is more susceptible to oxidation than gelatin-coated vitamin A (insoluble in water). Likewise, esterified vitamin E (tocopheryl acetate) is more stable than pure vitamin E (tocopherol). In general, the greater the water solubility of a vitamin, the greater its risk for oxidation. Thus, thiamin mononitrate (10% solubility) is more stable than thiamin monochloride (100% solubility).

Physical form also affects stability (BASF, 2000). There are vitamins that are stable in crystalline form (thiamin, pyridoxine), but most vitamins benefit from some form of protection. For example, spray-dried beadlets of vitamins A and D, fat-coated vitamin C and vitamin E, and choline chloride adsorbed in silica carrier, all possess far greater stability than their unprotected forms. Yet, some forms of vitamin protection may not be practical for feed manufacturing. Such examples include ethylcellulose coating and vitamin–starch spray-dried emulsions that decrease flowability due to increased adhesiveness.

Vitamins are exposed to oxidative conditions during thermal processing of feed. Thus, processes such as pelleting, extrusion, and expansion may have a detrimental impact on vitamin retention in the finished feed (van der Poel and Gadient, 1997). During thermal processing vitamins are exposed to high levels of temperature, humidity, pressure, and friction that dramatically increase the rate of oxidation. For example, pure vitamin C (ascorbic acid) retention after pelleting at about 68°C was only 65% and it was further reduced to only 25% when pelleting temperature reached 108°C. In contrast, ascorbyl phosphate (a more stable form of vitamin C) retention was almost 90% even at 108°C. Extrusion at 93 versus 143°C decreased retention of thiamin hydrochloride from 90 to 50%, but when thiamin mononitrate was used, retention was 94 and 77%, respectively (BASF, 2000). It is evident, therefore, that more stable vitamin forms must be used under aggressive thermal processing conditions.

Prolonged storage is another issue that affects vitamin stability. In containers with straight vitamins, stability is extremely high, especially when container design prevents exposure to oxygen and moisture. To this end, vitamin stability is rapidly lost in open containers. Most vitamins are expected to exhibit less than 0.1% monthly potency reduction in unopened containers for at least 12 months, whereas monthly losses in open containers approach 0.5% for most vitamins, with notable exceptions (BASF, 2000). For example, monthly reduction of menadione sodium bisulfate potency was 2 and 0% in open and unopened containers over a period of 6 months. Natural vitamin E (retinol) losses are also high (5 and 8% monthly in unopened and open containers), but become negligible in retinol acetate (less than 0.1%).

In vitamin premixes and complete diets, vitamin stability is markedly affected by contact with certain trace minerals and choline chloride that cause friction and accelerate oxidation. Copper, zinc, and iron are very reactive, whereas selenium, iodine, and manganese are almost inert. Free metal ions are most reactive, followed by sulfate, carbonate, and oxide salts, with chelated minerals being virtually inert. Thus, blends of vitamins and trace minerals are expected to exhibit reduced vitamin retention, especially during prolonged storage and (or) elevated temperature/humidity conditions (BASF, 2000). For example, riboflavin in a straight vitamin premix retained 93% of its potency after 6 months of storage. But, when the premix also included trace minerals, retention dropped to 71%. Choline chloride also reduced riboflavin retention from 99% to 95% after 6 months. Not all vitamins, however, are affected by trace minerals and choline chloride. For example, retention of folic acid after 6 months was 80% regardless of blending with trace minerals, and retention of retinol acetate remained constant with or without chlorine chloride. In diets and premixes for young pigs that contain pharmacological concentrations of zinc oxide and copper sulfate, vitamin retention becomes problematic, and thus these salts should be kept separately from vitamins.

A number of other factors affect vitamin stability. These include moisture concentration, light, acidity, abrasion, fat rancidity, carrier, enzymes, and medications. Each vitamin has unique properties; for a comprehensive review, refer to Combs (1998).

Prevention and (or) compensation are the main options to offset the negative effects of reduced vitamin stability during feed manufacturing. Vitamin stability is enhanced when:

1. Vitamin storage is minimum and under appropriate conditions;
2. Vitamins are not premixed with reactive ingredients; and

3. Vitamins bypass thermal processing (added as liquid after processing) or are processed under less aggressive conditions.

However, based on the relatively low requirement for formulation space (most vitamin premixes are included at less than 1% of the final formula) and relatively low cost (1–2% of total diet cost), overformulation is the most common method of compensating against potential vitamin losses. Margins of safety may range from 20 to 100% for the more expensive or toxic vitamins (e.g. vitamins A, D, and E), but may easily exceed 1000% for certain B vitamins. Guides to calculate vitamin fortification levels based on expected losses are furnished by most major vitamin suppliers. For example (BASF, 2000), it is calculated that retention of calcium pantothenate, furnished via a trace mineral premix previously stored for 2 months (87% retention), in a finished feed that was pelleted at 88°C (89% retention) and consumed 1 month after production (97% retention) was 75% ($0.89 \times 0.87 \times 0.97$). Thus, to compensate for potential losses, the dietary specification for calcium pantothenate must be increased by at least 34% (100/0.75–100).

Destruction of Anti-nutritional Factors

The major anti-nutritional factors in cereals commonly used in diets for young pigs (maize, wheat, oats, barley, and sorghum) include β-glucans, arabinoxylans, and tannins. Although selection of low-tannin varieties remains the only option for sorghum (Hancock and Behnke, 2001), proper enzyme supplementation may enhance the nutritional value of cereals with a high concentration of non-starch polysaccharides (Partridge, 2001), although results depend on cereal quality (Cadogan *et al.*, 2000) and particle size (Mavromichalis *et al.*, 2000).

Major anti-nutritional factors in protein-rich ingredients commonly used in diets for weaned pigs (soybeans, peas, lupines, rapeseed, sunflower seeds) include trypsin inhibitors, lectins, alkaloids, glucosinolates, and polyphenolic compounds (de Lange *et al.*, 2000). Fortunately, most of these anti-nutritional factors are heat-sensitive (Fig. 8.3) and, thus, thermal processing greatly diminishes their negative impact on animal performance (Zarkadas and Wiseman, 2000).

Ingredients derived from animals are usually rich in minerals (e.g. fishmeal, blood, meat-and-bone meal). Although excess minerals do not exhibit an anti-nutritional effect *per se*, they nevertheless are considered undesirable as they tend to dilute nutrient density of a diet and may also cause diarrheas. An excess microbial load in plasma protein was recently found to impair performance in weaned pigs (DeRouchey *et al.*, 2001), whereas irradiation of plasma protein yielded variable results (Cook *et al.*, 2002; see also Table 9.9).

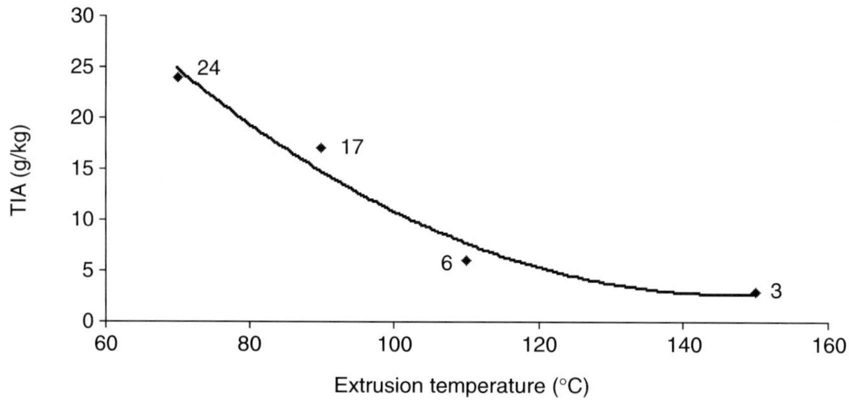

Fig. 8.3. Trypsin inhibitor activity (TIA) is reduced with increasing extrusion temperature. (From Zarkadas and Wiseman, 2000.)

Grinding and Particle Size

Grinding to reduce the particle size of raw materials is accomplished by roller or hammer mills. Roller mills use a combination of compaction and shearing forces to produce particles of uniform size, but irregular shape. Hammer mills use impact force to shatter material into particles of variable yet spherical size. Because of differences in physical characteristics, rolled ingredients are easier to handle as they flow better than ingredients ground with hammer mills. Roller mills are more expensive to install and maintain, but less demanding in energy inputs compared to hammer mills. Because roller mills require less energy to achieve the same particle size as hammer mills, they do not overheat processed ingredients, thus reducing moisture loss (i.e. shrink). It has been reported (Rexroth, 1985) that temperature increases of 2–6°C are common during hammer milling of maize. But, hammer mills provide more flexibility in the type of materials they can process, and they are also capable of reducing particle size further than most roller mills. In general, it is accepted that in most feed applications, which require a particle size reduction between 600 and 800 μm, roller mills reduce milling cost in terms of throughput per unit of energy (Hancock and Behnke, 2001), but this advantage is rapidly lost as particle size falls below 500 μm (Owens and Heimann, 1994).

It is often argued that the type of milling may also affect animal performance because of potential differences in nutrient digestibility. It is suggested (Reece *et al.*, 1985) that the spherical shape of hammer-milled ingredients inhibits enzyme penetration, and, thus, reduces nutrient digestibility. Studies with growing pigs (Wondra *et al.*, 1995a) revealed that the digestibility of organic matter, protein, and energy was increased by about 5% when maize was ground by a roller mill compared to maize ground by a hammer mill. Differences in nutrient digestibility caused by mill type diminished as particle size was reduced from 800 to 400 μm, and this effect was not associated with variation in particle size or growth performance.

Degree of fineness in ground material appears to have a more dramatic effect on nutrient digestibility and animal performance. It is well documented that a finer particle size improves performance in young pigs. Studies with oats (Lawrence, 1983) and barley (Goodband and Hines, 1988) indicated that finely ground cereals improved feed efficiency and rate of gain in weaned pigs. Similar improvements in performance were observed with maize (Fig. 8.4; Kim *et al.*, 1995), wheat (Fig. 8.5; Mavromichalis *et al.*, 2000), and sorghum (Healy *et al.*, 1994). It is speculated that as particle size

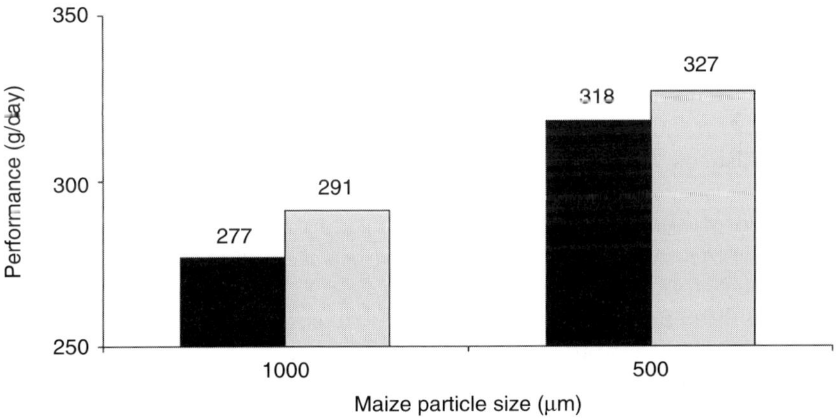

Fig. 8.4. Reducing particle size in maize improves piglet performance (■, weight gain; ▒, feed intake) post-weaning. (From Kim *et al.*, 1995.)

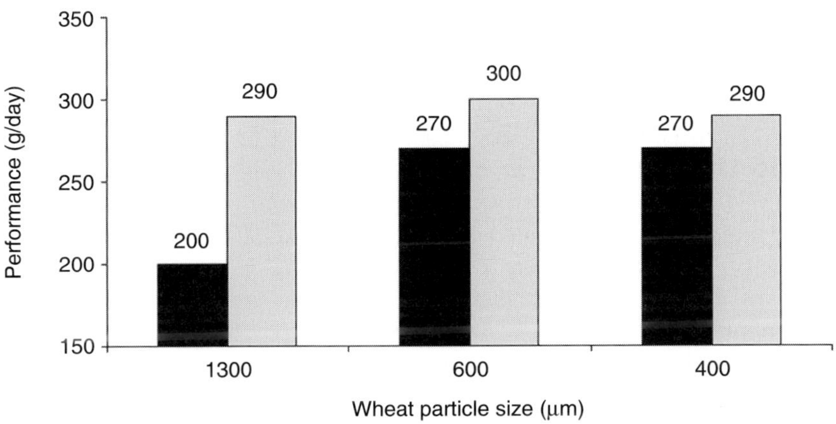

Fig. 8.5. Reducing particle size in wheat improves piglet performance (■, weight gain; ▒, feed intake) post-weaning. (From Mavromichalis *et al.*, 2000.)

decreases the surface available for enzymatic digestion increases, whereas increases in fluidity of digesta further enhance mixing of digesta and exposure to enzymes. Indeed, reducing particle size of maize from 800 to 400 μm increased the digestibility of dry matter (+3%), protein (+10%), and energy (+4%) in growing pigs (Wondra *et al.*, 1995a). From a comprehensive review of literature, Hancock and Behnke (2001) suggested 1.3% improvement in feed efficiency for each 100-μm reduction in particle size.

Reducing particle size not only increases energy consumption at the mill but it also reduces production throughput. Wondra *et al.* (1995b) demonstrated that as particle size of maize was reduced from 1000 to 400 μm, energy consumption increased and output drastically decreased. Reduction from 1000 to 600 μm resulted in a 40% increase in milling energy use and a 4% reduction in rate of production. At 400 μm, milling energy was increased by 200%, whereas output was reduced by 52%, again compared with grinding at 1000 μm. Thus, it is widely accepted today that a particle size of about 600 μm is an optimal compromise between animal and milling performance. Fine particle size may also reduce the flow characteristics of the feed, especially if dairy products, which are rather hygroscopic, make up a large fraction of the diet. Thus, for meal-type diets a particle size of about 700 μm is often considered optimal. Conversely, in pelleted diets finely ground ingredients (i.e. less than 600 μm) are desirable because they produce more durable pellets.

Recent attention to the particle size of soybean meal has yielded conflicting results. Particle size of soybean meal is rather coarse, with most samples around 900 μm. In one study (Fastinger and Mahan, 2001), reducing particle size from 900 to 600 μm improved digestibility of amino acids, but not that of energy, without further improvements as particle size was reduced to 150 μm. But, in a growth assay (Lawrence *et al.*, 2002), weaned pigs fed typical complex diets with coarse (900 μm) or fine (600 μm) soybean meal did not respond to differences in particle size. Clearly, more research is needed regarding optimal particle size in soybean meal and other plant protein sources.

Mixing Uniformity

Mixing uniformity, as estimated by the coefficient of variation of a specific nutrient or ingredient (usually chlorine from salt), is used to measure the degree of dispersion of ingredients throughout a batch of feed. It is often recommended that less than 10% CV indicates appropriate mixing, but recent data suggest that up to 20% CV may be adequate for most practical diets (Hancock and Behnke, 2001). In general, mixing uniformity increases with mixing time. Appropriate mixing time depends on mixer type and ingredient selection. Vertical mixers require considerably more time than horizontal mixers to achieve similar results (Fahrenholz, 1994). It is suggested that mixing times be at least 15 min for a vertical mixer, 7 min for a horizontal paddle mixer, and 4 min for a horizontal ribbon mixer (Hancock and Behnke, 2001). Also, a batch of feed composed of ingredients with uniform particles requires less time to mix than a batch of ingredients with greater variation in particle size. Best results are achieved when the mixer is loaded first with a portion of the major ingredients, then with minor ingredients and additives, and finally with the remaining portion of major ingredients. Liquids should be always added only after thoroughly mixing all dry ingredients.

The effects of feed undermixing on weaned pig performance were investigated (Traylor *et al.*, 1994) with a complex starter diet mixed for 0, 0.5, 2, and 4 min in a horizontal ribbon mixer (Table 8.6). As expected, pigs offered unmixed diets (ingredients were loaded in the mixer and then, without mixing, they were discharged into bags) had decreased growth performance compared to pigs offered mixed diets. Yet, performance was not greatly improved when diets were mixed for more than 0.5 min, although best performance was achieved with 4 min mixing time. In this study, the coefficient of variation decreased from 107 to 12% as mixing time increased from 0 to 4 min, respectively. Because no effects of undermixing were detected in finishing pigs (Traylor *et al.*, 1994; Wondra *et al.*, 1995b), it is suggested that mixing uniformity is of greater importance in young pigs, which take rather smaller meals especially during the first few weeks post-weaning (Holden, 1988).

Pelleting

Pelleting of complete diets involves steam-conditioning of the mixed mash, followed by compaction through die openings. The benefits of pelleting on feed quality are:

1. Reduced volume for transportation;
2. Reduced dust generation;
3. Less feed separation; and
4. Better flow characteristics compared to meal diets.

Table 8.6. Effect of feed mixing time on nursery pig performance[a]. (Adapted from Traylor *et al.*, 1994.)

Item	0 min	0.5 min	2 min	4 min	SEM[b]
Weight gain (g/day)	267	379	383	402	18
Feed intake (g/day)	598	711	701	720	22
Feed/gain	2.24	1.88	1.83	1.79	0.17

[a] A total of 120 pigs with an average initial weight of 5.5 kg.
[b] SEM, standard error of the mean. Statistical linear response in all parameters measured ($P < 0.01$).

In terms of animal performance, pellets offer the benefits of:

1. Reduced feed wastage;
2. Increased nutrient intake because of reduced volume; and
3. Improved nutrient digestibility due to thermal processing of starch and protein.

A combination of these factors usually improves growth rate and feed efficiency by about 5–15% in nursery pigs (Hancock and Behnke, 2001). Because the beneficial effects of pelleting are likely to decrease during the later phases of the nursery period, pelleting cost must be weighed against benefits in performance and, perhaps, reduced nutrient excretion. As a rule of thumb, for pelleting to be cost-effective, the percentage increase in feed cost due to pelleting must be less than the percentage improvement in feed efficiency.

During steam-conditioning, feed is exposed to relatively high levels of humidity and increased temperature. Usually, 2 to 6% moisture is added to the mash during conditioning at temperatures that range from 60 to 90°C for several seconds to more than 20 min (Fairfield, 1994). In general, for each degree change in moisture of the mash due to condensation of steam, temperature increases about 20°C. Extremely high temperatures also develop during pellet formation due to friction with the die walls as the conditioned mash is forced through die openings (Fairfield, 1994). Therefore, there is an increased risk of formation of Maillard reaction products during the entire process of pelleting. In piglet feeds, which are relatively rich in dairy products (lactose is a reducing sugar) and protein sources including free amino acids, the risk of reduced protein digestibility is genuine, but has received little attention from the scientific community. It is not surprising, therefore, that most diets for young pigs are heavily overformulated with amino acids.

Pelleting increases starch gelatinization from around 10–12% in the raw material, to approximately 25% during conditioning, to above 40% after pellet formation (Ziggers, 2003). Increased starch gelatinization improves pellet durability but it also increases pellet hardness.

Pellet quality has traditionally been associated with durability, a desirable trait in pelleted diets for young pigs. A pellet durability index over 90% (i.e. less than 10% fines in the diet) is used today as a target for nursery pelleted diets. A durable pellet is less likely to break during handling and transportation, and as a result, fewer fines are produced. An increased concentration of fine particles in feed not only increases the probability of feeder bridging, but also increases feed wastage (Table 8.7), especially in young pigs (Stark *et al.*, 1994). The most common way of increasing pellet durability is by increasing pellet hardness. Hard pellets are produced by a combination of ingredient selection, mash conditioning, and application of pellet binders. Field observations, however, suggest that weaned pigs exhibit an aversion to hard pellets by reducing feed consumption. When weaned

Table 8.7. Effect of fines in pelleted nursery diets on pig performance. (Adapted from Stark *et al.*, 1994.)

Item	Minimum fines	30% fines added	Difference (%)
Weight gain (g/day)	469[a]	454[b]	–3
Feed intake (g/day)	772	771	0
Feed/gain	1.65[a]	1.70[b]	+3

The trial was conducted from 7 to 21 days post-weaning.
[a,b]Means within a row with unlike superscript letters are different ($P < 0.05$).

pigs were offered hard versus soft pellets (Mavromichalis *et al.*, 2002), feed intake (–13%) and weight gain (–11%) were markedly reduced during the first 2 weeks post-weaning. Because soft pellets contained over 30% fines (Fig. 8.6), it is suggested that pellet durability index is not an adequate criterion of pellet quality for young pigs. Light pigs are the ones most likely to allow a mouthful of feed to soften with saliva before chewing and swallowing it. Mouth lesions found in small pigs are frequently attributed by nursery barn managers to hard pellets.

Another aspect of pellet quality is pellet size and more precisely pellet diameter (Fig. 8.7). There is a well-established notion that small pigs require small pellets to thrive. Yet, research indicates that piglets as young as 14–21 days old can easily cope with any pellet size ranging from 1 to 12 mm (Traylor *et al.*, 1996; Johnson *et al.*, 1999; Edge *et al.*, 2001), although wastage may be increased with pellets larger than 3–4 mm (Table 8.8). What remains unclear is whether pellet hardness interacts with pellet size. It is also most likely that as pellet size is reduced damage to amino acid bioavailability is increased due to increased die friction, but this has yet to be proven.

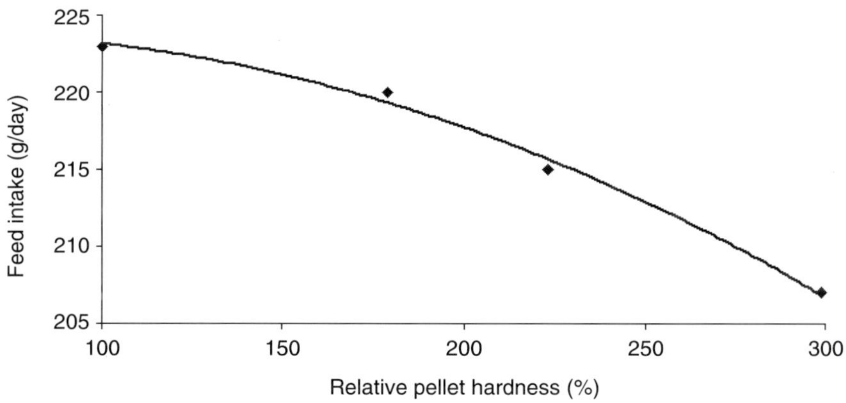

Fig. 8.6. Pellet hardness greatly reduces feed intake in young pigs. (From Mavromichalis *et al.*, 2002.)

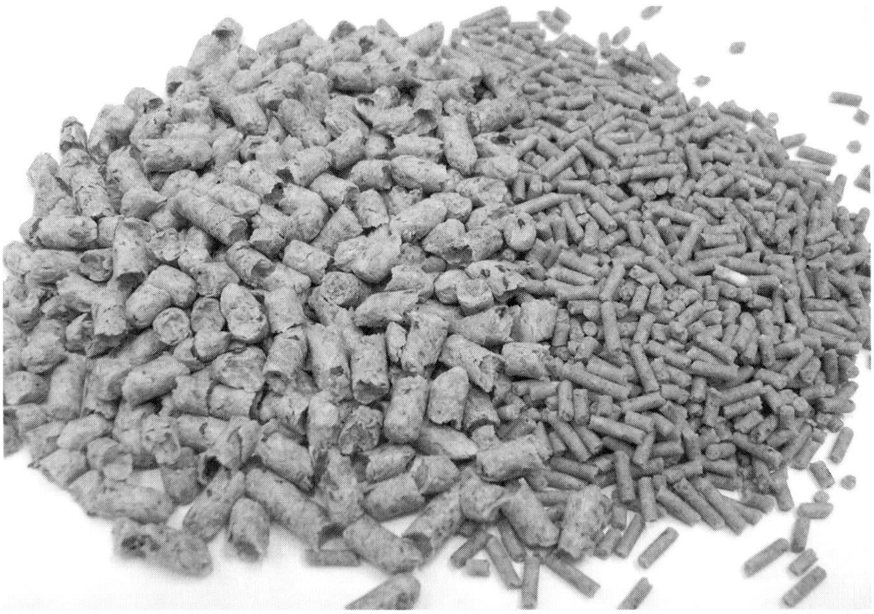

Fig. 8.7. Pellet size does not appear to affect feed intake in piglets.

Table 8.8. Effect of pellet diameter on nursery pig performance[a]. (Adapted from Traylor *et al.*, 1996.)

Item	Meal	2 mm	4 mm	6 mm	12 mm
Weight gain (g/day)	358	362	371	362	364
Feed intake (g/day)	537	510	516	541	532
Feed/gain	1.50	1.41	1.39	1.49	1.46

[a]Trial lasted 29 days post-weaning. There were no statistically significant differences between treatments.

Currently, commercial nursery diets are available in pellet sizes ranging from 2 to 4 mm for post-weaning diets, although mini-pellets (less than 2 mm) and larger pellets (4–5 mm) are also marketed.

Obviously, piglets do not pay attention to pellet color, but most producers do mind variability in pellet appearance. A darker pellet can be the result of either overprocessing or ingredient selection. Increased temperatures during pelleting may cause formation of Maillard products (browning reaction), which tend to darken the final product. Also, ingredients such as cooked cereals, fishmeal, and molasses, which are naturally darker than most unprocessed ingredients, tend to darken pellets. Black specks on pellets indicate either the inclusion of blood products or scorched ingredients, but they are not indicative of pelleting conditions. Pellets light in color are indicative of high levels of inclusion of raw ingredients such as maize, wheat, and minimally processed ingredients such as soybean meal and other protein sources. What must be of utmost concern to end users of pellets is excessive and frequent variation in pellet color and overall appearance, as this may be indicative of frequent changes in formulation and (or) inappropriate pelleting conditions.

Crumbles

Crumbles are produced by passing cool pellets between two rolls (Fig. 8.8). Earlier studies on the effects of crumbling on performance in young pigs are contradictory (Wu and Fuller, 1974; Pollmann *et al.*, 1983). Results are probably confounded by initial pellet hardness and amount of fines generated during crumbling. It is safe to assume that crumbles are preferable over hard pellets, especially for post-weaned pigs, but their benefits may be rapidly lost as fines increase due to excessive crumbling. Because there is additional cost in manufacturing crumbles, their potential benefits should be weighed against cost.

Crumbles may be beneficial as the first diet post-weaning or as a creep diet when they are offered on floor-mats. Piglets usually benefit from meal diets on mats because they are tacky and stick to their snouts, forcing piglets

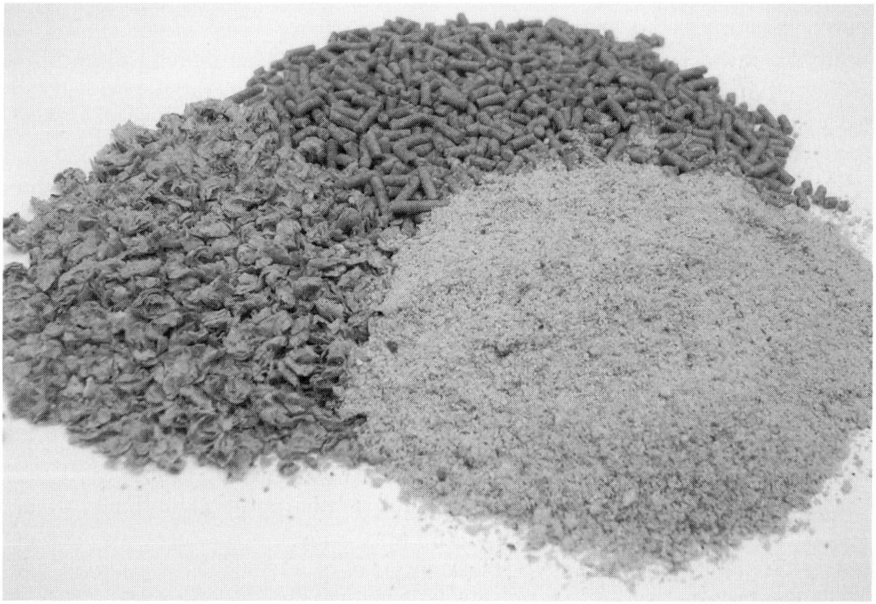

Fig. 8.8. Meal, pellets, and crumbles.

to lick and ingest them. Crumbles should offer the benefits of a meal and at the same time condition pigs to receiving pellets. Crumbling may also offer benefits when a portion of the diet (usually the specialty ingredients) is crumbled and then mixed with finely ground cereals and protein sources to be offered as a meal. Dairy products and other powdered ingredients usually reduce flowability of complete diets in meal form, and thus a mix of crumbles and finely ground ingredients flows easier and prevents feeder bridging.

Extrusion

Extrusion of ingredients and complete diets is a thermal processing method that involves progressively increasing pressure, friction, and attrition as the extruded material passes through the extruder barrel. Temperatures up to 160°C, at pressures of 15–40 atm, for as little as 30 s are typical for most commercial applications. An abrupt drop in pressure when the material exits the barrel dramatically increases product volume, as steam escapes instantly. Moisture reduction may reach up to 50% depending on the initial moisture content of the extruded material (Hancock and Behnke, 2001).

Extrusion offers numerous benefits in diet preparation for young pigs. Starch gelatinization, protein denaturation, destruction of certain anti-nutritional factors, microbial decontamination, and dehydration are the main benefits from extrusion technology. However, overprocessing may actually reduce the nutritive value of extruded products because of protein destruction (i.e. formation of Maillard products), starch retrogradation (i.e. starch resistant to digestion), and vitamin destruction (Ohh *et al.*, 2002). For example, poorly extruded full-fat soybeans, with urease activity three times higher than that of typical soybean meal, severely depressed growth performance in weaned pigs (5.2 kg) compared to soybean meal during the first week post-weaning (Piao *et al.*, 2000). Additionally, mildly extruded wheat (68% starch gelatinization) supported better growth performance than excessively extruded wheat (77% starch gelatinization) in 21-day-old pigs during the first three weeks post-weaning, although both were superior to untreated wheat (Jansen, 1992). In another study (Hongtrakul *et al.*, 1998), growth performance of weaned pigs (6.8 kg) actually decreased and then increased as starch gelatinization in extruded maize increased from 39 to 89%, perhaps because of excessive starch retrogradation in the intermediate levels of gelatinization (from added water during extrusion). Earlier studies also indicated that overprocessed maize (retrograded) may actually increase the incidence of diarrhea in young pigs (Aumaitre, 1976).

Proper extrusion of cereals improves starch digestibility (Fadel *et al.*, 1988; Carter and Liebholz, 1991), and marginally improves protein utilization (Noland *et al.*, 1976; Herkelman *et al.*, 1990). Thus, cereals with more naturally resistant starch and higher protein concentration, such as barley and wheat, benefit more from extrusion processing than cereals with more readily digested starch and lower levels of protein, such as maize and rice. Additionally, extrusion appears to increase solubility, and thus digestibility, of non-starch polysaccharides (Fadel *et al.*, 1988), which prevail in cereals such as rye, triticale, barley, and wheat and promote bacterial proliferation in the gastrointestinal tract (Pluske *et al.*, 2001). In terms of growth performance, cereal extrusion may enhance growth rate, depending on cereal source and processing conditions, but the most consistent effect is improved feed efficiency, due to enhanced energy and nutrient digestibility. For example, extrusion improved feed efficiency by 3% in weaned pigs (6.4 kg) fed diets based on maize or sorghum, but had no effect on growth rate or protein utilization (Chae *et al.*, 2000). Similar results were observed with extruded maize and wheat (Cho *et al.*, 2001). Extruded barley also improved weight gain and feed efficiency by about 14% in weaned pigs (6 kg) compared to raw barley (Medel *et al.*, 1999, 2000), but extruded maize actually reduced performance (perhaps due to overprocessing, 75% starch gelatinization). In conclusion, cereal extrusion improves starch digestibility and enhances feed efficiency, but excessive thermal processing may actually reverse any beneficial effects of extrusion.

In protein-rich ingredients, such as soybeans, peas, lupines, and rapeseed, the main effects of extrusion processing are mainly the destruction of anti-nutritional factors and any improvements in carbohydrate utilization are secondary (de Lange *et al.*, 2000; Zarkadas and Wiseman, 2000).

Expanding

Expanders are basically high-pressure conditioners with an annular gap that allows feed to expand instantly as it enters atmospheric pressure (Fairfield, 1994). Temperatures at the conditioning chamber may reach up to 120°C. Main benefits from expanding include: (i) improved pellet durability; (ii) ability to add up to 20% liquids; (iii) increased starch gelatinization; and (iv) reduction or elimination of undesirable microorganisms (Fairfield, 1994; Ziggers, 2003). The comparatively high cost of this equipment usually restricts its use only with high-fiber materials and when high levels of feed sanitation are required. It is generally recommended that only major ingredients be expanded to avoid destruction of vitamins and crystalline amino acids (O'Doherty *et al.*, 2002). However, when complete nursery diets are expanded (rarely) it is advisable for temperatures not to exceed 60°C or even lower when high levels of milk products are used (Ziggers, 2003).

Feed Storage and Preservation

The best measure against deterioration of feed quality is prompt incorporation of high-quality raw materials in diets that are rapidly consumed after manufacturing, all under strict conditions of hygiene and safety. But, when prolonged storage of finished products is expected, then feed preservatives are often used to guard quality. Moreover, feed sanitization by exposure to high temperatures or irradiation is frequently used to reduce microbial load and prolong the shelf-life of ingredients and finished products.

Storage

Proper storage of raw materials and finished products affects nutritive value in many ways. First, prolonged storage even under ideal conditions involves slow but continuous proliferation of bacteria, insects, and molds that naturally exist in most raw materials. At the very best, these pests consume nutrients, but they may also produce toxins (e.g. mycotoxins) that severely impair animal performance. Then, under hot and humid conditions not only the growth of pests accelerates, but also Maillard reaction products are rapidly formed, further reducing nutritive value. Additionally, objectionable flavors may develop mainly but not exclusively due to unavoidable lipid rancidity. Finally, several vitamins and enzymes that are sensitive to heat and oxygen rapidly lose potency, especially when mixed with oxidative trace minerals and exposed to high temperatures during storage.

Most raw materials have a shelf-life that ranges from several months to a year. Uncontaminated raw cereals and protein-rich ingredients may be stored even longer under appropriate conditions with minimal loss of nutritive value. But, complete diets and premixes usually have a shelf-life of about 3 months or less, depending on composition and storage conditions. Especially during the warm months of the year, it is advised to use complete diets and premixes within 2 months of production, if possible.

It is common practice in some operations to store bags of starter diets, frequently opened, inside the nursery barn, and often next to nursery pens. This practice exposes a diet rich in reducing sugars and amino acids to high levels of humidity and heat, commonly encountered in commercial nursery facilities. This has a severe impact on feed quality. For example, when a complex starter diet was stored in a typical nursery room for 7 days (28°C and 90% relative humidity), lysine bioavailability decreased by 10% (Mavromichalis and Baker, 2000), indicating the vulnerability of such diets. Comparable results should be expected when diets are stored in warm, humid warehouses for prolonged periods of time. The old advice of storing valuable products under dry and cool conditions remains valid.

Preservation

Elimination of salmonella in animal feed is a pressing issue, especially in production systems that do not use growth-promoting levels of antimicrobial agents, to safeguard animal health and food safety. To this end, steam-heating of finished feed has been applied with success. For example, it has been reported (Ziggers, 2002) that salmonella elimination was achieved by steam-heating meal diets to 85°C for 4 min in a heated mixer. Pelleting at 85°C also achieves reduction or even elimination of salmonella in finished products. However, a balance between feed sanitation and nutritive value should be achieved as overheating may reduce nutritive value. Thus, heat-sensitive materials that are naturally free of salmonella (vitamins, enzymes, etc.) may be added after heat treatment, and as always the extra cost of treatment should be weighed against benefits. Organic acids are also used effectively against salmonella proliferation in feeds (Best, 2001).

To prevent lipid oxidation in finished products, antioxidants are usually added. This is common practice in warm and humid climates, during the summer, and for products destined for export (long interval between production and consumption). Most common antioxidants include butylated hydroxyanisol, butylated hydroxytoluene, and ethoxyquin. Vitamins E and C are also examples of organic antioxidants often used in starter diets (McWilliams, 1997).

To prevent mold growth and production of mycotoxins, propionic acid is also frequently added in finished products. Because liquid propionic acid is highly corrosive, powdered propionic acid on carriers or buffered propionic acid products are preferred from a manufacturing standpoint. Usually, 0.1% propionic acid is enough to safeguard against mold growth under most conditions, but up to 0.5% may be essential in very humid climates. Because propionic acid is an organic acid, it may also act as an antimicrobial agent at the intestinal level, but such effects are usually observed at rather high concentrations. Of course, other organic acids (e.g. sorbic or benzoic) are often used instead of or in conjunction with propionic acid. The addition of clays and other mycotoxin binders does not check mold growth, but rather reduces the impact of toxins ingested by animals.

References

Adams CR (1972) Effect of environmental conditions on the stability of vitamins in feeds. In: *Effect of Processing on the Nutritional Value of Feeds*. National Research Council, National Academy of Sciences, Washington, DC.

Adrian J, Petit L, and Godon B (1962) Sur de nouvelles incidences nutritionelles de la reaction de Maillard. *Comptes Rendus de l'Academie des Sciences* 255:391–393.

Adrian J (1967) La reaction de Maillard. 4. Etude du compertement de quelques acides amines au cours du grillage d'aliments protidiques. *Annales de la Nutrition* 21:129–147.

Adrian J (1974) Nutritional and physiological consequences of the Maillard reaction. *World Review of Nutrition and Dietetics* 19:71–122.

Anderson-Hafermann JC, Zhang Y, and Parsons CM (1993) Effects of processing on the nutritional quality of canola meal. *Poultry Science* 72:326–333.

Aumaitre A (1976) Evaluation de divers traitements technologiques des cereales. *Annales de Zootechnie* 25:41–51.

Baker DH (1995) Vitamin bioavailability. In: *Bioavailability of Nutrients for Animals*, by Ammerman CB, Baker DH, and Lewis AJ (ed), 399–431. Academic Press, San Diego, CA.

BASF (2000) *Vitamins – One of the Most Important Discoveries of the Century* (6th edn). BASF-Animal Nutrition, Mount Olive, NJ.

Batterham ES, Andersen LM, Baigent RD, Darnell RE, and Taverner MR (1990) A comparison of the availability of ileal digestibility of lysine in cottonseed and soybean meals for grower/finisher pigs. *British Journal of Nutrition* 64:663–677.

Bensabat L, Frampton VL, Allen LE, and Hill RA (1958) Effect of processing on ε amino groups of lysine in peanut protein. *Journal of Agricultural and Food Chemistry* 6:778.

Berry CS (1986) Resistant starch: formation and measurement of starch that survives exhaustive digestion with amylolytic enzymes during the determination of dietary fiber. *Journal of Cereal Science* 4:301–314.

Best P (2001) Feeding against piglet diarrhoea. *Pig International* 31(6):19–21.

Bleyl DW, Schulze J, and Grutte FK (1980) Toxicological effects of steam-sterilized high lactose diets on conventional and gnotobiotic rats. *Archives of Toxicology Supplement* 4:431–434.

Cadogan DJ, Partridge GG, and Simmins PH (2000) Effect of xylanase addition in feed containing either pre-characterised wheat or wheat by-products on the performance of growing pigs. *Proceedings of the Annual Meeting of the British Society of Animal Science*, 21. York, UK.

Carter RR and Leibholz J (1991) Effects of extrusion of wheat on dry matter and starch digestibility in the young pig. In: *Manipulating Pig Production III*, by Batterham ES (ed), 86. Australasian Pig Science Association, Werribee, Australia.

Chae BJ, Kim YG, Han IK, Kim JH, Cho WT, Hancock JD, and Kim IH (2000) Effects of particle size and extrusion of maize and sorghum on ileal digestibility and growth performance in pigs weaned at 14 and 21 days of age. *Journal of Animal and Feed Sciences* 9:665–679.

Cho WT, Kim Y, Kim JD, Chae BJ, and Han IK (2001) Effects of feeding extruded corn and wheat grain on growth performance and digestibility of amino acids in early-weaned pigs. *Asian-Australian Journal of Animal Science* 14:224–230.

Collins NE, Moran ET Jr, and Stilborn HL (1999) Waxy corn improves pelleted feed quality, broiler performance, and meat yield. *Poultry Science* 78(Supplement 1):11.

Combs GF Jr (1992) *The Vitamins. Fundamental Aspects in Nutrition and Health* (2nd edn). Academic Press, San Diego, CA.

Cook DR, Ward MM, and Paton ND (2002) Effects of plasma grade, irradiation or formaldehyde treatment of plasma, or whole diet irradiation on growth performance of weaned pigs. *Journal of Animal Science* 80(Supplement 2):66.

de Lange CFM, Nyachoti CM, and Verstegen MWA (2000) The significance of antinutritional factors in feedstuffs for monogastric animals. In: *Feed Evaluation. Principles and Practice*, by Moughan PJ, Verstegen MWA, and Visser-Reyneveld MI (ed), 169–188. Wageningen Pers, Wageningen, The Netherlands.

DeRouchey JM, Hancock JD, Maloney CA, Park JS, Lee DJ, Cao H, Dean DW, and Hines RH (1999) Effects of rancidity in choice white grease on growth performance in nursery pigs. *Journal of Animal Science* 77(Supplement 1):195.

DeRouchey JM, Tokach MD, Nelssen JL, Goodband RD, Dritz SS, Woodworth JC, and Hastad CW (2001) Comparison of irradiated feed and food grade spray-dried animal plasma on nursery pig performance. *Report No. 880*:10–16. Agricultural Experiment Station and Cooperative Extension Service, Kansas State University, Manhattan, KS.

Edge HL, Dalby JA, Rowlinson P, and Varley MA (2001) The effect of pellet size on the voluntary food intake and performance of young pigs. *Proceedings of the British Society of Animal Science Annual Meeting*, 167. York, UK.

Erbersdobler H (1970) Zur schadigung des lysins bei der herstellung und lagerung von trokenmilch. *Milchwissenschaft* 25:280–284.

Fadel JG, Newman CW, Newman RK, and Graham H (1988) Effects of extrusion cooking of barley on ileal and fecal digestibilities of dietary components in pigs. *Canadian Journal of Animal Science* 68:891–897.

Fahrenholz C (1994) Proportioning and mixing cost center. In: *Feed Manufacturing Technology IV*, by McEllhiney RR (ed), 98–108. American Feed Industry Association, Arlington, VA.

Fairfield D (1994) Pelleting cost center. In: *Feed Manufacturing Technology IV*, by McEllhiney RR (ed), 111–130. American Feed Industry Association, Arlington, VA.

Fastinger ND and Mahan DC (2001) Effects of soybean meal particle size on amino acid and energy ileal digestibilities in grower-finisher swine. *Journal of Animal Science* 79(Supplement 2):83.

Fernandez SR and Parsons CM (1996) Bioavailability of digestible lysine in heat-damaged soybean meal for chick growth. *Poultry Science* 75:224–231.

Finot PA and Mauron J (1972) Blockage of lysine by the Maillard reaction. II. Chemical properties of the *N*-(1-deoxy-D-fructosyl) lysine and *N*-(1-deoxy-D-lactulosyl) derivatives of lysine. *Helvetica Chimique Acta* 55:1153–1164.

Goodband RD and Hines RH (1988) An evaluation of barley in starter diets for swine. *Journal of Animal Science* 66:3086–3093.

Hancock JD, Peo ER Jr, Lewis AJ, and Crenshaw JD (1990) Effects of ethanol extraction and duration of heat treatment of soybean flakes on the utilization of soybean protein by growing rats and pigs. *Journal of Animal Science* 68:3233–3243.

Hancock JD and Behnke KC (2001) Use of ingredient and diet processing technologies to produce quality feeds for pigs. In: *Swine Nutrition* (2nd edn), by Lewis AJ and Southern LL (ed), 469–497. CRC Press LLC, Boca Raton, FL.

Healy BJ, Hancock JD, Kennedy GA, Bramel-Cox PJ, Behnke KC, and Hines RH (1994) Optimum particle size of corn and hard and soft sorghum for nursery pigs. *Journal of Animal Science* 72:2227–2236.

Henry KM, Kon SK, Lea CH, Smith JAB, and White JCD (1946) Deterioration on storage of dried skim milk. *Nature (London)* 158:348–349.

Herkelman KL, Rodhouse SL, Veum TL, and Ellersieck MR (1990) Effect of extrusion on the ileal and fecal digestibilities of lysine in yellow corn in diets for young pigs. *Journal of Animal Science* 68:2414–2424.

Holden PJ (1988) Diagnosing feed mixing problems in swine herds. *Agri-Practice* 9(4):3.

Hongtrakul K, Goodband RD, Behnke KC, Nelssen JL, Tokach MD, Bergstrom JR, Nessmith WB Jr, and Kim IH (1998) The effects of extrusion processing of carbohydrate sources on weanling pig performance. *Journal of Animal Science* 76:3034–3042.

Horvatic M and Vedrina-Dragojevic I (2000) Changes in available methionine and tryptophan contents during cereal flake production. *Journal of the Science of Food and Agriculture* 80:502–506.

Hoseney RC (1994) *Principles of Cereal Science and Technology* (2nd edn). American Association of Cereal Chemists, Inc., St Paul, MN.

Jansen HD (1992) Flaking and extrusion of wheat. Nutrient changes estimated *in vitro* and in pigs. *Muhle-Mischfuttertechnic* 129:706–707.

Johnson GH, Baker DH, and Perkins EG (1977) Nutritional implications of the Maillard reaction: the availability of fructose–phenylalanine to the chick. *Journal of Nutrition* 107:1659–1664.

Johnson TE, Stephas EL, and Miller BL (1999) Evaluation of the effect of feeding a micro-pellet to an early weaned pig. *Journal of Animal Science* 77(Supplement 1):64.

Kim IH, Hancock JD, Cabrera MR, Hines RH, Rantanen MM, and Behnke KC (1995) Particle size (1,000 vs 500 microns) affects nutritional value of simple and complex diets for weanling pigs and broiler chicks. *Report No. 746*:89. Kansas State University, Manhattan, KS.

Kim SW and Easter RA (2001) Nutritional value of fish meals in diets for young pigs. *Journal of Animal Science* 79:1829–1839.

Lawrence KR, Hastad CW, Goodband RD, Tokach MD, Nelssen JL, Dritz SS, and Webster MJ (2002) Effects of soybean meal particle size on growth performance of nursery pigs. *Journal of Animal Science* 80(Supplement 2):60.

Lawrence TLJ (1983) The effects of cereal particle size and pelleting on the nutritive value of oat-based diets for the growing pig. *Animal Feed Science and Technology* 8:91–98.

Lea CH and Hannan RS (1949) The effect of activity of water, of pH and of temperature on the primary reaction between casein and glucose. *Biochimica et Biophysica Acta* 3:313–325.

Lea CH and Hannan RS (1950) Biochemical and nutritional significance of the reaction between proteins and reducing sugars. *Nature (London)* 165:438–439.

Lewis VM and Lea CH (1950) A note on the relative rates of reaction of several reducing sugars and sugar derivatives with casein. *Biochimica et Biophysica Acta* 4:532–534.

Mahan DC and Newton EA (1993) Evaluation of feed grains with dried skim milk and added carbohydrate sources on weanling pig performance. *Journal of Animal Science* 71:3376–3382.

Maillard LC (1912) Reaction generale des acides amines sur les sucres. Ses consequences biologiques. *Comptes Rendus des Seances de la Societe de Biologie et de ses Filiales* 72:599–601.

Maillard LC (1916) Synthese des matieres humiques par action des acides amines sur les sucres reducteurs. *Annales de la Chimique* 6:258–317.

Mavromichalis I and Baker DH (2000) Effects of pelleting and storage of a complex nursery pig diet on lysine bioavailability. *Journal of Animal Science* 78:341–347.

Mavromichalis I, Hancock JD, Senne BW, Gugle TL, Kennedy GA, Hines RH, and Wyatt CL (2000) Enzyme supplementation and particle size of wheat in diets for nursery and finishing pigs. *Journal of Animal Science* 78:3086–3095.

Mavromichalis I, Cook DR, Ward MM, and Paton ND (2002) Effect of pellet hardness on growth performance of weaned pigs. *Journal of Animal Science* 80(Supplement 2):60.

McEllhiney RR (1994) *Feed Manufacturing Technology IV*. American Feed Industry Association, Arlington, VA.

McWilliams M (1997) *Foods – Experimental Perspectives* (3rd edn). Prentice-Hall, Inc., Upper Saddle River, NJ.

Medel P, Salado S, de Blas JC, and Mateos GG (1999) Processed cereals in diets for early-weaned piglets. *Animal Feed Science and Technology* 82:145–156.

Medel P, Garcia MC, Lazaro R, de Blas JC, and Mateos GG (2000) Particle size and heat treatment of barley in diets for early-weaned piglets. *Animal Feed Science and Technology* 84:13–21.

Moughan PJ, Gall MPJ, and Rutherford SM (1996) Absorption of lysine and deoxyketosyl lysine in an early-Maillard browned casein by the growing pig. *Journal of Agricultural and Food Chemistry* 44:1520–1525.

Nielsen HE, Weck D, Finot PA, Liardon R, and Hurrell RF (1985) Stability of tryptophan during food processing and storage. 1. Comparative losses of tryptophan, lysine and methionine in model systems. *British Journal of Nutrition* 53:281–292.

Noland PR, Campbell DR, Gage RK Jr, Sharp RN, and Johnson ZB (1976) Evaluation of processed soybeans and grains in diets for young pigs. *Journal of Animal Science* 43:763–769.

O'Doherty JV, Glynn SG, and Murphy D (2002) The influence of fibre level and fat supplementation in expander-processed diets on grower-finisher pig performance. *Journal of the Science of Food and Agriculture* 82:1036–1043.

Ohh SH, Han KN, Chae BJ, Han IK, and Acda SP (2002) Effects of feed processing methods on growth performance and ileal digestibility of amino acids in young pigs. *Asian–Australasian Journal of Animal Sciences* 15:1765–1772.

Owens JM and Heimann M (1994) Material processing cost center. In: *Feed Manufacturing Technology IV*, by McEllhiney RR (ed), 81–90. American Feed Industry Association, Arlington, VA.

Partridge GG (2001) The role and efficacy of carbohydrase enzymes in pig nutrition. In: *Enzymes in Farm Animal Nutrition*, by Bedford MR and Partridge GG (ed), 161–198. CABI Publishing, Wallingford, UK.

Patil AR, Murray SM, Hussein HS, and Faheyg C Jr (1998) Quantification of starch fractions in selected starchy feed ingredients. *Journal of Animal Science* 76(Supplement 1):168.

Piao XS, Kim JH, Jin J, Kim JD, Cho WT, Shin IS, and Han IK (2000) Effects of extruded full fat soybean in early-weaned piglets. *Asian–Australasian Journal of Animal Sciences* 13:645–652.

Plakas SM, Lee TC, and Wolke RE (1988) Bioavailability of lysine in Maillard browned protein as determined by plasma lysine response in rainbow trout (*Salmo gairdneri*). *Journal of Nutrition* 118:19–22.

Pluske JR, McDonald DE, Pethick DW, Mullan BP, and Hampson DJ (2001) Nutritional management of the gastrointestinal tact to reduce enteric diseases in pigs. *Recent Advances in Animal Nutrition in Australia* 13:127–134.

Pollmann DS, Behnke KC, and Allee GL (1983) The effect of diet complexity and physical form on the performance of starter pigs and feed processing efficiency. *Animal Feed Science and Technology* 8:99–106.

Reece FN, Lott BD, and Deaton JW (1985) The effects of feed form, grinding method, energy level, and gender on broiler performance in a moderate (21°C) environment. *Poultry Science* 64:1834–1839.

Rexroth DW (1985) Material processing cost center. In: *Feed Manufacturing Technology III*, by McEllhiney RR (ed), 137—150. American Feed Industry Association, Arlington, VA.
Robbins KR and Baker DH (1980) Evaluation of the resistance of lysine sulfite to Maillard destruction. *Agricultural and Food Chemistry* 28:25–28.
Scott ML (1972) Effect of processing on the availability and nutritional value of vitamins. In: *Effect of Processing on the Nutritional Value of Feeds*, by National Research Council (ed), 119–130. National Academy of Sciences, Washington, DC.
Sgarbieri VC, Amaya J, Tanaka M, and Chichester CO (1973) Response of rats to amino acid supplementation of brown egg albumin. *Journal of Nutrition* 103:1731–1738.
Stark CR, Behnke KC, Hancock JD, Traylor SL, and Hines RH (1994) Effect of diet form and fines in pelleted diets on growth performance of nursery pigs. *Journal of Animal Science* 72(Supplement 1):214.
Traylor SL, Hancock JD, Behnke KC, Stark CR, and Hines RH (1994) Uniformity of mixed diets affects growth performance in nursery and finishing pigs. *Journal of Animal Science* 72(Supplement 2):59.
Traylor SL, Behnke KC, Hancock JD, Sorrell P, and Hines RH (1996) Effects of pellet size on growth performance in nursery and finishing pigs. *Journal of Animal Science* 74(Supplement 1):67.
van Barneveld RJ, Batterham ES, and Norton BW (1991) Utilization of ileal digestible lysine from heat-treated filed peas by growing pigs. In: *Manipulating Pig Production III*, by Batterham ES (ed), 184. Australasian Pig Science Association, Werribee, Australia.
van Barneveld RJ, Batterham ES, and Norton BW (1994) The effect of heat on amino acids for growing pigs. 1. A comparison of ileal and feacal digestibilities of amino acids in raw and heat-treated field peas (*Pisum sativum* cultivar Dundale). *British Journal of Nutrition* 72:221–241.
van der Poel AFB and Gadient M (1997) Effects of expander processing on the recovery of feed additives. In: *Expander Processing of Animal Feeds*, by van der Poel AFB (ed), 49–56. Wageningen Feed Processing Centre, Wageningen, The Netherlands.
Wiseman J, Pickard J, and Zarkadas L (2001) Starch digestion in piglets. In: *The Weaner Pig – Nutrition and Management*, by Varley MA and Wiseman J (ed), 65–80. CAB International, Wallingford, UK.
Wondra KJ, Hancock JD, Behnke KC, Hines RH, and Stark CR (1995a) Effects of particle size and pelleting on growth performance, nutrient digestibility, and stomach morphology in finishing pigs. *Journal of Animal Science* 73:757–763.
Wondra KJ, Hancock JD, Behnke KC, and Stark CR (1995b) Effects of mill type and particle size uniformity on growth performance, nutrient digestibility, and stomach morphology in finishing pigs. *Journal of Animal Science* 73:2564–2573.
Wu JF and Fuller MF (1974) A note on the performance of young pigs given maize-based diets in different physical forms. *Animal Production* 18:317–320.
Zarkadas LN and Wiseman J (2000) Inclusion of differently processed full-fat soya bean in diets for piglets. *Proceedings of the British Society of Animal Science Occasional Meeting 'The Weaner Pig – Nutrition and Management'*, 45–46. University of Nottingham, Nottingham, UK.

Zhang Y and Parsons CM (1994) Effects of overprocessing on the nutritional quality of sunflower meal. *Poultry Science* 73:436–442.

Zhang Y and Parsons CM (1996) Effects of overprocessing on the nutritional quality of peanut meal. *Poultry Science* 75:514–518.

Ziggers D (2002) Hygienising meals batch by batch with Thermidor. *FeedTech* 6(9/10):22–23.

Ziggers D (2003) Expanding and structurizing feed benefits pig performance. *Feed Tech* 7(6):8–11.

Feeding Programs

9

Introduction

This chapter reviews the basic nutritional philosophies in feeding young pigs and presents examples of common feeding programs according to major production systems around the world. More often than not, generic programs based for convenience on a central nutritional philosophy are adjusted to account for specific requirements or restrictions on nutrients and (or) ingredients. For example, such programs could target minimizing post-weaning digestive upsets or replacing traditional ingredients with less expensive alternatives. Others could aim at reducing nutrient excretion in the environment or meeting specific welfare requirements.

It should be emphasized that all feeding programs presented throughout this book should be considered only as examples. Recommendations are for illustration purposes only and should not be applied to specific farm situations without consulting a qualified nutritionist and (or) a veterinarian. Conditions not accounted for in these examples may require a totally different approach.

European Approach

Contemporary applied piglet nutrition follows two major schools of thought, namely the European and North American approaches (Mavromichalis and Varley, 2003). The European nutritional philosophy calls for complex ingredients in nutrient-dense diets to promote rapid weight gain and improve feed efficiency, especially during the post-weaning period. The main goal of this approach is to maximize profit per pig because most producers in Europe are rather limited in the number of pigs they can raise in a specific geographic area. The North American nutritional philosophy calls for less complex diets with slightly reduced nutrient density, with more emphasis on minimizing the cost of production per unit of body weight gain. Here, the goal is to maximize profit per group of pigs or per pig space on an annual basis, because the turnaround time of facilities dictates profitability. Systems that utilize features from both schools of thought are becoming increasingly popular. Such a 'hybrid' program would utilize, for example, European-type diets immediately after weaning to ease the transition to solid diets, followed by North American-type diets for the rest of the nursery period to minimize feed cost. Regardless of which nutritional philosophy is followed, available ingredients, regulations, and, most importantly, production methods and goals (zootechnical or financial) eventually shape the design of a specific feeding program.

Weaning age

In Europe, most pigs are weaned between 21 and 28 days of age (6–8 kg body weight), although weaning at a later age is not uncommon (Evans, 2001). For example, where antimicrobial growth promoters are not used (e.g. the EU) or in less intensive production systems (e.g. Eastern Europe) most pigs are weaned between 28 and 35 days of age. Current EU legislation (2006) regulates minimum weaning age at 28 days. To avoid underage pigs within a farrowing batch (usually with a 7-day spread of age), some producers tend to wean a few days later than their stated target.

To preserve sow condition with later weaning and to promote piglet growth, most suckling pigs receive a high-quality creep diet (Partridge, 1989). Quite often, they continue to receive the same or a very similar diet after weaning for about 1 week or even longer. Because 'all-in all-out' production systems are not widespread in Europe (yet), due to the relatively small size of most units, continuous-flow nurseries are the norm. Hence, feed budgets are usually based on time rather than on amount of feed per pig, to facilitate feeding pigs of disparate ages within the same barn. A typical feed budget is presented in Fig. 9.1, for illustration purposes. Variations should be expected even within the same farm.

Major ingredients

In Europe, most commercial piglet diets are based on wheat and (or) barley (Partridge, 1989; Hardy, 1992). These cereals are often thermally processed (i.e. cooked), because research has demonstrated that cooked cereals are more digestible and can enhance feed intake and growth, at least in the early nursery period (Campbell, 1989). Cooked (usually steam-flaked) decorticated

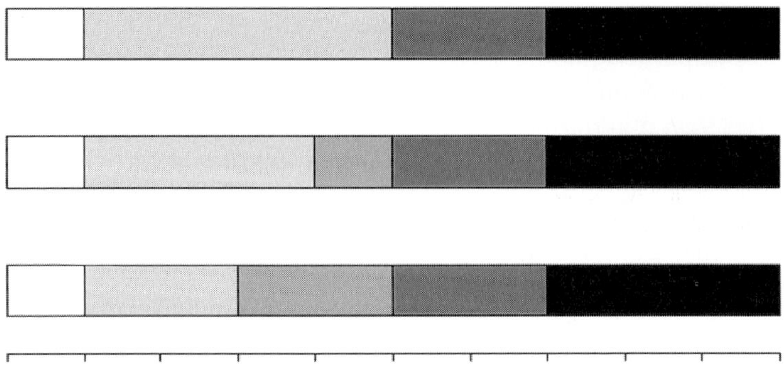

Fig. 9.1. Example of a typical feeding program (□, milk only; ▒, milk+creep; ▒, nursery 1; ▒, nursery 2; ■, nursery 3) for late-weaned pigs (Europe).

oats and sugarbeet pulp are often used in piglet diets to provide a source of fermentable fiber that promotes a healthy gut microflora. Triticale is sporadically available, but unless of high quality (i.e. with low arabinoxylans content) it is not preferred for piglet diets. Rye and whole oats are seldom used if at all, especially in the first diets post-weaning. Maize, either imported or grown on European plains, is considered a choice ingredient for piglet diets, but it is usually too expensive in other regions. Sorghum (low in tannins) is also imported in limited quantities. Finally, imported tapioca is used mainly in The Netherlands. Cereals make up about 30–70% of piglet diets depending on target weight (see Table 9.1).

Dairy ingredients traditionally abound in Northwest Europe, but prices fluctuate widely and can be rather prohibiting in other parts of the continent. Therefore, the concentration of milk products varies widely by region. Skim milk (often denaturated) is the preferred source of lactose and milk protein, but whey and its derivatives are usually available at more competitive prices. Products termed 'milk replacers' are also available in the European market as replacements of straight dairy ingredients. These products are usually blends of dairy ingredients and other highly digestible sources of sugars and proteins, usually of plant origin. Dairy products make up 10–30% of most piglet diets, again depending on target weight.

Before 2005, feed legislation in the EU banned animal-derived products (except for milk) from pig diets. This included products such as meat meal, meat-and-bone meal, animal blood, and animal plasma. Although fishmeal is legally permitted in pig diets, most European feed manufacturers refrain from using fishmeal to avoid cross-contamination in their plants. Animal protein sources used to make up 10–15% of most piglet diets (Fowler, 1997), as an excellent source of highly digestible amino acids. Today, they have been

Table 9.1. Example diets from Europe[a].

	Body weight range (kg)[c]				
Ingredients (%)[b]	4–6	6–8	8–12	12–20	20–30
Cereals (wheat, barley, maize, oat groats, wheat milling by-products, tapioca)	20–30	30–40	40–50	50–60	60–70
Oils (soybean oil, sunflower oil, coconut oil)	0–10	0–8	0–6	0–4	0–2
Sugarbeet products (molasses, sugarbeet pulp)	0–10	0–10	0–10	0–10	0–10
Dairy ingredients (skim milk, whey, lactose, casein)	20–40	10–20	5–15	0–5	0
Animal proteins (fishmeal, meat meal, blood products)	5–15	5–10	0–10	0–5	0
Plant proteins (refined plant proteins, e.g. soy, potato, wheat; soybean meal and extruded soybeans; rapeseeds, peas, sunflower meal)	10–30	15–30	20–30	20–30	20–30
Nutrients[d]					
Net energy (MJ/kg)	12.00	11.50	11.00	10.50	10.00
Crude protein (%)[e]	23.00	22.00	21.00	20.00	19.00
Total lysine (%)	1.65	1.55	1.45	1.35	1.25
True ileal digestible lysine (%)	1.50	1.40	1.30	1.20	1.10
Calcium (%)	1.00	0.90	0.80	0.70	0.60
Total phosphorus (%)	0.90	0.80	0.70	0.60	0.50
Digestible phosphorus (%)	0.45	0.40	0.35	0.30	0.25
Sodium (%)	0.40	0.35	0.30	0.25	0.20
Zinc from zinc oxide (ppm)[f]	3000	3000	3000	–	–
Copper from copper sulfate (ppm)[f]	–	–	–	125	125

[a] These examples are not complete diets and should be used only as guides.
[b] Inclusion percentages refer to ingredient groups, but ingredients within each group may change by phase.
[c] In programs with more or fewer phases, ingredient and nutrient levels should be adjusted accordingly.
[d] This is a partial list of nutrients for illustration purposes. Actual values may vary around these levels.
[e] Legislation or veterinary advice may impose lower upper limits in crude protein concentration.
[f] In the EU, pharmacological additions of zinc and copper are likely to be discontinued in the near future.

replaced largely by plant proteins, usually at a high cost. Recent developments in feed regulations now allow controlled use of animal blood and plasma in pig diets, but only in facilities dedicated to non-ruminant feed production.

The major source of plant proteins in Europe is soybeans, which are mainly imported in the form of soybean meal (Cole and Sprent, 2001).

Soybean proteins (concentrates and isolates) are also used (mostly in post-weaning diets due to cost) to prevent possible gastrointestinal allergenic reactions. For the same reason, extruded soybeans are preferred over traditional soybean meal (Zarkadas and Wiseman, 2000), but its availability is often limited. Other sources of plant proteins include peas, fava beans, rapeseed, sunflower seeds, and other minor legumes. These ingredients are always thermally processed to diminish their strong anti-nutritive properties and enhance amino acid digestibility (Cole and Sprent, 2001). Plant proteins make up to 30% in most piglet diets.

Nutrient levels

European diets for young pigs are traditionally rich in energy and protein (ITP, 2002). The theory behind this practice is that nutrient-dense diets may compensate for the low feed intakes invariably observed after weaning (Campbell, 1989). However, European diets remain nutrient-dense throughout the nursery period, because rapid growth rates and low feed/gain are favored. In addition, several ingredients have a wide disparity between total and available/digestible nutrient content, thus requiring a generous margin of safety when diets are formulated on a total nutrients basis. The latter is of concern with most agro-industrial by-products frequently used in Europe. Nutrient levels in Table 9.1 are examples of diets most likely to be encountered in Northwest Europe.

Feed preparation

Depending on the region and economics, producers purchase either complete diets from local feed manufacturers (e.g. Eastern Europe) or premixes that require home-mixing with major ingredients (e.g. Southern Europe). When complete diets are purchased, feed is usually in pelleted form to improve feed efficiency and reduce freight cost. Premixes vary in size from the simple vitamin/trace mineral packs to concentrates that require only cereals to complete the diet. Although the level of trust between producers and feed manufacturers is generally satisfactory, even small producers in some regions are forced to home-mixing as their only way to quality feed.

Recent advancements in liquid feeding and nutrition have enabled producers to extend this practice to nursery pigs (Brooks *et al.*, 1999). Liquid feeding is often combined with a nearby source of cheap by-products, such as liquid whey or potato and wheat by-products. A premix (or balancer) is often purchased to balance liquid by-products with home-grown cereals. Automated systems are always recommended for offering liquid diets to young pigs.

Feed budgets

European nutritionists and producers prefer to feed each diet for longer before switching to the next stage diet, compared to their American counterparts. Although this invariably increases feeding cost, it ensures that pigs adapt well to their post-weaning environment before challenging them nutritionally with simple diets. This is especially important in the era of antimicrobial-free diets. In Europe, pigs are also kept to nutrient-dense diets longer in the nursery period to sustain rapid growth rates and high efficiency of feed utilization (to maximize profit per pig). Therefore, it is not uncommon for pigs to finish the nursery period on a diet containing 1.5% lysine and 5% whey and (or) fishmeal (ITP, 2002). However, there is a trend, driven mostly by economics, to challenge pigs nutritionally earlier than before, especially when health is above average.

A typical European program calls for one or two diets from weaning at 6–8 kg to 12 kg body weight, with diets usually being pelleted and of high complexity at this stage. Pigs are fed 5–7 kg feed, with an expected feed/gain close to 1.2. After 12 kg body weight, pigs receive one to three diets depending on exit weight (which varies from 20 to 30 kg), but feed efficiency is higher (over 1.5) because cereals and protein sources used at this stage are of lower digestibility. The target is to produce a 30-kg pig at 70 days of age with feed/gain ratio around 1.5.

North American Approach

Relatively inexpensive cereals (wheat, maize, sorghum) and plant proteins (i.e. canola and soybeans) abound on the American continent. In the USA particularly, growing pigs are fed almost exclusively on maize and soybean meal diets fortified with minerals and vitamins. This abundance of cheap energy and protein sources creates pressure for nursery programs to use such resources as soon as possible after weaning to minimize feed cost (Mavromichalis and Baker, 1998). However, with early weaning widely practiced in North America, ingredient-complex and nutrient-dense diets are normally used post-weaning, albeit at reduced amounts compared to European standards.

Weaning age

The majority of pigs in North America are weaned between 14 and 18 days of age, at least in most commercial units of substantial size. The introduction of segregated early weaning (Alexander *et al.*, 1980), which is based on the health advantages of off-site housing, has reduced weaning age from 21–28 days in the 1980s (Patience *et al.*, 1989) to almost 10–14 days in the early

1990s (Maxwell and Carter, 2000). However, a balance between sows' reproductive performance, feeding and management requirements of weaned pigs, and overall profitability currently dictates a more delayed weaning age at 14–18 days. At this age, pigs weigh about 4–6 kg, being thus about 2 kg lighter than the average pig weaned in Europe.

Although traditional farrow-to-finish units are still popular throughout the continent, specialized nursery facilities are becoming extremely common, especially among contract growers (Fig. 9.2). This facilitates the contracting of a large number of pigs from a single source (usually a sow mega-farm) and the design of a farm-specific feeding program. In these facilities, health status is also above average due to strict biosecurity and 'all-in all-out' practices. On the negative side, large nursery units are frequently short on labor and, thus, mechanized feeding from bulk bins is favored over bagged products.

Major ingredients

Wheat is the main cereal in Canada (Patience *et al.*, 1995), whereas producers in the USA use mainly yellow maize (corn). Sorghum is available in the southern USA and Mexico, but maize again is the main pig staple in

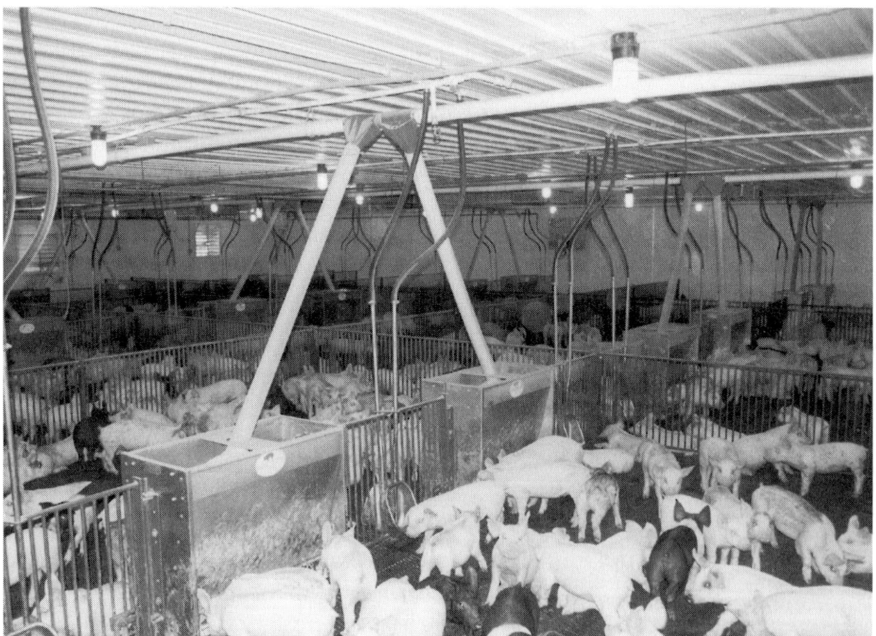

Fig. 9.2. A modern nursery facility now common in most parts of the world.

Central and Latin America. Cereals are used in their raw form (i.e. uncooked), with the exception of decorticated steam-flaked oats, which are favored as an aid against incidents of diarrhea (Nelssen *et al.*, 1999). European-type diets (with cooked cereals) adapted to local ingredients and market conditions are becoming increasingly popular, especially for the first couple of stages post-weaning (Mavromichalis and Varley, 2003).

Whey and its derivatives are the main dairy ingredients, usually added at 10–30% in most piglet diets, followed by lactose and sparingly skim milk, which is rather expensive (Maxwell and Carter, 2000). Blends of milk by-products (such as lactose, whey proteins, and buttermilk) are frequently standardized to the specifications of skim milk to be used as less expensive alternatives.

Fishmeal (64% crude protein), poultry by-products, and blood-derived products (such as animal plasma, red blood cells, and blood meal) are also in wide use (Thacker, 1999). Meat-and-bone meal, however, is not used by some feed manufacturers as a precaution against possible cross-contamination with ruminant products. Animal products make up to 15% of piglet diets depending on target body weight, cost, and quality.

Soybean meal, which ranges in crude protein from 44 to 48%, is the major protein source, especially after 7 kg body weight. Before that, the use of soybean meal is restricted to around 20% (Nelssen *et al.*, 1999; Maxwell and Carter, 2000). Refined soybean proteins are used only in post-weaning diets, as they tend to be rather expensive. Alternatively, extruded soybeans are favored for pigs below 7 kg, at least as a partial replacement to soybean meal. In Canada, canola (i.e. rapeseed variety – very low in glucosinolates) and soybean meal are the main sources of protein (Patience *et al.*, 1995). It appears that the use of animal plasma, which promotes early feed intake, combined with antibiotics and zinc oxide (or copper sulfate) that control scours, enables greater reliance on less refined plant proteins (see Table 9.2).

Nutrient levels

Most nursery diets designed on North American standards contain less energy compared to an average diet designed on European standards. This reflects the widespread belief in North America that because young pigs do not digest supplemental lipids very efficiently, such ingredients should not be used at all. Thus, amino acid levels are also comparatively lower than in Europe, especially during the later stages of the nursery period (NRC, 1998a). In the USA, for example, it is not uncommon for pigs between 12 and 20 kg body weight to receive a diet with 1.20% total lysine and 9.5 MJ NE/kg. In comparison, a similar pig in the UK would receive a diet with at least 1.40% total lysine and at least 11 MJ NE/kg. In general, however, the ratios of lysine to energy are relatively similar (Table 9.3).

Table 9.2. Example diets from North America[a].

	Body weight range (kg)[c]				
Ingredients (%)[b]	4–6	6–8	8–12	12–20	20–30
Cereals (maize, sorghum, wheat, oat groats, wheat and maize milling by-products)	20–30	30–40	40–50	50–60	60–70
Fats and oils (soybean oil, lard, poultry fat, animal–vegetable blends, tallow)	5	5	5	5	5
Dairy ingredients (whey and derivatives, skim milk, lactose, cheese by-products, dairy blends)	30–40	10–30	5–10	0	0
Animal proteins (animal plasma, blood meal, fishmeal, poultry meal, egg proteins)	10–20	10–15	5–10	5	0
Plant proteins (extruded soybean and canola seeds; refined plant proteins, e.g. soy, potato, wheat; soybean and canola meals)	5–10	10–20	20–30	25–35	25–35
Nutrients[d]					
Net energy (MJ/kg)	11.50	11.00	10.50	10.00	9.50
Crude protein (%)	24.00	23.00	22.00	21.00	20.00
Total lysine (%)	1.60	1.50	1.40	1.30	1.20
True ileal digestible lysine (%)	1.45	1.35	1.25	1.15	1.05
Calcium (%)	0.90	0.85	0.80	0.75	0.70
Total phosphorus (%)	0.80	0.75	0.70	0.65	0.60
Digestible phosphorus (%)	0.40	0.37	0.35	0.32	0.30
Sodium (%)	0.45	0.40	0.35	0.30	0.25
Zinc from zinc oxide (ppm)	3000	2000	1000	–	–
Copper from copper sulfate (ppm)[e]	–	–	–	250	250

[a] These examples are not complete diets and should be used only as guides.
[b] Inclusion percentages refer to ingredient groups, but ingredients within each group may change by phase.
[c] In programs with more or fewer phases, ingredient and nutrient levels should be adjusted accordingly.
[d] This is a partial list of nutrients for illustration purposes. Actual values may vary around these levels.
[e] Copper sulfate is often used throughout the nursery period in addition to or as a replacement for zinc oxide.

Feed preparation

Most pigs in the American continent receive a minimum of 0.5 kg pellets after weaning, although 1–2 kg pellets are favored in smaller operations with more available labor (Mavromichalis and Varley, 2003). The first diet post-weaning is usually purchased from feed manufacturers and it is fed by hand. Following the first diet, most feeding programs call for a sequence of three to

Table 9.3. Lysine/energy ratios suitable for diets in Europe and North America (from Tables 9.1 and 9.2)[a].

Body weight (kg)[b]	True ileal digestible lysine/net energy ratio (g/MJ)[c,d,e]
4–6	1.26
6–8	1.22
8–12	1.18
12–20	1.14
20–30	1.10

[a] These are guidelines for illustration purposes only.
[b] In programs with more or fewer phases, nutrient levels are adjusted proportionately.
[c] To convert values to total lysine basis, divide values by 0.90.
[d] To convert to values metabolizable or digestible energy basis, multiply values by 0.74 or 0.71, respectively.
[e] To convert values from g/MJ to g/Mcal, multiply values by 4.184.

five diets in meal form manufactured either on site or at a nearby local feed mill. These diets are usually delivered and fed in bulk. Home-mixing in small operations requires blending of a premix with maize, soybean meal, and (occasionally) fat. Larger units have more ingredients available on site (e.g. minerals, dairy ingredients, fishmeal, etc.) and, thus, they rely on premixes of relatively smaller inclusion rates to complete their nutrition program.

Liquid feeding is sporadic and often troublesome because of the lack of local expertise. Quite often it is connected with locally available by-products, with dairy ingredients (e.g. whey and ice cream) being predominant.

Feed budgets

From weaning at 4–6 kg until about 12 kg, pigs receive two or three diets, depending on weaning weight and management practices (Fig. 9.3). The first diet is usually high in animal plasma (around 5%) and dairy ingredients (20–30%), along with pharmacological doses of zinc oxide (3000 ppm) and other specialty ingredients (e.g. egg yolk antibodies, flavors, probiotics, organic acids, etc.). The following diet(s) contain progressively lower concentrations of specialty ingredients and nutrients (Nelssen *et al*., 1999). Feed efficiency at this stage is about 1.2, with 7 to 10 kg feed being fed.

After 12 kg body weight, pigs are considered able to cope with simple maize and soybean meal-based diets (fortified with minerals and vitamins). At most, 1% fishmeal or another animal-derived source of protein may be used to boost performance, especially in low-health operations. Again two

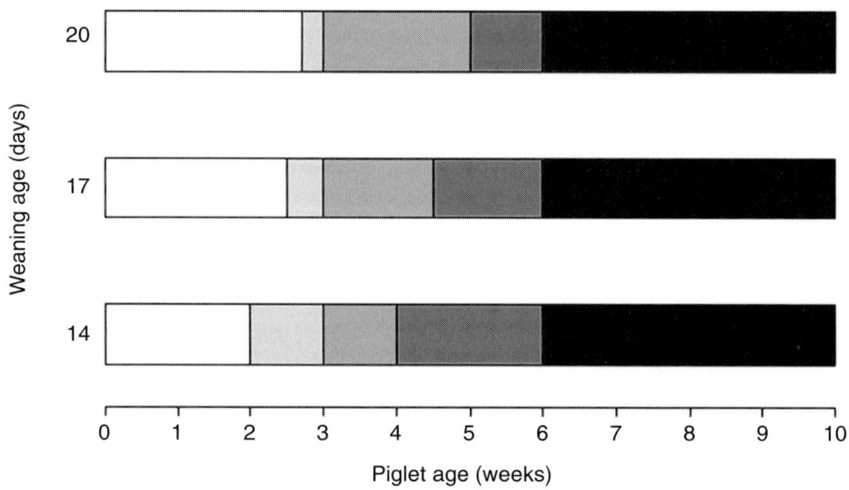

Fig. 9.3. Example of a typical feeding program (□, milk only; ▒, nursery 1; ▒>, nursery 2; ▓, nursery 3; ■, nursery 4) for early-weaned pigs (USA).

or three diets (usually in meal form) are fed until pigs exit the nursery, at a body weight that varies from 20 to 30 kg. Feed efficiency ranges from 1.5 to over 2.0 in this stage (depending, of course, among other factors on exit weight). Feeding pelleted diets throughout the nursery period, which is favored in Northwest Europe, is usually not cost-effective, because the cost of pelleting often outweighs the expected 5–10% increase in growth performance, unless the producer also owns the pellet mill.

Like their European counterparts, American producers aim to produce a 30-kg pig at 70 days of age with a feed efficiency around 1.5, but at less cost (Mavromichalis and Varley, 2003).

Feeding Without Antimicrobials

The use of antimicrobial agents (summarily termed under the familiar name of antibiotics) at growth-promoting levels was first banned in Sweden in 1986 (Stein, 2002). This action was taken to prevent increasing resistance of bacteria to antibiotics used in human medicine. Assuming that resistant genes from bacteria in pigs were able to cross into the genome of human bacteria (from contact with pigs, their products and excreta), there was concern that certain human bacterial diseases could not be treated effectively with antibiotics similar to those used for promoting animal growth. Following the ban, the use of antibiotics for therapeutic purposes increased dramatically (mainly for the treatment of post-weaning diarrhea), but overall use was markedly reduced. In the nursery period, mortality increased by 1.5% and feed intake by 3–5 kg (Stein, 2002). In response, production practices changed to conform to antibiotic-free diets, with increasing weaning age (up to 5 weeks) being the most notable.

That antibiotics fed for prolonged periods of time increase the resistance of certain bacteria in pigs has been a concern since the introduction of antibiotics in 1950s (Holmberg *et al.*, 1984; Dupont and Steele, 1987). However, the risk imposed on public health was largely unknown. Recent research has proven beyond doubt that bacteria do develop resistance to antibiotics (Salyers, 2002) and that the human populace in contact with such resistant bacteria may harbor resistant genes in their own microflora (Fedorka-Cray *et al.*, 2002; Witte *et al.*, 2002). What remains to be assessed is whether this poses any real health concerns for humans, especially when the risk from the outrageous use of antimicrobial substances in human medicine is ignored (Hardy, 2002). A recent report (NRC, 1998b) based on available scientific literature indicated that such risk has not been documented.

Nevertheless, based on political pressure, Denmark imposed a voluntary ban on the use of all antibiotics in 1998, which became a national law in 2000. Similar bans were also imposed in The Netherlands and Switzerland. In these countries, in agreement with the Swedish experience, the use of antimicrobial substances increased substantially in the nursery phase for therapeutic purposes (Stein, 2002). In finishing pigs and sows, the antibiotic ban had trivial, if any, effects on performance and overall health.

In the rest of the EU, four antibiotics were allowed until 1 January 2006 for use in animal diets as growth promoters. These were rumensin, salinomycin, avilamycin, and flavomycin (Stein, 2002), but a complete ban has been effective since then. In the USA, an industry-wide plan for the judicious use of antibiotics is in effect to achieve a balance between human health safety and efficiency of pig production (Cromwell, 2002).

Alternatives

It is apparent that today no single technology, feed additive, or management practice can promote growth in young pigs as cost-effectively as most antibiotics, especially in production systems where health status is below average. Research and field experience have demonstrated that a synergy of practices is needed to promote growth at least as effectively as most antibiotics (Gourmelen *et al.*, 2002). Feed and (or) production costs, however, are invariably higher in antibiotic-free programs because the technology is still under development.

The most common approach in replacing feed-grade antibiotics calls for other additives that mimic the effects of antibiotics. Thus, compounds with bacteriostatic and bacteriocidal activity are added in existing diets to depress microbial load and reduce diversity of the microflora at the gastrointestinal level. Such additives include zinc oxide, copper sulfate, certain organic acids, and several spice/herbal extracts. This approach is more appropriate for production systems unable to modify their husbandry practices to reduce dependence on antibiotic-like additives.

A more systematic approach that is gaining popularity in Europe calls for substantial changes in both production practices and diet formulation (Wallgren and Melin, 2001). In summary, production methods aim to minimize exposure of pigs to pathogenic microorganisms and improve immune status. Thus, higher levels of biosecurity, later weaning age, and improved feed intake patterns post-weaning are becoming crucial components of an overall antibiotic-free strategy. In addition, formulas for post-weaned pigs are being re-designed to promote proliferation of beneficial bacteria at the gastrointestinal level that compete vigorously for nutrients with pathogenic bacteria. This method, also called 'competitive exclusion', requires a strong understanding of gut microbiology and high standards of production.

Under commercial conditions, elements from both approaches are often combined to achieve desired performance goals at optimal cost. Common practices employed in the absence of antibiotics are described below.

Improved health status

Because antibiotics are most effective in low-health herds (Cromwell, 2002), it is expected that improving health by tightening biosecurity, adopting all-in, all-out procedures, enhancing cleaning/disinfecting procedures, and stabilizing sow herd health will reduce dependence on antibiotics. Research and field experience have clearly demonstrated that the effect of antibiotics diminishes notably under high-health conditions (Table 9.4).

Increased weaning age

Increasing weaning age allows piglets to build a robust immune and digestive system that will cope better with post-weaning challenges (Cranwell

Table 9.4. Summary of performance improvement expected in young pigs from feed-grade antibiotics. (Adapted from Cromwell, 2002.)

	Improvement over non-medicated control (%)	
	Weight gain	Feed/gain
Review 1 (12,000 pigs; 7–26 kg)		
High health (128 trials)	+17	–7
Low health (32 trials)	+28	–15
Review 2 (3321 pigs; 8–20 kg)		
High health (nine trials)	+13	–5
Low health (67 trials)	+26	–10

et al., 1995; Madec *et al.*, 1998). This is especially true when piglets are allowed to develop active immunity (past the third week of age) while suckling on the sow. Also, later weaning may offer the advantage of prolonged exposure to creep feed that could further enhance overall condition (Sprent *et al.*, 2000).

Enhanced nutrient digestibility

Unabsorbed nutrients from diets of low digestibility become substrate for bacterial proliferation. A large microbial load not only drains nutrients from the animal (hence the growth-promoting effects of antibiotics), but also harbors large numbers of potentially pathogenic bacteria such as colibacilli, salmonella, and clostridia. Nutrient digestibility is of paramount importance during the first week post-weaning when feed intake is usually depressed (Mavromichalis and Varley, 2003).

Ingredient selection in post-weaning diets greatly influences nutrient digestibility. Diets based on rice and animal proteins (highly digestible) support firmer stools and greater performance than diets based on wheat and plant protein sources (Montagne *et al.*, 2003a). This protective effect of a diet based on cooked rice and animal proteins may also be partially attributed to reduced digesta viscosity that hinders bacterial proliferation (McDonald *et al.*, 2001).

Stimulated feed intake

Feed intake plays a critical role in the maintenance of gut health after weaning. Even a short period of feed deprivation increases gut permeability to antigenic proteins (such as those present in soybean meal) and susceptibility to bacterial attachment (McCracken *et al.*, 1999). This often leads to diarrhea from hypersensitivity reaction to antigenic proteins in legumes and (or) from endotoxins produced by attached bacteria such as *E. coli*.

Reduced dietary protein

Bacteria require protein to grow and multiply. By reducing dietary protein and (or) increasing its digestibility, bacterial proliferation and scouring can be markedly reduced (Goransson *et al.*, 1995). Pigs fed low-protein diets (less than 21%) have been shown to be less prone to *E. coli*-induced post-weaning diarrhea (Prohaszka and Baron, 1980). At the same time, it is important to offer a well-balanced profile of digestible amino acids to ensure maximal lean deposition. Dietary protein concentration should not be lowered below 4 percentage units to avoid deficiencies in valine and isoleucine, which cannot be supplemented currently in crystalline form.

Increased dietary fiber

Diets for early weaned pigs contain minimal fiber because excess fiber dilutes nutrient energy and impairs digestibility. However, a certain amount of dietary crude fiber (3–5%) stimulates proliferation of a healthy microflora that can compete with pathogenic bacteria (Mosenthin *et al.*, 1999; Pluske *et al.*, 2003). Thus, many diets without antibiotics are often supplemented with a source of highly fermentable fiber, usually from sugarbeet pulp (5–10%) or barley (up to 30%) in Europe, or oats (10–20%) and wheat bran (5–10%) in North America.

Organic acids

Most pathogenic bacteria, such as salmonella and colibacilli, are acid-intolerant. Thus, acidification of the gastrointestinal tract by means of dietary organic acids may halt or even reverse microbial growth (Mroz, 2003). Furthermore, organic acids that reach the small intestine in undissociated form enter bacteria cells and kill them. Research and field experience dictate that blends of organic acids cover a broader spectrum of pathogenic bacteria and, therefore, they tend to be more effective than single organic acids (Lee *et al.*, 2002; Partanen *et al.*, 2002).

Plant extracts

Certain herbal extracts have antimicrobial and (or) antiviral properties, whereas spices are known for both their antimicrobial and digestive-enhancing properties. Cinnamon, oregano, clove, and garlic are among the most commonly used extracts in commercial products. Research is currently underway to identify extracts and concentrations appropriate for young pigs (Lis-Balchin, 2003). It is also suggested that plant extracts combined with organic acid blends are more effective than either additive alone.

Enzymes

Enzymes have no direct antibacterial properties. However, enzymes that break down anti-nutritional factors, such as non-starch polysaccharides, may be beneficial in antibiotic-free programs because they reduce the availability of substrate (undigested feed) to microbes (Bedford and Apajalahti, 2001). Enzymes are more beneficial in diets based on wheat, barley, and rye, rather than maize or sorghum (Partridge, 2001). Soybean-based diets may also benefit from enzyme supplementation, especially during the late nursery period, but less research is available on this aspect (Kim *et al.*, 2001).

Probiotics (direct-fed microbials)

Feeding beneficial bacteria is also an alternative strategy in antibiotic-free programs (Simon *et al.*, 2003). Most commercial preparations include one or multiple species of lactobacillus and (or) bifidobacterium. Pelleting reduces the effectiveness of these products, and, thus, heat-stable preparations should be used. Selected strains must also be acid-resistant so that they can be combined with organic acids.

Prebiotics

These are non-digestible, yet fermentable, sugars used to promote proliferation of beneficial bacterial populations in the gastrointestinal tract (Patterson and Burkholder, 2003). Inulin, transgalactose, and fructose oligosaccharides are among the most popular prebiotics. Product quality is of paramount importance in selecting prebiotics, as research results have been extremely variable.

Yeast derivatives

Yeast cells are naturally equipped with surface mannan oligosaccharides that can bind bacteria such as *E. coli* and salmonella (Spring *et al.*, 2000). *In vitro*, bacteria bound to yeast oligosaccharides are unable to attach to gut enterocytes and are, thus, rendered harmless for the host animal. *In vivo* research with pigs, however, has failed to yield consistent results or elucidate the conditions under which such an approach is effective in practice (Davis *et al.*, 2002).

Egg immunoglobulins

Spray-dried eggs high in immunoglobulins (produced from hens hyperimmunized against certain *E. coli* strains) are often used against diarrhea (Owusu-Asiedu *et al.*, 2002), especially in cases of F18 or K88 serotypes. Field observations indicate that pigs suffering from gut edema may benefit the most from this nutritional intervention.

Nucleotides

Commercial preparations of nucleotides are derived mainly from yeast cultures. In laboratory animals (e.g. rats) dietary nucleotide supplementation is involved in promoting gut maturation (Uauy *et al.*, 1990) and in repair of intestinal function after diarrhea (Nunez *et al.*, 1990). Research with pigs is limited (Bustamante *et al.*, 1994) and controversial, but certainly merits further exploration.

Plasma and minerals

Although re-allowed in the EU only recently (2005), animal plasma may have a role in antimicrobial-free programs because it enhances feed intake post-weaning and provides a readily available source of immunoglobulins. The effects of plasma are more pronounced under conditions of increased environmental and health stress (Coffey and Cromwell, 1995; Stahly *et al.*, 1995). Pharmacological doses of zinc oxide (up to 3000 ppm) and copper sulfate (up to 250 ppm) are also valuable additions in the absence of antibiotics, as they enhance growth and check diarrhea (Hill *et al.*, 2000, 2001).

Protection against *Escherichia coli* K88

Canadian researchers (Owusu-Asiedu *et al.*, 2003) recently tested the efficacy of antibiotic alternatives in the face of an *E. coli* (strain K88) challenge. Products used included animal plasma, egg yolk antibodies, zinc oxide, and fumaric acid. A negative control diet without additives was included in the experimental design along with a positive medicated control (carbadox). A total of 90 pigs (10 days of age) were used in a 14-day assay with five replicates per treatment. Pigs were challenged with *E. coli* after 7 days on trial.

Anti-K88 and anti-F18 antibody titers in diets with plasma were 1800 and 1500 mg/dl, respectively. In diets with yolk antibodies these titers were 1800 and 900 mg/dl, respectively. In all other diets, titers were negligible. Before infection, all pigs were healthy without scours. After infection, pigs with no protective agents in the feed (negative control) had depressed growth rate and developed severe diarrhea followed by marked mortality (40%). Remarkably, all feed additives provided the same level of protection, in terms of scour prevention and growth performance, against infection (Table 9.5). It would be interesting to further evaluate any synergistic effects.

Feeding to Combat Diarrhea

Diarrhea is the most common cause of depressed performance in recently weaned piglets. The origins of diarrhea can be pathogenic, nutritional, or both through secondary complications. Pathogenic scours (e.g. *E. coli*, salmonella), as identified by proper diagnostics, require veterinary intervention to cure symptoms and eliminate the source of offending microorganisms. Usually a medication regimen along with changes in biosecurity, animal flow, and husbandry procedures are required to eliminate pathogenic diarrheas. Nutritional diarrheas usually follow or precede pathogenic complications, and thus, a combination of nutritional and medical interventions is often required. Obviously, a properly designed nutritional program should prevent nutritional diarrhea.

Table 9.5. Efficacy of alternatives for antibiotics in diets for young pigs[a,b]. (Adapted from Owusu-Asiedu *et al.*, 2003.)

	Not medicated[c]	Antibiotic alternative				Medicated[d]
		Plasma	Egg	ZnO	Acid	
Weight gain (g/day)	101	157	151	159	155	153
Feed intake (g/day)	141	213	208	215	212	222
K88 shedding (%)	81	29	23	42	31	21
Scours score (3 = diarrhea)	2.2	0.5	0.3	0.6	0.5	0.2
Mortality (%)	40	7	7	13	7	13

[a] A total of 90 weaned pigs (10 days old) in five replicates were used in a 14-day growth trial.
[b] Pigs were infected with *Escherichia coli* seven days after the onset of the trial.
[c] Performance of the negative control (non-medicated) versus all other treatments was significantly lower ($P < 0.05$).
[d] No differences were observed among antibiotic alternatives and medicated treatment.

Nutritional diarrhea originates from three main faults in the design of a feeding program. First, diets that fail to initiate vigorous feed intake immediately post-weaning cause hunger, followed by overeating when pigs associate dry feed with nourishment. Even short-term starvation is capable of diminishing the digestive and immune capabilities of the gastrointestinal system. Thus, when pigs overeat after a period of malnutrition, digestion is incomplete, resulting in excess amounts of substrate (energy and protein) available for proliferation of opportunistic pathogenic microorganisms (e.g. *E. coli* or salmonella). Second, diets of relatively low quality, which are often used to reduce feed cost, not only discourage the development of an early appetite, but their intrinsic low digestibility also results in more undigested material becoming available for bacterial proliferation in the lower gastrointestinal tract. Third, certain ingredients (e.g. soybean meal) contain anti-nutritional factors (e.g. storage proteins glycin and β-conglycin) that may cause gastrointestinal inflammation when combined with a low feed intake, and impair the structure of the gastrointestinal epithelium.

It is also suggested that diets with a high concentration of simple sugars and minerals may disturb the osmotic balance across the enteric epithelium, causing excessive water secretion in the lumen and loose stools. For instance, by changing the amount of sugars (sucrose and corn syrup solids), dietary osmolality was manipulated between 250 and 700 mOsm/kg (Case *et al.*, 1981). Absorption of water and carbohydrates from the small intestine in piglets increased, and thus the chances for diarrhea were minimized, as osmolality increased at similar dietary electrolyte balance. Dietary maltodextrin increases water absorption, whereas glucose increases water secretion in the gastrointestinal tract (Weber and Ehrlein, 1998), indicating that sugar oligomers are more effective than monomers in preventing secretory diarrhea. Secretory diarrhea may not be detrimental to animal performance and health as pigs are able to compensate by drinking more water. Nevertheless, it is a disturbing sight for human operators and it should be prevented, as it is rather difficult and expensive to differentiate from other forms of diarrhea. For this purpose, the addition of water-absorbing materials (fiber, clay) in feed, or reformulation to avoid sugar and mineral excesses, is often recommended.

Escherichia coli survey

Post-weaning *E. coli* diarrhea has been long associated with low-digestibility diets, because undigested nutrients in the gut favor proliferation of enterotoxigenic strains of *E. coli* that cause hypersecretion of intestinal fluids and electrolytes in the lumen of the gut (Hopwood and Hampson, 2003). This invariably leads to diarrhea, malnutrition, poor growth, and occasionally death.

Results from a comprehensive survey in Canada (Cardinal *et al*., 2002) including 34 commercial farms, of which 17 were reporting *E. coli* problems, indicated that the majority of diarrhea incidents occurred between 3 and 10 days post-weaning. However, cases as late as 23 days post-weaning were not uncommon. In farms where *E. coli* diarrhea was prevalent in nursery pigs, diets were found to contain higher levels of vegetable protein sources (+12%), namely soybean meal and canola meal (Table 9.6). Also, pigs that suffered from diarrhea were fed diets higher in calcium (+25%) and magnesium (+6%), both of which increase alkalinity in the gut (*E. coli* thrives in alkaline conditions). Moreover, zinc oxide use was 21% less in diets for pigs that were reported suffering from diarrhea. Finally, electrolyte balance was relatively reduced in diets for scouring pigs (–8%). Although this study does not establish a clear cause–effect relationship between dietary composition and *E. coli* diarrhea, it provides at least an indication that improper diet formulation can predispose pigs to diarrhea, intensify symptoms, or delay recovery.

Table 9.6. Canadian survey on dietary links to *Escherichia coli* diarrhea[a]. (Adapted from Cardinal *et al*., 2002.)

Dietary specification	Farms with diarrhea	Farms without diarrhea
Soybean and canola meal (kg/t)	241.0	214.5
Calcium (%)	1.26	1.01
Magnesium (%)	0.18	0.17
Zinc (ppm)	2182	2778
Electrolyte balance (mEq/kg)	250	272

[a]A total of 34 commercial farms, of which 17 reported diarrhea problems.

Nutritional links to edema disease

Edema disease, a complicated enteric disorder caused by enterotoxemic *E. coli* strains, continues to puzzle veterinarians and nutritionists regarding prevention and treatment of affected animals. A Dutch research group (Nabuurs *et al.*, 2001) examined affected and healthy pigs from the same herd and concluded that although edema disease is closely associated with the presence of *E. coli* (O139K82 strain in this case), dietary factors may also contribute or aggravate this intestinal disorder. Affected pigs exhibited symptoms of metabolic acidosis, evidenced by higher blood and intestinal acidity. The researchers speculated that toxins produced by *E. coli* in the gastrointestinal tract may have a greater chance to cross the intestinal barrier in pigs suffering from metabolic acidosis, because increased intestinal acidity is associated with enhanced permeability. Therefore, nutritional intervention strategies to reduce acidosis in the face of an edema disease outbreak may be beneficial. More studies are required, however, to verify these results and define appropriate nutritional intervention strategies before practical recommendations can be made.

Intervention strategies

It should be emphasized that nutritional interventions after the onset of diarrhea should be made in consultation with the attending veterinarian and nutritionist. Because scientific experiments with infected pigs raised alongside healthy pigs in the same room are extremely challenging and expensive, practical experience rather than scientific evidence is usually the basis for deriving most recommendations (Goransson, 2001). Farms experiencing high incidents of post-weaning diarrhea often implement the following measures (with variable results).

Prevention

For bacterial diarrheas, measures prescribed for antibiotic-free diets are certainly applicable. For viral diarrheas, however, vaccination is most helpful, although antibacterial measures are strongly recommended to prevent secondary bacterial complications.

Restricted feeding

This practice is particularly popular in Europe. Weaned pigs are offered a limited amount of feed (about 2–3% of body weight) during the first week post-weaning, with increasing allowances of feed until pigs attain *ad libitum* levels during the second week (Goransson, 2001). The theory behind this practice is that restricted feed intake will limit bacterial growth in the gastrointestinal tract, especially when available diets are of rather low digestibility and antibiotics are not used. Although this practice has the potential of clearing or preventing post-weaning diarrhea, it nevertheless deprives pigs of vital nutrients during the most crucial period of their life. Thus, this method of diarrhea control may have negative effects on lifetime performance and should be used only as a last resort. A recent field study from Denmark (Johansen *et al.*, 2000), where restricted feeding is the norm, revealed that restricted feeding is not always effective against diarrhea as previously thought.

Reduced anti-nutritional factors

Soybeans and most legumes contain anti-nutritional compounds that have the potential of triggering the immature digestive immune system of the weaned piglet, with inflammation and diarrhea usually following ingestion of high doses of such anti-nutritional factors (Li *et al.*, 1990). Thermal processing of offending ingredients usually prevents intestinal inflammation, but in pigs suffering with severe diarrhea elimination of such ingredients is strongly recommended.

Increased dietary bulkiness

Moderate levels of fiber (2–3%) enhance movement of digesta through the gastrointestinal system, increase digesta water retention, and facilitate defecation. Addition of fiber in nursery diets is believed to increase excretion of pathogenic microorganisms, prevent attachment of bacteria to the enteric epithelium, and establish a healthy gut microflora (Mosenthin *et al.*, 1999; Montagne *et al.*, 2003b). Excess dietary fiber (over 3–5%), however, severely dilutes nutrient density and deprives both the animal and the beneficial hosted microorganisms from vital nutrients. Although adding fiber to combat diarrhea is a rather drastic measure, it is often employed as a last resort against severe diarrhea that has already affected the enteric epithelium and reduced digestive capacity in young pigs. Rolled oats (5–20%), sugarbeet pulp (5–10%), alfalfa meal (3–5%) and wheat bran (5–10%) are the most common sources of fiber.

Feed quality issues

Ensuring that feed-borne pathogens do not reach young pigs is a sound way of preventing unnecessary cases of diarrhea. To this end, ingredient selection is of paramount importance, as is a rigid quality assurance program. Finished complete feeds are often heat-treated to reduce bacterial load. For example, in Denmark there is a requirement for all piglet pelleted feeds to be heated at least at 83°C (Best, 2001). Recent evidence also suggests that a coarse feed texture and meal form is more protective against proliferation of *E. coli* and salmonella compared with finely ground or pelleted diets (Jensen *et al*., 2003).

Danish experience

In Denmark, pelleted feeds are preferred for their improved feed efficiency, but fiber is also favored in the form of coarsely ground, untreated whole or flaked cereals such as barley, oats, and wheat. These cereals are often incorporated in the original (complete) formula after pelleting. For example, complete pellets may be loaded in a truck compartment at the feed mill along with 25% barley, with motion movement and unloading to bins providing all necessary mixing (Best, 2001). This is recommended especially for post-weaned pigs suffering or susceptible to severe cases of diarrhea. These high-fiber and bulky diets are usually low or even devoid of soybean meal during the first couple of weeks post-weaning (Olsen and Maribo, 1999).

In a field trial involving 22 replicates per treatment (Olsen and Maribo, 1999), a control pelleted diet (2.2% fiber) was tested against a high-fiber

Table 9.7. Diets used in a Danish experiment to test the effects of fiber on post-weaning diarrhea[a]. (Adapted from Olsen and Maribo, 1999.)

	Control (%)	Anti-diarrhea (%)
Wheat	65.63	20.90
Barley bran	–	36.00
Soybeans, toasted	13.60	–
Oats, dehulled	–	20.00
Fishmeal	5.00	8.00
Milk–soy protein blend	–	8.00
Fat	4.75	3.60
Molasses	2.00	–
Potato protein concentrate	4.89	–
Organic acids	–	0.50
Vitamins/minerals/amino acids	+	+
Nutrient analysis		
Net energy (MJ/kg)	10.90	11.08
Crude protein (%)	22.30	18.00
Total lysine (%)	1.45	1.44
Calcium (%)	0.85	0.78
Total phosphorus (%)	0.75	0.68
Crude fiber (%)	2.20	4.90

[a] These are incomplete experimental diets and should not be used without proper balancing of all nutrients.

(4.9%) pelleted diet (Table 9.7). In the first couple of weeks post-weaning (from 4 to 6 weeks of age), 25% of control pigs were treated for diarrhea. In contrast, only 7% of pigs receiving the high-fiber diet were treated for diarrhea. Growth performance was not affected by dietary treatment, indicating the often perplexing effects of diarrhea on growth (Table 9.8). It should be noted, however, that growth performance in the control pigs was below average industry standards. Also, the anti-diarrhea diet was lower in protein, extremely low in soybean proteins, and it was supplemented with organic acids. Thus, the diarrhea-controlling effect cannot be attributed to the higher fiber concentration alone, but more likely to an effective combination of strategies as outlined above.

Diets without Animal Plasma

The introduction of animal plasma in the early 1990s revolutionized piglet nutrition, especially in North America where diets were fairly simple in ingredient composition (Gatnau and Zimmerman, 1990). The success of animal plasma-based diets is attributed to invariably higher feed intake (up to 50%), especially in early-weaned piglets, during the first couple of weeks post-weaning. The magnitude of response to animal plasma, however, depends on the level of baseline performance (i.e. performance achieved with diets devoid of animal plasma; van Dijk *et al*., 2001). Thus, factors that ensure rapid development of early post-weaning appetite (e.g. high health, proper feeding techniques) tend to diminish the response to animal plasma. It is also suggested (Toplis and Miller, 1999) that the effects of animal plasma diminish as the overall quality of the diet increases. Nevertheless, during the last decade, the use of animal plasma in most commercial post-weaning diets has dropped from over 7% to below 5% as animal husbandry techniques and nutrition science continue to improve.

Despite its strong benefits, animal plasma currently faces many challenges. Suitable solutions often result in comparable performance,

Table 9.8. Performance of pigs fed a high-fiber diet under Danish field conditions (2 weeks post-weaning)[a]. (Adapted from Maribo and Olsen, 1999.)

	Control diet	Anti-diarrhea diet
Weight gain (g/day)	203	216
Feed intake (g/day)	246	281
Feed/gain	1.21	1.30
Pigs treated for diarrhea (%)	25	7

[a] Note that growth performance of the control pigs was relatively poor compared to industry standards.

especially when the overall growth period is concerned (Toplis and Miller, 1999). In many cases, however, reduced performance, especially during the first week post-weaning, may be the only alternative to animal plasma in diets for young pigs.

Price

Animal plasma is relatively expensive and can account for up to 30% of ingredient cost in complex diets. Although consumption of such diets is relatively small (1–3 kg per pig) and the contribution of the cost of animal plasma to overall (wean to market) feed cost is trivial (less than 1%), expensive diets remain unattractive, especially to least cost-oriented producers. Alternative products (e.g. other sources of immunoglobulins) with often debatable efficacy are priced at or slightly less than the cost of animal plasma, making substitution for cost savings questionable.

To reduce the impact of animal plasma on feed cost, its inclusion level may be titrated to farm-specific levels barely enough to elicit a feed intake response post-weaning. This depends, of course, on production practices. For example, in a high-health farm exercising appropriate feeding management, use of animal plasma may be halved compared to diets designed for less favorable conditions. It is also prudent to contain the use of animal plasma-based diets only during the first week post-weaning or until pigs appear to consume feed vigorously. Obviously, production practices that enable pigs to better express their genetic potential in terms of growth performance reduce dependence on animal plasma.

Availability

In the EU, the use of animal plasma (among other animal-derived ingredients) is currently regulated and although theoretically it can be used in piglet diets, manufacturing restrictions prohibit some plants from using it. Nevertheless, animal plasma was never as popular in Europe as it is in North America. Animal plasma, however, can certainly be of great benefit with the current ban on antimicrobial growth promoters and strict regulations on zinc oxide and copper sulfate. Research has demonstrated that animal plasma may be beneficial under disease stress (Coffey and Cromwell, 1995; Quigley *et al.*, 2003), although it is not clear yet whether this response is associated with higher feed intake or improved immunological support.

Replacements for animal plasma are usually sources of immunoglobulins either from milk (Miller and Toplis, 2000) or eggs (Owusu-Asiedu *et al.*, 2002, 2003). Commercial products based on cow colostrum contain 15–30% immunoglobulins, whereas egg proteins from hyperimmunized hens contain also about 15% immunoglobulins. Other products with claims of replacing animal plasma (e.g. nucleotides, yeast derivatives) can be as expensive as animal plasma, but their efficacy is currently debatable. It appears that the best strategies for replacing animal plasma are: (i) heavier reliance on traditional milk products, which are good sources of immunoglobulins; and (ii) absence or restriction of offending ingredients that may cause intestinal inflammation (e.g. unrefined plant proteins rich in anti-nutritional factors), at least during the first couple of weeks post-weaning.

Contamination

Recent academic research (DeRouchey *et al.*, 2001) indicated that irradiation of animal plasma greatly reduced its microbial load and enhanced pig performance compared with non-irradiated plasma (Table 9.9). Such a response, however, was not replicated under commercial conditions with a common source of animal plasma (Cook *et al.*, 2002). Today reliable suppliers provide ample evidence of the highest standards used in producing animal plasma and of the absence of pathogenic organisms. Nevertheless, irradiation does reduce overall microbial load in animal plasma.

Despite all reassurances, several pig producers and their consultants refuse to use animal plasma based on their own evaluation of available data. Therefore, they request diets devoid of any blood products. These diets usually contain maximum levels of zinc oxide and (or) copper sulfate, higher levels of dairy products and minimum levels of soybean meal. Refined plant proteins (e.g. soy protein isolate, potato protein), fishmeal, egg by-product, and crystalline amino acids are also increased to compensate for the contribution of highly digestible amino acids from animal plasma. Anecdotal evidence suggests that performance loss is not noticeable when the overall growth period is concerned.

Table 9.9. Feeding irradiated plasma to nursery pigs yields variable results.

	Treatment	
Report	Control	Irradiated
DeRouchey *et al.* (2001)[a]		
Weight gain (g/day)	232	262
Feed intake (g/day)	204	213
Cook *et al.* (2002)[b]		
Weight gain (g/day)	174	159
Feed intake (g/day)	165	149

[a] Plasma irradiation improved performance ($P < 0.05$) during the first 7 days post-weaning.
[b] Plasma irradiation decreased performance ($P < 0.10$) during the first 5 days post-weaning.

Replacing Fish and Meat Meals

Fishmeal and products of the rendering industry (i.e. meat and meat-and-bone meals) have long been a source of highly digestible amino acids in pig diets at relatively competitive prices. Fishmeal of high quality is often used at 5–10% in diets for post-weaned pigs (Cole and Sprent, 2001), whereas meat meal may be used at similar concentrations if of low ash (mainly calcium) content. Yet, like most ingredients, these raw materials are not without problems.

In the aftermath of the bovine spongiform encephalopathy (BSE) outbreak, the use of meat meal in pig diets has virtually ceased worldwide, with notable exceptions, of course. Although fishmeal can still be used freely in pig diets many feed manufacturers (and even some pig producers) have opted not to use any at all to avoid contamination of manufacturing lines.

The continuous blooming of the worldwide aquaculture industry, with its heavy reliance on fishmeal for aquafeeds, and the increasing limits to fishing quotas, forecast dwindling supplies and increasing prices for high-quality fishmeal. It is estimated that by 2010, aquaculture feeds will use around 50% of global fishmeal production (Naylor *et al*., 2000). Moreover, although some regions of the world (e.g. Australia) are fortunate not to encounter BSE disease, they are either too far away from main producing areas (i.e. Latin America and Northern Europe) of high-quality fishmeal or produce local fishmeal of rather low quality. Such areas usually rely more on meat meal and poultry by-products.

Fishmeal of low quality is often found contaminated with salmonella, especially after prolonged storage under hot and humid conditions. Also, increasing ash content (sand and bones) due to poor fishing and processing practices greatly diminishes the nutritive value of fishmeal. Finally, prolonged storage of fish before processing produces unfavorable compounds (biogenic amines) in the final product, which greatly diminish fishmeal acceptance by animals (FAO, 1986).

Alternatives to fish and meat meals

Meat meal can be readily replaced by fishmeal (and vice versa), but when these ingredients are either unavailable or too expensive, other ingredients with a high protein concentration are naturally sought. On a cost basis, blood, egg, poultry, and cheese products are suitable replacements. But, emphasis should be placed on quality, because replacing high-quality fishmeal with a cheaper alternative of lower quality will impact animal performance and overall profitability of production.

If animal-derived ingredients are to be totally excluded, possible alternatives include dairy ingredients, which are most suitable for post-weaning diets. Skim milk, whey protein concentrates, and even casein are often used, but they invariably increase diet cost compared to fishmeal. Refined vegetable proteins (e.g. from soy and peas), extruded legumes (e.g. soybean and canola seeds), wheat gluten (low in lysine), and brewer's yeast may also replace fishmeal, at least partially. These ingredients usually reduce diet cost, but may also reduce animal performance if not properly used.

Crystalline amino acids are frequently used to replace part of fishmeal, but dietary crude protein concentration should not be reduced by more than 2–4 percentage units from that of the original diet. Diets without fishmeal may become limiting in branched-chain amino acids (especially in valine and isoleucine). Potential sources of these amino acids are potato protein and soy proteins. Also, addition of a small amount of sodium bicarbonate (e.g. 0.5%) may be required to buffer increased acidity from crystalline amino acids (especially from L-lysine HCl). Diets used in the first couple of weeks post-weaning, however, should not be supplemented with sodium bicarbonate as pigs suffer from anhydrochloria during this time.

Finally, diets with lower nutrient density may be employed when fishmeal or other sources of highly digestible protein are not available. In this case, energy density must be adjusted accordingly. This recommendation should be used only as a last measure since it will invariably lead to reduced performance, because young pigs cannot compensate by eating more of a lower density diet.

Wheat versus Maize

The question whether maize can replace wheat is often asked in major wheat-producing areas (e.g. Canada, Europe) where there is considerable experience in feeding wheat. Similarly, producers in major maize-producing areas (e.g. the USA, Latin America) frequently ask whether wheat can replace maize. Such concerns usually emerge when alternative cereals are priced competitively (due to oversupply or lower quality).

There is ample evidence (Cho *et al.*, 2001) suggesting that properly balanced diets using similar quality wheat or maize will yield similar results, at least in terms of animal performance (Table 9.10). Obviously, replacing good-quality wheat (or maize) with moldy maize (or wheat rich in arabinoxylans) will fail to produce similar results. Therefore, more emphasis should be placed on quality than nutrient composition when comparing cereals.

When replacing wheat for maize the following should be taken into consideration:

- Wheat has less energy (95% of that in maize), more protein (11–12 versus 7–8%), and higher phosphorus bioavailability (50 versus 14%) than maize (ITP, 2002). Thus, a one-to-one substitution based on weight will produce severe nutrient imbalances.

Table 9.10. Feeding wheat or maize to nursery pigs[a,b]. (Adapted from Cho *et al.*, 2001.)

Performance	Maize		Wheat	
	Raw	Cooked	Raw	Cooked
Days 0–7 post-weaning				
Weight gain (g/day)	142	137	141	129
Feed intake (g/day)	193	199	188	172
Days 0–21 post-weaning				
Weight gain (g/day)	286	283	285	304
Feed intake (g/day)	488	430	460	447

[a] A total of 160 pigs (14 days of age and 4.3 kg) were used in four replicates per treatment.
[b] Cereal source and thermal processing had no effects on growth performance.

- Wheat contains certain anti-nutritional factors (arabinoxylans) that could be detrimental to animal performance at high concentrations. In this case, a wheat-specific enzyme (xylanase) is recommended for piglet diets (Partridge, 2001).
- Finely ground wheat increases pellet durability (but pellets also become harder), decreases feed flow in bins and feeders, and may increase incidents of ulceration in susceptible pigs (Mavromichalis *et al.*, 2000).
- Finally, there is some evidence to suggest that wheat (and barley) support a healthier microflora than maize-based diets, especially in the absence of feed-grade antibiotics (Drew *et al.*, 2002).

In conclusion, local availability, quality, and price should be the main factors determining use of wheat or maize in most parts of the world (Patience *et al.*, 1995). Properly balanced diets that take into account the strong and weak features of each ingredient support excellent performance throughout the world. However, when replacing wheat or maize with other cereals of lower nutrient density and higher concentrations of fiber and anti-nutritional factors, such as barley and rye, performance may suffer without serious alterations in diet design.

Programs for Breeders

Breeders of replacement animals often desire specific nutrition programs that enable pigs to fully express their genetic potential. Such programs are characterized by increased nutrient density and ingredients of enhanced complexity. Thus, they tend to be more expensive than common programs for terminal-market pigs. Goals in nursery feeding programs for breeders are usually one or more of the following.

Rapid growth

This is usually achieved by ensuring pigs start rapidly on feed after weaning. Diets rich in highly digestible ingredients such as animal plasma, dairy ingredients, and fishmeal usually elicit such response. These post-weaning diets are then followed by diets with elevated levels of amino acids and energy that allow high-health pigs to grow close to their genetic potential.

There are no strict guidelines regarding the degree of nutrient density and ingredient complexity that must applied, although some breeders offer their own dietary specifications or preferences. It is generally suggested, however, that incremental steps of 10% be tested until performance ceases to respond to further supplementation. Another strategy is to offer diets designed for commercial pigs (such as those described in this book) for longer periods of time, which can extend from a few days (in the initial stages post-weaning) to a couple weeks or longer (in the later stages of the nursery period). Again, no strict guidelines are available, but rather these allowances should be determined by trial and error for each specific operation.

Appearance

Most breeders are particularly interested in animal appearance. Thus, bloom, baby fat, and shiny overcoat are highly sought after in breeding animals. A liberal feeding regimen ensures sufficient fat deposition when pigs start eating immediately after weaning. If this is not easily achieved with dry diets, then liquid milk replacers may prevent the loss of pre-weaning 'baby fat'. A shiny coat may be achieved by a balanced nutrition program enhanced with oil or fat. Because most post-weaning diets contain 5–8% added oil or fat, this should be adequate under normal feed intake patterns. Supplemental zinc and linseed oil (1–2%) are also excellent hair coat conditioners.

Health

Naturally, scouring pigs are strongly disliked by breeders and their visiting customers. Scours in replacement animals not only reduce their marketability but may also depress growth rates. Unhealthy animals often fail to develop in time for breeding purposes. Prevention of health challenges through feed is usually in the form of additives (with variable results) and medications. Elimination or reduction of ingredients that could potentially be associated with pathogenic organisms, such as most animal-derived ingredients, is also required by many breeders. Finally, steps to control feed-borne salmonella and *E. coli* transmission, and inhibition of mold growth should be included in a well-designed program for quality assurance.

References

Alexander TJL, Thornton K, Boon G, Lysons RJ, and Gush AF (1980) Medicated early weaning to obtain pigs free from pathogens endemic in the herd of origin. *Veterinary Records* 106:114–119.

Bedford MR and Apajalahti J (2001) Microbial interactions in the response to exogenous enzyme utilization. In: *Enzymes in Farm Animal Nutrition* (2nd edn), by Bedford MR and Partridge GG (ed), 299–314. CABI Publishing, Wallingford, UK.

Best P (2001) Feeding against piglet diarrhoea. *Pig International* 31(6):19–21.

Brooks PH, Geary TM, Morgan DT, and Campbell A (1999) New developments in liquid feeding. *Pig Journal* 36:43–64.

Bustamante, SA Sanches N, Crosier J, Miranda D, Colombo G, and Miller MJ (1994) Dietary nucleotides: effects on the gastrointestinal system in swine. *Journal of Nutrition* 124:149S–156S.

Campbell RG (1989) The nutritional management of weaner pigs. In: *Manipulating Pig Production II*, by Barnett JL and Hennessy DP (ed), 170–175. Australasian Pig Science Association, Werribee, Australia.

Cardinal F, D'Allaire SD, and Fairbrother JM (2003) Feed composition in herds with and without postweaning *Escherichia coli* diarrhoea in early-weaned piglets. In: *Perspectives in Pig Science*, by Wiseman J, Varley MA, and Kemp B (ed), 491–492. Nottingham University Press, Nottingham, UK.

Case GL, Phillips RW, Lewis LD, and Connolly B (1981) Effects of osmolality of liquid nutrient diets on plasma equilibration of water and carbohydrate in Yucatan miniature swine. *American Journal of Clinical Nutrition* 34:1861–1867.

Cho WT, Kim Y, Kim JD, Chae BJ, and Han IK (2001) Effects of feeding extruded corn and wheat grain on growth performance and digestibility of amino acids in early-weaned pigs. *Asian–Australian Journal of Animal Science* 14:224–230.

Coffey RD and Cromwell GL (1995) The impact of environment and antimicrobial agents on the growth response of early weaned pigs to spray dried plasma. *Journal of Animal Science* 73:2532–2539.

Cole M and Sprent M (2001) Protein and amino acid requirements of weaner pigs. In: *The Weaner Pig – Nutrition and Management*, by Varley MA and Wiseman J (ed), 45–63. CABI Publishing, Wallingford, UK.

Cook DR, Ward MM, and Paton ND (2002) Effects of plasma grade, irradiation or formaldehyde treatment of plasma, or whole diet irradiation on growth performance of weaned pigs. *Journal of Animal Science* 80(Supplement 2):66.

Cranwell PD, Tarvid MA, and Harrison RG (1995) Weight at weaning, causes and consequences. In: *Manipulating Pig Production V*, by Hennessy DP and Cranwell PD (ed), 174. Australasian Pig Science Association, Werribee, Australia.

Cromwell GL (2002) Why and how antibiotics are used in swine production. *Animal Biotechnology* 13:7–27.

Davis ME, Maxwell CV, Brown DC, de Rodas BZ, Johnson ZB, Kegley EB, Hellwig DH, and Dvorak RA (2002) Effect of dietary mannan oligosaccharides and (or) pharmacological additions of copper sulfate on growth performance and immunocompetence of weanling and growing/finishing pigs. *Journal of Animal Science* 80:2887–2894.

DeRouchey JM, Tokach MD, Nelssen JL, Goodband RD, Dritz SS, Woodworth JC, and Hastad CW (2001) Comparison of irradiated feed and food grade spray-dried animal plasma on nursery pig performance. *Report No. 880*:10–16. Agricultural Experiment Station and Cooperative Extension Service, Kansas State University, Manhattan, KS.

Drew MD, van Kessel AG, Estrada AE, Ekpe ED, and Zijlstra RT (2002) Effect of dietary cereal on intestinal bacterial populations in weaned pigs. *Canadian Journal of Animal Science* 82:607–609.

Dupont HL and Steele JH (1987) Use of antimicrobial agents in animal feed: implications for human health. *Review of Infectious Diseases* 9:447–460.

Evans M (2001) Practical management and housing of the young weaned pig. In: *The Weaner Pig – Nutrition and Management*, by Varley MA and Wiseman J (ed), 299–307. CABI Publishing, Wallingford, UK.

FAO (1986) The production of fish meal and oil. *Fisheries Technical Paper No. 142*. Food and Agriculture Organization of the United Nations, Rome.

Fedorka-Cray PJ, Englen MD, Gray JT, Hudson C, and Headrick ML (2002) Programs for monitoring antimicrobial resistance. *Animal Biotechnology* 13:43–55.

Fowler V (1997) Fishmeal can provide insurance in pig diets. *Pig Farming* 8:20–21.

Gatnau R and Zimmerman DR (1990) Spray dried porcine plasma (SDPP) as a source of protein for weanling pigs. *Journal of Animal Science* 68(Supplement 1):374.

Goransson L, Lange S, and Lonroth I (1995) Post-weaning diarrhoea: focus on diet. *Pig News and Information* 16(3):89N–91N.

Goransson L (2001) Alternatives to antibiotics – the influence of new feeding strategies for pigs on biology and performance. In: *Recent Developments in Pig Nutrition 3*, by Wiseman J and Garnsworthy PC (ed), 39–50. Nottingham University Press, Nottingham, UK.

Gourmelen C, Royer E, and Rugraff Y (2002) *Facteurs de croissance et produits alternatifs en alimentation porcine*. Institut Technique du Porc, Rennes, France.

Hardy B (1992) Diets for young pigs. In: *Neonatal Survival and Growth*, by Varley MA, Williams PEV, and Lawrence TLJ (ed), 99–107. Occasional Publication No. 15. British Society of Animal Science, Midlothian, UK.

Hardy B (2002) The issue of antibiotic use in the livestock industry: what have we learned? *Animal Biotechnology* 13:129–147.

Hill GM, Cromwell GL, Crenshaw TD, Dove CR, Ewan RC, Knabe DA, Lewis AJ, Libal GW, Mahan DC, Shurson GC, Southern LL, and Veum TL (2000) Growth promotion effects and plasma changes from feeding high dietary concentrations of zinc and copper to weanling pigs (regional study). *Journal of Animal Science* 78:1010–1016.

Hill GM, Mahan DC, Carter SD, Cromwell GL, Ewan RC, Harrold RL, Lewis AJ, Miller PS, Shurson GC, and Veum TL (2001) Effect of pharmacological concentrations of zinc oxide with or without the inclusion of an antibacterial agent on nursery pig performance. *Journal of Animal Science* 79:934–941.

Holmberg SD, Osterholm MT, and Senger KA (1984) Drug-resistant Salmonella from animals fed antimicrobial agents. *New England Journal of Medicine* 311:617–622.

Hopwood DE and Hampson DJ (2003) Interactions between the intestinal microflora, diet and diarrhoea, and their influences on piglet health in the immediate post-weaning period. In: *Weaning the Pig: Concepts and Consequences*, by Pluske JR, Le Dividich J, and Verstengen MWA (ed), 199–218. Wageningen Academic Publishers, Wageningen, The Netherlands.

ITP (2002) *Tables d'alimentation pour les porcs* (13th edn). Institut Technique du Porc, Paris.

Jensen BB, Holberg O, Mikkelsen LL, Hedemann MS, and Canibe N (2003) Enhancing intestinal function to treat and prevent intestinal disease. *Proceedings of 9th International Symposium on Digestive Physiology in Pigs (Volume 1)*, 103–119. University of Alberta, Canada.

Johansen M, Jorgensen L, and Hansen CF (2000) Restricted feeding for prevention of *E. coli* associated diarrhea in weaned pigs. *16th International Pig Veterinary Society Congress (Volume 1)*, 20. Australia.

Kim SW, Mavromichalis I, and Easter RA (2001) Supplementation of α-1,6-galactosidase and β-1,4-mannanase to improve soybean meal utilization by nursery pigs. *Journal of Animal Science* 79(Supplement 1):106.

Lee YL, Cesario T, Owens J, Shanbrom E, and Thrupp LD (2002) Antibacterial activity of citrate and acetate. *Nutrition* 18:665–666.

Li DF, Nelssen JL, Reddy PG, Blecha F, Hancock JD, Allee GL, Goodband RD, and Klemm RD (1990) Transient hypersensitivity to soybean meal in the early-weaned pig. *Journal of Animal Science* 68:1790–1799.

Lis-Balchin M (2003) Feed additives as alternatives to antibiotic growth promoters: botanicals. *Proceedings of the 9th International Symposium on Digestive Physiology in Pigs (Volume 1)*, 333–352. University of Alberta, Canada.

Madec F, Bridoux F, Bounaix S, and Jestin A (1998) Measurement of digestive disorders in the piglet at weaning and related risk factors. *Preventative Veterinary Medicine* 35:53–72.

Mavromichalis I and Baker DH (1998) The complex diet for nursery pigs – its evolution in the USA. *Pig Progress* 14(9):45–47.

Mavromichalis I, Hancock JD, Senne BW, Gugle TL, Kennedy GA, Hines RH, and Wyatt CL (2000) Enzyme supplementation and particle size of wheat in diets for nursery and finishing pigs. *Journal of Animal Science* 78:3086–3095.

Mavromichalis I and Varley MA (2003) Transition feeding systems for weaned pigs. In: *Perspectives of Pig Science*, by Wiseman J, Varley MA, and Kemp KBF (ed), 405–456. Nottingham University Press, Nottingham, UK.

Maxwell CV Jr and Carter SD (2000) Feeding the weaned pig. In: *Swine Nutrition* (2nd edn), by Lewis AJ and Southern LL (ed), 691–723. CRC Press LLC, Boca Raton, FL.

McCracken BA, Spurlock ME, Roos MA, Zuckermann FA, and Gaskins HR (1999) Weaning anorexia may contribute to local inflammation in the piglet small intestine. *Journal of Nutrition* 129:613–619.

McDonald DE, Pethick DW, Mullan BP, and Hampson DJ (2001) Increasing the viscosity of the intestinal contents alters small intestinal structure and intestinal growth, and stimulates proliferation of enterotoxigenic *Escherichia coli* in newly-weaned pigs. *British Journal of Nutrition* 86:487–498.

Miller HM and Toplis P (2000) Supplement containing immunoglobulins fed post weaning promotes nursery pig performance. *Proceedings of the Annual Meeting of the British Society of Animal Science*, 164. York, UK.

Montagne L, Lockwood FS, Lalles JP, Hampson DJ, and Pluske JR (2003a) Cereal and protein sources influence the proliferation of enterotoxigenic *Escherichia coli* in the gastrointestinal tract of piglets after weaning. *Proceedings of the 9th International Symposium on Digestive Physiology in Pigs (Volume 2)*, 183–185. University of Alberta, Canada.

Montagne L, Pluske JR, and Hampson DJ (2003b) A review of interactions between dietary fibre and the intestinal mucosa, and their consequences on digestive health in young non-ruminant animals. *Animal Feed Science and Technology* 108:95–117.

Mosenthin R, Hambrecht E, and Sauer WC (1999) Utilization of different fibers in piglet feeds. In: *Recent Advances in Animal Nutrition*, by Garnsworthy PC and Wiseman J (ed), 227–256. Nottingham University Press, Nottingham, UK.

Mroz Z (2003) Organic acids of various origins and physico-chemical forms as potential alternatives to antibiotic growth promoters for pigs. *Proceedings of the 9th International Symposium on Digestive Physiology in Pigs (Volume 1)*, 267–293. University of Alberta, Canada.

Nabuurs MJA, van de Weijgert EJHM, Grootendorst AF, and Niewold TA (2001) Oedema disease is associated with metabolic acidosis and small intestinal acidosis. *Research in Veterinary Science* 70:247–253.

Naylor RL, Goldburg RJ, Primavera JH, Kautsky N, Beveridge MCM, Clay J, Folke C, Lubchenco J, Mooney H, and Troell M (2000) Effect of aquaculture on world fish supplies. *Nature* 405:1017–1024.

Nelssen JL, Dritz SS, Tokach MD, and Goodband RD (1999) Nutritional programs for segregated early weaning. In: *Diseases of Swine* (8th edn), by Straw BE, D'Allaire S, Mengeling WL, and Taylor DJ (ed), 1045–1055. Iowa State University, Ames, IA.

NRC (1998a) *Nutrient Requirements of Swine* (10th edn). National Academy Press, Washington, DC.

NRC (1998b) *The Use of Drugs in Food Animals: Benefits and Risks*. National Academy Press, Washington, DC.

Nunez MC, Ayudarte MV, Morales D, Suarez MD, and Gil A (1990) Effect of dietary nucleotides on intestinal repair in rats with experimental chronic diarrhea. *Journal of Parenteral and Enteral Nutrition* 14:598–604.

Olsen LE and Maribo H (1999) Commercial feed and feed products for piglets. *Report No. 433*. The Federation of Danish Pig Producers and Slaughterhouses, Copenhagen.

Owusu-Asiedu A, Baidoo SK, Nyachoti CM, and Marquardt RR (2002) Response of early-weaned pigs to spray-dried porcine or animal plasma-based diets supplemented with egg-yolk antibodies against enterotoxigenic *Escherichia coli*. *Journal of Animal Science* 80:2895–2903.

Owusu-Asiedu A, Nyachoti CM, and Marquardt RR (2003) Egg yolk antibody, zinc oxide, and fumaric acid supplementation provides passive control to *Escherichia coli* (K88) infection in early-weaned pigs fed pea protein isolate-containing diets. *Proceedings of the 9th International Symposium on Digestive Physiology in Pigs (Volume 1)*, 232–234. University of Alberta, Canada.

Partanen K, Siljander-Rasi H, Alaviuhkola T, Suomi K, and Fossi M (2002) Performance of growing-finishing pigs fed medium- or high-fibre diets supplemented with avilamycin, formic acid or formic acid–sorbate blend. *Livestock Production Science* 73:139–152.

Partridge IG (1989) Alternative feeding strategies for weaner pigs. In: *Manipulating Pig Production II*, by Barnett JL and Hennessy DP (ed), 160–169. Australasian Pig Science Association, Werribee, Australia.

Partridge GG (2001) The role and efficacy of carbohydrase enzymes in pig nutrition. In: *Enzymes in Farm Animal Nutrition* (2nd edn), by Bedford MR and Partridge GG (ed), 161–198. CABI Publishing, Wallingford, UK.

Patience JF, Thacker PA, and de Lange CFM (1989) *Swine Nutrition Guide*. Prairie Swine Center, Saskatchewan, Canada.

Patience JF, Thacker PA, and de Lange CFM (1995) *Swine Nutrition Guide* (2nd edn). Prairie Swine Center, Saskatchewan, Canada.

Patterson JA and Burkholder KM (2003) Prebiotic feed additives: rationale and use in pigs. *Proceedings of the 9th International Symposium on Digestive Physiology in Pigs (Volume 1)*, 319–331. University of Alberta, Canada.

Pluske JR, Black B, Pethick DW, Mullan BP, and Hampson DJ (2003) Effects of different sources and levels of dietary fibre in diets on performance, digesta characteristics and antibiotic treatment of pigs after weaning. *Animal Feed Science and Technology* 107:129–142.

Prohaszka L and Baron D (2001) The predisposing role of high dietary protein supplies in enteropathogenic *E. coli* infection of weaned pigs. *Zentralblatt für Veterinarmedizin* 27:222–232.

Quigley JD, Campbell JM, Crenshaw JD, Russell LE, and Polo FJ (2003) Effects of spray-dried animal plasma on intestinal health of weaned pigs challenged with *Escherichia coli*. *Proceedings of the 9th International Symposium on Digestive Physiology in Pigs (Volume 2)*, 75–77. University of Atlanta, Canada.

Salyers A (2002) An overview of the genetic basis of antibiotic resistance in bacteria and its implications for agriculture. *Animal Biotechnology* 13:1–5.

Simon O, Vahjen W, and Scharek L (2003) Micro-organisms as feed additives – probiotics. *Proceedings of the 9th International Symposium on Digestive Physiology in Pigs (Volume 1)*, 295–318. University of Alberta, Canada.

Sprent M, Cole MA, and Varley MA (2000) The use of supplementary creep feed for pre-weaned piglets on subsequent performance. *Proceedings of the British Society of Animal Science Occasional Meeting 'The Weaner Pig – Nutrition and Management'*, 42. University of Nottingham, Nottingham, UK.

Spring P, Wenk C, Dawson KA, and Newman KE (2000) The effects of dietary mannanoligosaccharides on cecal parameters and the concentrations of enteric bacteria in the ceca of Salmonella-challenged broiler chicks. *Poultry Science* 79:205–211.

Stahly TS, Cook DR, Swenson SG, Williams NH, and Zimmerman DR (1995) Growth responses of pigs to dietary plasma protein (PP) additions as influenced by pig antigen exposure and PP source. *Journal of Animal Science* 73(Supplement 1):81.

Stein HH (2002) Experience of feeding pigs without antibiotics: European perspective. *Animal Biotechnology* 13:85–95.

Thacker PA (1999) Nutritional requirements of early weaned pigs: a review. *Pig News and Information* 20:13N–24N.

Toplis P and Miller HM (1999) Postweaning benefits of porcine plasma. *Proceedings of the British Society of Animal Science Annual Meeting*, 173, Scarborough, UK.

Uauy RG, Stringel, Thomas R, and Quan R (1990) Effect of dietary nucleotides on growth and maturation of the developing gut in the rat. *Journal of Pediatric Gastroenterology and Nutrition* 10:497–503.

van Dijk AJ, Everts H, Nabuurs MJA, Margry RJCF, and Beynen AC (2001) Growth performance of weanling pigs fed spray-dried animal plasma: a review. *Livestock Production Science* 68:263–274.

Wallgren P and Melin L (2001) Weaning systems in relation to disease. In: *The Weaner Pig – Nutrition and Management*, by Varley MA and Wiseman J (ed), 309–316. CABI Publishing, Wallingford, UK.

Weber E and Ehrlein HJ (1998) Glucose and maltodrextrin in enteral diets have different effects on jejunal absorption of nutrients, sodium, and water and on flow rate in mini pigs. *Deutsche Tierärztliche Wochenschrift* 105:446–449.
Witte W, Klare I, and Werner G (2002) Molecular ecological studies on spread of antibiotic resistance genes. *Animal Biotechnology* 13:57–70.
Zarkadas LN and Wiseman J (2000) Inclusion of differently processed full-fat soya bean in diets for piglets. *Proceedings of the British Society of Animal Science Occasional Meeting 'The Weaner Pig – Nutrition and Management'*, 45–46. University of Nottingham, Nottingham, UK.

10 Creep Feeding

Introduction

It is interesting to note that although the practice of creep feeding was developed when pigs were housed mainly outdoors, it is still employed today even though most commercial pigs are reared in enclosed facilities. Before intensive pig production was introduced, sows were kept in pasture or dry lots and they farrowed in groups while roaming relatively freely with their litters. Because weaning took place usually after 6 weeks of age, there was a pressing need to provide piglets with supplemented feed to support the declining supply of sow's milk. Such feeds were offered in creep areas or pens (hence, the term creep feeding), which had openings large enough only for piglets to enter, thus preventing sows effectively from entering the creep area to consume the expensive 'creep' feed (Mohler, 1922).

The Practice Today

Today, most lactating sows are housed indoors with relatively restricted freedom for movement, and, thus, no special creep areas are needed in farrowing stalls. Yet, the practice of providing supplemental feed to piglets during the lactation period is still called creep feeding and the diets creep feeds. Of course, in modern housing systems that allow sows to intermix freely with their litters, creep areas have been revived.

Creep feeding is more common in parts of the world where weaning age is over 3 weeks of age, and especially in Europe where creep feeding has a long tradition. With recent EU regulations calling for weaning at 4 weeks or older, the emphasis on creep feeding has increased (King and Pluske, 2003).

In areas where weaning is before 3 weeks of age, creep feeding is practiced sporadically depending on specific farm preferences and experiences. It is notable that in North America, creep feeding has been almost discontinued with the advent of very early weaning at 15–17 days of age.

Although providing a liquid form of diet to suckling piglets is indeed creep feeding, such practice is called liquid feeding (or feeding a milk replacer). Traditionally, the term creep feeding has been reserved for dry feeding. Gruel feeding is another form of supplemental nutrition that can be described under liquid, dry, or creep feeding, but for lack of any better classification it is examined here, under creep feeding.

Benefits

The question whether creep feeding is worth investing the money and effort required to make it effective has been pondered constantly in the past (Pluske *et al.*, 1995). As results from such practice depend entirely on the amount of feed eaten and time of exposure to such feed before weaning, it is important to consider them in the context of production schemes under commercial conditions.

In production systems practicing prolonged lactation periods (over 6 weeks) creep feeding is a necessity to protect the condition and health of the lactating sow, especially if she cannot isolate herself from her litter. In such systems, it is a common observation that sows after the third week of lactation start to lose body condition quickly unless piglets are introduced to creep feeding (Patience *et al.*, 1995). It is about this time also that milk production starts to decline naturally, while nutrient demand from piglets continues to increase. Thus, the sooner piglets start consuming supplemental feed, the better the condition of the sow at the end of the lactation.

In late-weaning production systems, where pigs are weaned around their fourth week of age, the main benefit of creep feeding is the increased weaning weight as pigs have time to consume enough feed to make such a difference notable. Indeed, in a recent trial involving piglets weaned under commercial conditions around their fourth week of age, British researchers (Sprent *et al.*, 2000) indicated that creep-fed piglets were about 1 kg heavier at weaning compared to counterparts receiving no supplemental nutrition while on the sow (Fig. 10.1). This observation is supported by most studies involving late-weaned pigs (Friend *et al.*, 1970; Aherne *et al.*, 1982) that consumed enough feed pre-weaning, but not by others (Okai *et al.*, 1976; Hampson and Kidder, 1986) in which creep feed intake was low or highly variable between and among litters. Assuming that the feed conversion rate in young pigs is around or even below 1:1 (feed/gain), we can easily assess that the benefits of creep feeding in terms of enhanced weaning weight are proportional to the amount of creep feed consumed (except of course when feed wastage is excessive).

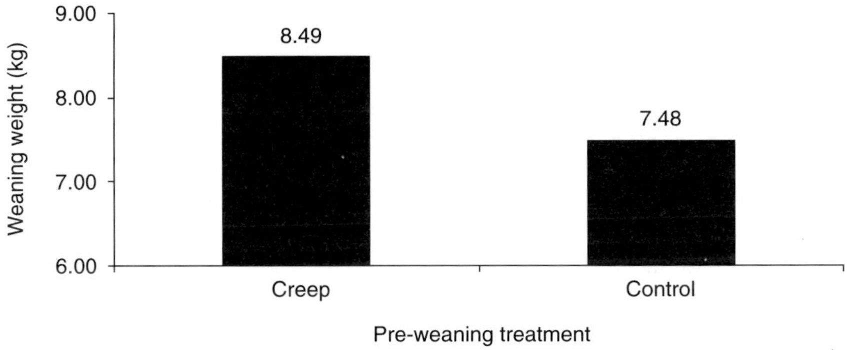

Fig. 10.1. Creep feeding enhanced weaning weight at 4 weeks of age by around 1 kg ($P < 0.05$). (From Sprent *et al.*, 2000.)

In production systems weaning between 3 and 4 weeks of age, intake of creep feed is usually not sufficient to enhance weaning weight in any substantial way, and this has been demonstrated consistently (Okai *et al.*, 1976; Barnett *et al.*, 1989). But, the induction of digestive enzymes in preparation for handling dry feed after weaning (Cranwell, 1977; Corring, 1980) is often considered enough of a benefit to allow for creep feeding. Indeed, it has been clearly demonstrated in earlier studies that creep feeding induces maturation of the digestive system and enhances the production of enzymes (amylases and proteases) suitable for digesting the complex nutrients usually found in post-weaning diets (Friend *et al.*, 1970; Hampson and Kidder, 1986; Kelly, 1990). The consequences of such pre-weaning education of the digestive system are believed to be: (i) reduced digestive upsets (Hampson, 1986); and (ii) enhanced feed intake and growth post-weaning. This, of course, is related to the level of creep feed intake before weaning (Pluske *et al.*, 1995).

When weaning age is below 3 weeks, the only possible benefit of creep feeding can be that of getting piglets accustomed to recognize dry feed as nourishment, as feed intake is usually insufficient to cause any substantial changes in digestive system and weaning weight parameters. Such benefit is not well documented and is based largely on anecdotal evidence and farm-specific experiences. Success is naturally quite variable as feed intake at such young age is also extremely variable and unpredictable (Pluske *et al.*, 1995).

Creep Feeds

All diets described in Chapters 5 and 9 are suitable as creep feeds for piglets of the appropriate weight. More dense diets, or formulas especially rich in lactose (up to 50%), would be even better, especially for piglets weaned very early.

For piglets weaned before the third week of age, the first diet (4–6 kg body weight) described in Table 9.1 is rather suitable as a creep feed. For piglets weaned between the third and fourth week of age, the next diet (6–8 kg body weight) would be adequate, but for piglets weaned after the fourth week of age, two creep diets should be offered. The first feed can be one of the two diets described above, whereas the second feed should be the diet piglets will consume immediately after weaning (this can be the diet for 8–12 kg body weight). Offering an expensive diet for too long would be cost-prohibitive, whereas offering a later diet to very young pigs would certainly induce digestive upsets.

The form of creep feed has received little scientific attention. It is generally believed that very young pigs benefit more from creep feed in meal form because they might have difficulty chewing pellets if they are too hard. The usually sticky nature of a powdery creep feed may also enhance the speed by which piglets accept this diet as it tends to stick in their snouts while exploring it and, thus, it forces them to lick and ingest it. Nevertheless, meal diets are usually not favored by producers as they tend to cake due to their high content of milk products. Wastage of creep feed is usually higher with meal; with the exception of pellets offered on sleeping mats without rims as piglets enjoy rolling them over the edges. Regardless of the form of creep feed selected for suckling pigs, it is important to use the same form for the first feed offered post-weaning to facilitate the establishment of early appetite.

There are no feed additives specifically designed for creep feeds (King and Pluske, 2003). Nevertheless, it is often advised to include a probiotic/prebiotic combination to enhance the early establishment of a beneficial microflora. It is also recommended that the taste/aroma of the creep feed be similar of that in the feed offered immediately post-weaning. To this effect, it is often suggested that the same creep feed be used for the first 2 or 3 days in the post-weaning nursery facility. It has also been suggested (Madsen, 1977) that the same flavor be used in the sow lactation diet, piglet creep feed and first post-weaning diet to enhance piglet feed intake (some flavors may be transferred from sow's feed to milk and thus impart a flavor preference to piglets that could last well after weaning).

How Much to Feed?

The answer to this question is rather simple: as much as possible. For all practical purposes, however, a minimum allowance should be established, at least for the task of placing a feed order.

Piglets weaned before the third week of age may consume about 100 g/piglet under the best management conditions, and it is a rare case when a farm succeeds in feeding more than 250 g/piglet (actual consumption excluding wastage). It is therefore suggested that no more than 50 g/piglet be allowed for the first time a unit runs a trial with creep feeding, with subsequent amounts adjusted according to gained experience.

Piglets weaned between 3 and 4 weeks of age should consume around 500 g/piglet, because this ensures proper development of the digestive system (English, 1999). Piglets consuming less than this amount might be susceptible to developing an allergic hypersensitivity reaction to certain feed antigens that manifests itself negatively after weaning (Miller *et al.*, 1984), especially when piglets start consuming large amounts of dry feed.

Piglets weaned later than 4 weeks of age should consume at least 500 g/piglet of the first creep feed, and then be offered the first post-weaning diet for consumption *ad libitum* to prevent overfeeding of the expensive first creep feed. If the reaction of piglets to the second, less-complex diet is negative (feed refusal, scours), then it is recommended that the first diet be fed longer and the amount offered be increased to 750 or even 1000 g/piglet; again actual figures should be based on trial and error.

From the above, it is rather apparent that no solid advice based on concrete scientific evidence is available such that it can be used without skepticism under all possible conditions. Thus, the recommendations above should be used only as starting points in developing a farm-specific creep feeding program, if any can be justified at all!

Management

Practical experience indicates that the success of creep feeding depends largely on the management of the practice, with different human operators having quite variable results even within the same building. It is often surprising that some young pigs will not consume a highly digestible and palatable creep diet, or for the same purpose a warm liquid milk replacer, even though they have the genetic potential for growth beyond that conferred by the supply of sow's milk. Thus, enticing piglets to consume creep feed is as important, or even more important, as selecting the proper formula or brand of feed. The following are offered for consideration based again more on practical experience rather than hard scientific evidence, which is currently unavailable:

- Only the most palatable and digestible diets available should be used, albeit this can be quite expensive, because these factors govern almost exclusively feed intake in young pigs.
- Creep feeds should be stored in a cool and dry place to preserve their nutritive value and organoleptic properties. Clearly, such feeds should not be stored inside the nursery barn next to animal pens. Care should be taken to prevent contamination by rodents and insects.
- Creep feeding should start as soon as possible after the first week of age, with feed allowance gradually increasing to match piglet appetite, taking care to avoid wastage or leftover feed.

- Feed should be offered on a little-and-often basis. This prevents feed from being spoiled and triggers piglets to explore the new feed more vigorously. Feeding three times per day is often recommended as optimum.
- Creep feeding should be done between sow feedings and not concurrently. Sows almost always nurse their litters right after eating, and, thus, piglets might refuse to eat dry feed in expectance of a better meal.
- Nevertheless, a limited amount of creep feed may be offered at the time of feeding the sow as some piglets might try to imitate the feeding behavior of the sow, or prefer a lesser meal to fierce rivalry from stronger littermates.
- At the time of creep feeding any leftover feed should be discarded (fed to the sow) to ensure piglets will continue to explore the new feed with interest.
- When creep feeders and floor-mats (when feed is offered on them) are found soiled they should be cleaned before adding more creep feed. If piglets continue to soil them, it is advisable to change the position of the feeder.
- Creep feeders should be placed near (but not below) the piglets' water drinker, ideally near the head of the sow so that piglets can imitate her feeding behavior.
- Placing feed directly under a heating lamp will rapidly spoil the feed, but placing the feeder too far away from heating lamp might reduce the number of visits piglets pay to it, especially during cold weather.
- Creep feeders that allow communal feeding are deemed more successful than feeders that can accommodate only a few piglets at a time (Appleby *et al.*, 1991).

Gruel Feeding

Despite the advent of high-quality creep diets some pigs still fail to recognize dry feed as a proper form of nourishment. In these cases, it is suggested that creep feed be offered as gruel to enhance acceptance. Although this discussion regards pre-weaned piglets, the same procedures outlined here are also suitable for piglets that fail to thrive after weaning and end up as runts or 'fallbacks'.

British researchers recently showed in repeated studies that gruel feeding improves intake of dry matter and growth performance of piglets (Toplis *et al.*, 1999; Blanchard *et al.*, 2000). For example, piglets that were offered gruel feed before weaning were about 10% heavier 35 days after weaning compared to control pigs that received no supplemental diet while suckling.

Although provision of a liquid milk replacer greatly enhances intake of dry matter and weaning weight (Azain *et al.*, 1996), this practice is seldom feasible to implement on a large scale due to high cost and labor requirements. Gruel feeding, on the other hand, is both practical and economical and it can be equally effective in increasing dry matter intake. Gruel feeding requires minimal investment in equipment, but some investment in labor is essential if it is to be done properly. Lock-down feeders are usually sufficient, although any shallow container can be used (Fig. 10.2). Any high-quality creep or pre-starter diet can be used for both gruel and dry feeding.

Pigs should receive gruel no more than three times per day; otherwise they may fail to consume dry feed, which should be offered *ad libitum* in dry feeders from the first day. Feeding gruel for 3 to 5 days is usually enough for most piglets to recover and associate dry feed with nourishment, but specific cases may call for longer periods of gruel feeding (up to 10 days for sick pigs is not uncommon).

A gradual change from gruel-supplemented nutrition to all-dry diets is recommended. To this end, gruel consistency must be gradually thickened to allow pigs to adapt to dry formulas. It is also advisable to use the same formula fed as gruel in dry form (meal or pellets) to accelerate the transition from gruel to dry feeding. Table 10.1 provides an example of a 5-day program with gruel feeding. In this program, the gruel consistency changes

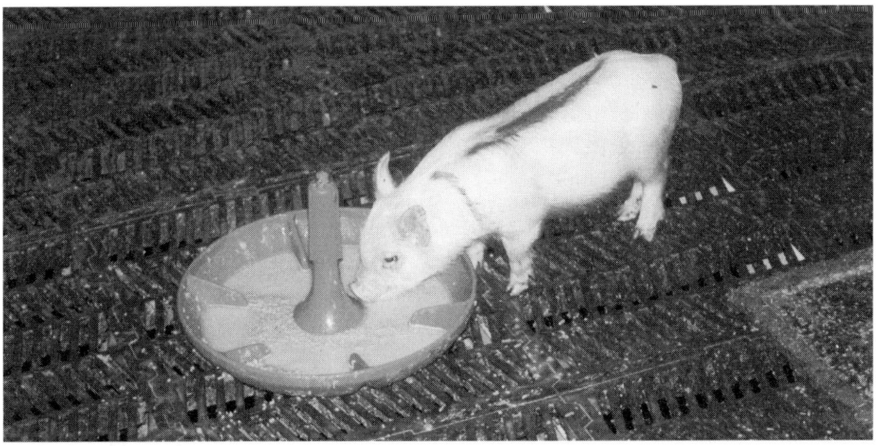

Fig. 10.2. Gruel feeding in a US commercial nursery barn.

Table 10.1. Example of a 5-day program for feeding gruel to piglets before or after weaning.

Day	Mix (water/feed)	Feedings (per day)
1	3:1	3
2	2:2	3
3	2:2	2
4	1:3	2
5	1:3	1

gradually within the first three days, but a more 'liquid' gruel may be fed longer if piglets start refusing a thicker consistency.

The gruel must always be prepared fresh for each meal in a bucket or any other suitable container and then distributed in lock-down feeders or bowls. A simple container may be fixed with an electric stirring device to facilitate rapid and easy preparation of gruel in larger batches. Alternatively, feed taken from self-feeders can be mixed in lock-down feeders with water from drinkers in each individual pen. Pigs should receive only enough gruel to consume in a single feeding episode of about 10–20 min. Leftovers should be cleaned before offering fresh gruel. At least one lock-down feeder for every ten piglets is recommended to ensure sufficient consumption of gruel by all pigs.

Sometimes, especially during the first couple of days of gruel feeding, pigs may drink the liquid and leave a paste of feed at the bottom of the feeder. This indicates pigs are particularly thirsty and an alternative way of providing water must be investigated. If this continues to happen, it is a good idea to check drinkers to ensure they function properly and provide enough flow for all piglets to satisfy their thirst. Otherwise, replenishing the feeder with more water usually results in consumption of all feed.

References

Aherne FX, Danielson V, and Nielsen HE (1982) The effects of creep feeding on pre- and post-weaning pig performance. *Acta Agricultura Scandinavia Section A* 32:155–160.

Appleby MC, Pajor EA, and Fraser D (1991) Effects of management options on creep feeding by piglets. *Animal Production* 53:361–366.

Azain MJ, Tomkins T, Sowinski JS, Arentson RA, and Jewell DE (1996) Effect of supplemental pig milk replacer on litter performance: seasonal variation in response. *Journal of Animal Science* 74:2195–2202.

Barnett KL, Kornegay ET, Risley CR, Lindemann MD, and Schurig GG (1989) Characterization of creep feed consumption and its subsequent effects on immune response, scouring index and performance of weanling pigs. *Journal of Animal Science* 67:2698–2708.

Blanchard PJ, Toplis P, Taylor L, and Miller HM (2000) Liquid diets prior to weaning enhance performance of weaned piglets. *Proceedings of the Annual Meeting of the British Society of Animal Science*, 119. York, UK.

Corring T (1980) The adaptation of digestive enzymes to the diet: its physiological significance. *Reproduction, Nutrition, Development* 20:1217–1235.

Cranwell PD (1977) Acid and pepsin secretion in young pigs reared solely by the sow or supplemented with solid food and weaned at 21 d. *Proceedings of the Nutrition Society* 36:142A.

English P (1999) The importance of a high weaning weight and milk intake. *Pig Progress* 15(1):27–30.

Friend DW, Gorrill DL, and MacIntyre TM (1970) Performance and proteolytic enzyme activity of the suckling piglet creep-fed at one or three weeks of age. *Canadian Journal of Animal Science* 50:349–354.

Hampson DJ (1986) Influence of creep feeding and dietary intake after weaning on malabsorption and occurrence of diarrhoea in the newly weaned pig. *Research in Veterinary Science* 41:63–69.

Hampson DJ and Kidder DE (1986) Influence of creep feeding and weaning on brush border enzyme activities in the piglet small intestine. *Research in Veterinary Science* 40:24–31.

Kelly D (1990) Effect of creep feeding on structural and functional changes of the gut of early weaned pigs. *Research in Veterinary Science* 48:350–356.

King RH and Pluske JR (2003) Nutritional management of the pig in preparation for weaning. In: *Weaning the Pig – Concepts and Consequences*, by Pluske JR, Le Dividich J, and Verstegen MWA (ed), 37–51. Wageningen Academic Publishers, Wageningen, The Netherlands.

Madsen FC (1997) Development of feed preference in young swine. *Feedstuffs* 39(5):25.

Miller BG, Newby TJ, Stokes CR, Hampson DJ, Brown PJ, and Bourne FJ (1984) The importance of dietary antigen in the cause of postweaning diarrhea in pigs. *American Journal of Veterinary Research* 45:1730–1733.

Mohler J (1922) *Hogs in Kansas* (2nd edn). Kansas State Board of Agriculture, Topeka, KS.

Okai DB, Aherne FX, and Hardin RT (1976) Effects of creep and starter composition on feed intake and performance of young pigs. *Canadian Journal of Animal Science* 56:573–586.

Patience JF, Thacker PA, and de Lange CFM (1995) *Swine Nutrition Guide* (2nd edn). Prairie Swine Center, Saskatchewan, Canada.

Pluske JR, Williams IH, and Aherne FX (1995) Nutrition of the neonatal pig. In: *The Neonatal Pig: Development and Survival*, by Varley MA (ed), 187–235. CAB International, Wallingford, UK.

Sprent M, Cole MA, and Varley MA (2000) The use of supplementary creep feed for pre-weaned piglets on subsequent performance. *Proceedings of the British Society of Animal Science Occasional Meeting 'The Weaner Pig – Nutrition and Manegement'*, 42. University of Nottingham, Nottingham, UK.

Toplis P, Blanchard PJ, and Miller HM (1999) Creep feed offered as a gruel prior to weaning enhances performance of weaned piglets. In: *Manipulating Pig Production VII*, by Cranwell P (ed), 129. Australasian Pig Science Association, Werribee, Australia.

11 Liquid Feeding

Introduction

Back in 1922, hogs raised on small-scale (family) farms were often given a 'slop' consisting of dry cereals and other ingredients mixed with water and (or) dairy by-products such as whey and buttermilk. This kind of nutrition was considered superior to an all-dry diet; perhaps because grinding of cereals was not practiced to any great extent (Mohler, 1922).

In the 1950s and 1960s, the expansion of industrial milk processing factories for the production of dairy products such as cheese, yogurt, and butter created a superfluity of liquid by-products that were often given free of charge to farmers willing to incur transportation costs for removal from the factory. Such opportunities increased interest in liquid feeding practices under large-scale commercial operations and also enhanced the understanding of the practice and its problems (Gadd, 2003).

As recently as the 1990s, the benefits of liquid feeding, even when the added liquid was only water, were firmly established in terms of animal growth performance and health, not only for growing-finishing pigs but also for sows and piglets (Brooks, 1999; Brooks *et al.*, 1999).

Today, liquid feeding is a highly sophisticated practice employed in progressive operations, but it still lacks the popularity of the simpler dry feeding methods, mostly because of the greater cost of acquiring a liquid feeding system.

The Practice Today

In most commercial farms practicing liquid feeding (Fig. 11.1), a computerized system is used to mix and deliver feed. Mixing recipes are entered into a computer, which in turn is connected to storage bins and one or more mixing tanks. When feed is required, ingredients are automatically delivered to and mixed with water and (or) liquid by-products to the desired dry matter concentration in a mixing tank equipped with a stirring mechanism. Pneumatic conveyors then deliver the soup to individual pens as required based on electronic depth sensors in each trough (Fig. 11.2). With such a system, it is also possible to deliver different diets to different pens within a room according to body weight and (or) age of pigs (data previously entered in the computer). One of the great benefits of such computerized systems is that feed intake is monitored on a daily basis and this offers a tool in detecting forthcoming problems.

Benefits

The most obvious benefit from liquid feeding is increased feed intake. It has been clearly demonstrated in repeated trials (Table 11.1) that pigs consume on average 12% more dry matter when offered liquid rather than dry diets (Jensen and Mikkelsen, 1998), with increases up to 33% not being

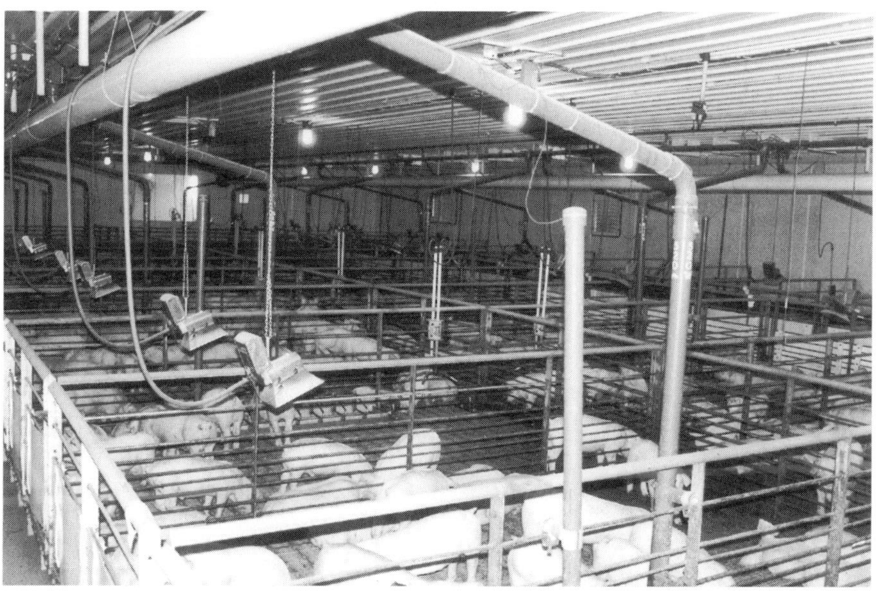

Fig. 11.1. Liquid feeding system in a commercial nursery facility.

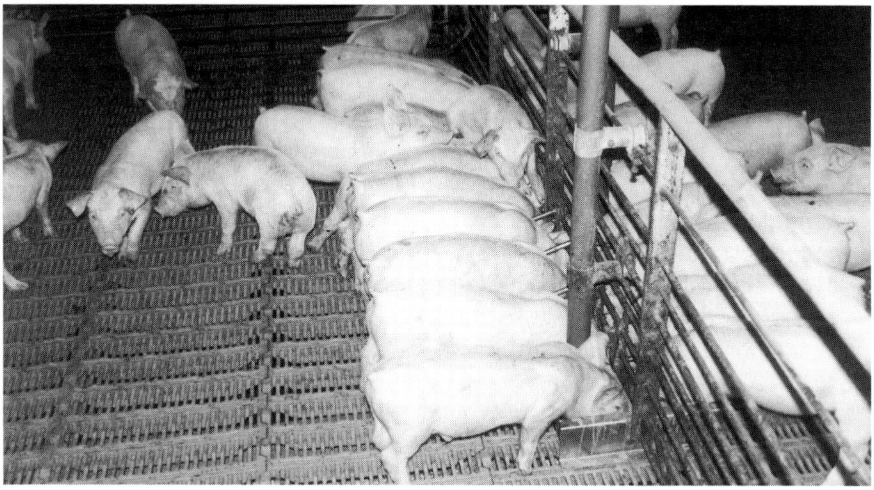

Fig. 11.2. Close-up of a feeding trough equipped with a depth sensor.

Table 11.1. Comparative performance differences according to feed presentation form in piglets. (Adapted from Jensen and Mikkelsen, 1998.)

	No. of trials	Weight gain (%)		Feed/gain (%)	
		Average	Range	Average	Range
Liquid versus dry	10	+12	–8 to 34	–4	–33 to 10
Fermented liquid versus dry	4	+22	9 to 44	–11	–44 to 6
Fermented liquid versus liquid	3	+13	6 to 23	–1	– to 1

uncommon. Efficiency of feed utilization has been found to be inferior for liquid feed, perhaps due to excessive wastage, which today is addressed via management and trough design interventions.

Other benefits, largely based on field observations and to a lesser degree on scientific evidence, include reduced dust in the facilities with associated respiratory health benefits, reduced incidences of salmonella (Gadd, 2003), ability to utilize liquid and semi-liquid by-products (see below), reduced animal aggression and particularly belly-nosing (Brooks *et al.*, 2001), and improved gut health as evidenced by reduced scours, especially with properly fermented liquid feeding (see below).

Disadvantages

Obviously, the most serious concerns over liquid feeding in general are initial cost and demand for on-farm professional training. Assuming financial and technical difficulties are overcome, the neophyte user is then faced with not insignificant issues that must be addressed even before the first batch of pigs enters the building.

Fermentation

Although controlled fermentation can be advantageous, the opposite can have quite detrimental effects on animal health. This is perhaps the major complaint from newly established liquid feeding systems. Uncontrolled fermentation often results in increased populations of *E. coli*, salmonella, yeasts, and other possible pathogens. To this effect acidification with lactic acid to pH 4 is often recommended (Canibe *et al.*, 2002) as well as treatment with 300 ppm chlorine dioxide (Demeckova *et al.*, 2001). It should be noted that each mixing and delivery system is provided with specific procedures for cleaning and disinfection that must be followed strictly to ensure animal health and feed nutritive value.

Dry matter

Another crucial issue in liquid feeding is the dry matter concentration of the soup. The rule of thumb is three parts water for each part dry feed or approximately 25% dry matter. Many older delivery systems were unable to deliver a thicker mix, whereas a less dense soup was undesirable because of increased effluent production. Research has clearly demonstrated that piglets can effectively use liquid diets even with 15% dry matter (Fig. 11.3) without

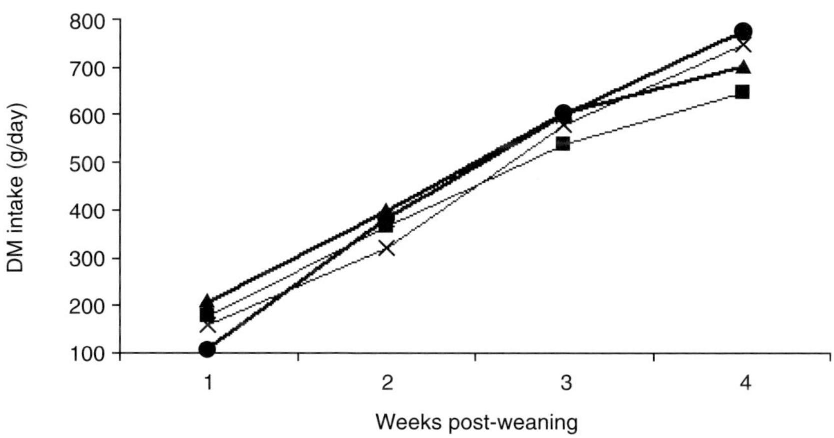

Fig. 11.3. Piglets sustained high dry matter (DM) intake from liquid diets even when density (▲, 25%; ■, 22%; ●, 18%; ×, 15%) dropped considerably. (Adapted from Geary *et al.*, 1996.)

any loss in performance (Geary *et al.*, 1996), although a soup with 25% dry matter is strongly recommended for the first week post-weaning (Brooks *et al.*, 2001).

Effluent production

Experience indicates that pigs consuming liquid diets produce more effluent, especially when fed liquid by-products rich in protein and (or) salt. This can be a desirable effect as the slurry becomes thinner and can be handled more easily or, in contrast, an undesirable effect as more effluent must be disposed of at greater cost. Nevertheless, it is recommended (Brooks *et al.*, 2001) that soup dry matter be kept above 20% to control effluent production.

Water availability

It is strongly recommended to provide pigs with free access to fresh non-saline water, even when liquid diets contain no liquid by-products and (or) normal sodium levels. Pigs require water at variable quantities according to individual body weight and growth rate, room temperature, and health.

Feed refusal

It is occasionally reported that, during the first few days post-weaning, pigs previously unfamiliar with liquid feed may refuse to eat, despite no obvious faults with the feed. This is often resolved by placing some dry feed in lock-down feeders close to the liquid feed troughs for a couple of days or until pigs start consuming liquid feed.

Liquid By-products

The recycling of liquid by-products from the human food industry through feeding to animals, and especially pigs, has increased considerably during the past couple of decades (Scholten *et al.*, 1999). Most agro-industrial by-products are rich in carbohydrates, but protein- and (or) fat-rich by-products are not uncommon. The most common liquid by-products are described below.

Cheese whey

Most likely the major dairy by-product throughout the world, cheese whey is readily available in most milk-producing areas and it is especially attractive to farmers near cheese factories. It has around 5% dry matter, 12–13% crude protein (in dry matter), and 60–70% lactose (in dry matter). The salt (sodium) content may be variable and can limit its use as a feed ingredient.

Due to its low dry matter content, intake might be limited in piglets due to small stomach physical capacity. Diets based on liquid whey seldom require further dilution with water.

Liquid wheat starch

A by-product of the extraction of starch and gluten from wheat, liquid wheat starch contains about 25% dry matter, 50–60% sugars and starch (in dry matter), and 10–12% crude protein (in dry matter). Excessive intake of sugars may cause secretory diarrhea.

Potato steam peel

This is the residue from the process of peeling potatoes using pressure and high temperature. It contains about 14% dry matter, 13% crude protein (in dry matter), and 40–50% starch and sugars (in dry matter). Solanine, an anti-nutritional factor in potatoes, might be problematic especially for young pigs.

Molasses

This semi-liquid ingredient is a well-known by-product from the production of sugar from sugarbeet and cane. It contains about 75% dry matter, 3–8% crude protein (as fed), and 46–48% sugars (as fed). It is widely used by the feed industry in dry feeds and its price is not always competitive for use in liquid feeding systems. Nevertheless, in liquid feeding molasses may participate in higher dietary concentrations than currently feasible in dry diets. Its only disadvantage can be a high potassium concentration that is often associated with secretory scours.

Skim or whole milk

Occasionally, skim or whole milk is offered at competitive prices. These batches are usually expired milk or milk unfit for human consumption. It is suggested that if there is a question regarding its microbiological quality, it is best not to use it at all. Otherwise, milk is an excellent source of nutrients for piglets. Whole milk contains about 12% dry matter, 28% crude protein (in dry matter), and 40% lactose (in dry matter). Skim milk contains about 9–10% dry matter, 38% crude protein (in dry matter), and 53% lactose (in dry matter).

Ice cream mix

A fat-rich by-product that is usually a blend of residual ice cream lots and other dairy ingredients, ice cream mix contains about 28% dry matter, 8%

protein (in dry matter), 20% fat (in dry matter), and over 60% lactose (dry matter). Its inclusion level should be determined based on its energy/lipid contribution. It can be of highly variable composition and quality, which necessitates constant monitoring.

Problems with by-products

Feeding liquid by-products is not without its shortcomings. First, quality and composition can be extremely variable. Without a vigorous quality control system, diets based on liquid by-products are frequently overformulated, which subsequently erodes any cost savings from the practice of feeding them. To this end, a price system based on major components (for example, dry matter in whey or fat in ice cream mix) can be of some benefit, although a more thorough quality control system is required. Second, many liquid by-products are prone to fermentation, especially during the summer months. This can be beneficial if it results in the proliferation of lactobacteria, but does not always go as intended. Thus, fermentation is often avoided by the addition of an organic acid to reduce pH to about 4. Third, pigs consuming liquid by-products, and especially liquid whey, are prone to bloating, overeating, overdrinking, and excessive urination, all of which are indications of nutrient imbalances (too much sodium) and (or) the presence of certain anti-nutritional factors. Fourth, supply of such by-products at the source (factory) might be interrupted abruptly, leaving pigs hungry unless emergency diets are in place. Fifth, although feeding liquid by-products with a bucket or even a hose directly in the trough and (or) through nipple drinkers are practices still used today, these methods are suitable only for very small operations, and usually lead to severe nutrient imbalances.

Balancing diets with liquid by-products

Liquid diets based on agro-industrial by-products can be balanced in two different ways. It is strongly recommended, however, to consult first with a nutritionist experienced in liquid feeding systems.

Fixed dry matter concentration

In this method, the required dry matter content is established based on previous experiences and (or) capabilities of the feed delivery system. Most systems should be able to handle liquid diets with 25% dry matter (3:1 water/feed ratio), although new systems can handle thicker mixes. At the defined dry matter concentration, the inclusion of the liquid by-products is determined based on the dry matter concentration of dry feed (about 90% dry matter in most starter diets). Then, the contribution in nutrients from the liquid by-product(s) is deducted from the composition of the dry feed and the latter is finally balanced using a computer formulation program.

Variable dry matter concentration

In this method, all nutrient profiles for ingredients and dietary specifications are entered on a dry matter basis in a typical least-cost formulation program. A diet is then formulated/balanced with dry matter concentration being a constraint factor (set for example from 24 to 26%). The balanced formula is then converted into an as-fed basis (usually by hand) and this final formula is used as the mixing recipe. Most computerized liquid feeding systems accept mixing recipes on a dry matter basis as they are capable of doing the conversions internally.

Fermented Liquid Feeding

In recent years, there has been considerable interest in feeding fermented liquid feed to pigs (Canibe *et al.*, 2002). In brief, liquid diets such as those described under liquid feeding practices are allowed to ferment for a certain period of time in the mixing tank before being fed to pigs. Of course, this is an elaborate process requiring careful monitoring and considerable experience, but the benefits appear to outweigh any disadvantages, at least in most cases.

Research (Jensen and Mikkelsen, 1998; van Winsen *et al.*, 2001) has demonstrated that fermented liquid feed significantly decreases coliform counts and incidences of salmonella in the gastrointestinal tract of pigs. This is the effect of the reduced pH of fermented liquid feed (pH 3–4) compared to unfermented liquid feed (pH 6–8). It has also been indicated that soaking of feed for at least 9 h improves digestibility of phosphorus (Larsen *et al.*, 1999) and it might also improve feed palatability.

A review of trials regarding the effects of feeding liquid diets to pigs (Jensen and Mikkelsen, 1998) indicated that feeding fermented liquid feed improves weight gain on average by 22 and 13% over dry and unfermented liquid feed, respectively (Table 11.1). Surprisingly, in both cases feed efficiency has always been found to be inferior (–4 and –11% for liquid and fermented liquid feeding, respectively) compared to dry feeding, which can be attributed to increased wastage (perhaps due to unresolved distribution problems at the time of collating the review) and (or) reduced protein quality (especially lysine) in fermented feed.

The negative aspects of fermented liquid feeding focus around the need for considerable experience before this practice can be applied successfully (Canibe *et al.*, 2002; Gadd, 2003). For example, insufficient fermentation can actually lead to increased pathogen populations in feed. Fluctuations in temperature greatly affect the fermentation process, as does the introduction of cold water, especially during the winter months (Brooks, 1999). In addition, the problem of reduced protein quality because of bacterial use of dietary amino acids and (or) formation of Maillard reaction products during fermentation definitely increase feed cost as they are currently being addressed via overformulation. Finally, feed medication cannot be practiced with fermented liquid feeding as it greatly affects the proliferation of beneficial bacteria during fermentation.

The process

The whole idea of fermenting liquid feed is based on the fact that lactobacteria and yeasts occurring in cereals proliferate naturally if feed is soaked in water for a certain period of time under the right temperature (Jensen and Mikkelsen, 1998). The end result is a feed rich in lactic and acetic acids with a reduced pH (Russell *et al.*, 1996), all of which are considered beneficial for gastrointestinal health (van Winsen *et al.*, 2001). Table 11.2 presents a comparison of chemical and microbiological differences between dry, liquid, and fermented liquid feed. It is evident that during fermentation the microbial and chemical composition of the feed is altered significantly (Canibe *et al.*, 2002).

Studies carried out in Denmark and the UK demonstrated that the optimum conditions for fermenting liquid pig feed are 8 h of fermentation at 20°C (Brooks *et al.*, 2001; Canibe *et al.*, 2002). For the fermentation process to continue it is imperative that at least 50% of fermented feed be used as 'seed' for the next batch of feed. This dictates that the mixing/fermentation

Table 11.2. Microbial and chemical composition of dry, liquid, and fermented liquid feed. (Adapted from Canibe *et al.*, 2002.)

	Dry	Liquid	Fermented liquid
Bacteria (log cfu/g)			
Lactobacteria	4.3	6.8	9.3
Coliforms	3.7	5.3	3.0
Nutrients (in dry matter)			
Gross energy (MJ/kg)	18.8	19.0	19.2
Crude protein (%)	18.6	18.2	19.0
Lysine (%)[a]	5.6	4.5	4.0
Starch (%)	45.4	44.9	44.5
Carbohydrates (%)[b]	66.7	63.7	59.9

cfu, colony-forming units.

[a] The reduction in lysine reflects deamination for microbial proliferation in fermented liquid feed.

[b] The reduction in total carbohydrates from fermentation is due to reduced low-molecular-weight sugars and fiber.

tank capacity be at least double of what is required for one normal feeding episode. These conditions will produce feed with a maximum pH value of 4.5 and very low levels of coliform bacteria. Lower temperatures favor the development of yeasts and cold-resistant coliform bacteria that become increasingly resilient to low pH (Geary *et al.*, 1996).

It should be noted that during the first hours of fermentation (starting without 'seed'), the number of coliform bacteria actually increases. But, given enough time their density drops quickly as the concentration of lactic acid increases to levels that first inhibit growth and then eliminate colibacteria. It is estimated that it takes at least 3 days for the fermentation process to reach stability and be suitable for feeding to piglets (Canibe *et al.*, 2002).

To aid initiation of the fermentation process and enhance stability, it is often suggested that a 'starter culture' be used during the first three days (Geary *et al.*, 1999; Canibe *et al.*, 2001). This includes bacteria species beneficial to the fermentation process, such as *Lactobacillus alimentarious*, *Pediococcus acidilactici*, and *Lactobacillus plantarum*, usually found as commercial products. Although such a preparation definitely adds to the strength of the process, it offers no further benefits once the system reaches stability.

Milk Replacers

The provision of a liquid supplement based on milk products to piglets during suckling or immediately after weaning is also a form of liquid feeding, although this practice requires mainly manual labor rather than elaborate delivery systems. Products used under this context are often called milk replacers, but they should not be confused with commercial dry products (also called milk replacers in certain parts of the world) that are used as cheaper alternatives to dairy ingredients in dry feed formulas.

Applications

It is currently accepted that under most commercial conditions it is still more efficient and definitely safer to allow a sow to suckle her litter instead of artificially rearing the piglets with milk replacers. Therefore, milk replacers are used mainly in a supportive role, especially when the sow's milk supply is inadequate or in shortage.

Supplementing the sow

The most common use of milk replacers is for supplementing piglets on the sow. Such cases include sows with depressed milk production due to health problems (e.g. metritis/mastitis/agalactia), reduced appetite, stressful environmental conditions, or simply with not enough teats to support a relatively large litter. It has also been indicated that milk replacers are capable of sustaining piglet weaning weight during summer months (Fig. 11.4) when sow feed intake and subsequently milk yield are usually depressed (Azain *et al.*, 1996). Today, systems capable of automated delivery of milk replacer in the farrowing crate are available to reduce labor requirements.

Orphan and surplus piglets

Rearing orphan or surplus piglets away from the sow is another area where milk replacers can be of great benefit. Piglets should receive colostrum from a foster sow or from frozen supplies at least for the first day of age (Veum and Odle, 2001). A warm milk replacer may then be offered in open troughs or specific milk replacer feeders until pigs reach 12–14 days of age. From the second week of age, a high-quality piglet diet suitable for the age and body weight of the piglets must also be offered for *ad libitum* consumption (on a little-and-often basis). Fresh water should always be available for *ad libitum* consumption. It is estimated that approximately 2–4 kg of milk replacer powder (reconstituted to 20% dry matter) and at least 2 kg of dry feed are needed, depending on required weaning age. A typical feeding program is illustrated in Table 11.3.

After weaning

A liquid milk replacer is often made available to piglets right after weaning for a short period of time to aid them overcome the weaning process. This is particularly effective for small-for-age piglets and piglets weaned at an early age (12–14 days old). Table 11.4 demonstrates that offering a milk replacer

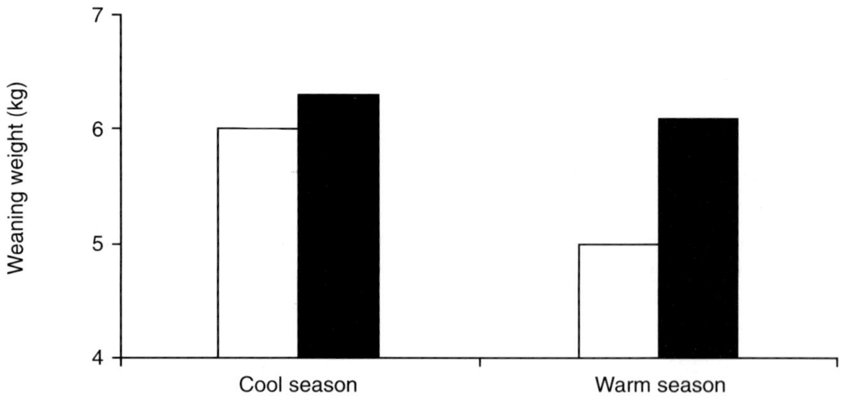

Fig. 11.4. The greatest benefit from milk replacers (□, control; ■, milk replacer) comes during warm months. (Adapted from Azain *et al.*, 1996.)

Table 11.3. Example feeding program for neonatal piglets raised on milk replacer.

Days of age	Milk replacer[a] (ml/day)	Dry feed (g/day)
1	Colostrum[b]	–
2–3	500	–
4–7	750	Milk powder[c]
8–12	1000	50 g minimum
13–18	750	100–200 g
19–21	500	200 g minimum

[a] Liquid with around 20% dry matter.
[b] At least 100 g/piglet and milk replacer *ad libitum*.
[c] Sprinkled on floor-mats or offered on small lock-down feeders for *ad libitum* consumption.

Table 11.4. Effect of offering milk replacer before and (or) after weaning on body weight development in piglets. (Adapted from Azain, 1998.)

Milk replacer pre-weaning	–	–	+	+	–	–	+	+
Milk replacer post-weaning	–	+	–	+	–	+	–	+
Body weight (kg)	6.1	6.1	6.0	6.1	8.9	8.9	9.5	9.3
Day 10 post-weaning	8.5	8.7	8.7	9.0	11.7	11.6	12.7	12.6
Day 45 post-weaning	12.8	12.5	13.7	14.5	13.2	13.0	14.3	14.8

before and (or) after weaning may slightly increase weaning weight and early post-weaning growth. Such practice, however, has a far-reaching carryover growth effect that becomes more evident as pigs grow heavier. This enhanced later growth is thought to be due to enhanced early nutrient intake (Zijlstra *et al.*, 1996; Kim *et al.*, 2001), both locally (enteral) and systemically (whole-body).

Australian experience

Australian researchers (Dunshea *et al.*, 1999) fed liquid skim milk before and shortly after weaning to enhance weaning weight and assist in the transition to dry feed. From day 10 after birth and until weaning on day 20, pigs that were offered supplemental skim milk grew significantly faster (291 versus 223 g/day) than pigs with access only to sow's milk. Sow live weight change and backfat loss were not affected by dietary treatments, which indicates the potential for piglets to grow beyond the milking capacities of their dams. After weaning, pigs on the skim milk regimen were allowed a 2-day period of adjustment, in which time they were fed only skim milk. Consumption of dry matter (257 versus 30 g/day) and growth rates (213 versus –30 g/day) were greater when compared to pigs that received no skim milk before weaning and only dry pellets after weaning. Thereafter, pellets were gradually introduced into skim milk over a period of 5 days to ensure a smooth transition from the liquid to an all-dry diet. Piglets on the skim milk regimen were 33% and 10% heavier at 41 and 120 days of age, respectively, compared to pigs that had access only to sow's milk during suckling and dry pellets after weaning.

Choosing the right milk replacer

The ideal milk replacer would of course be cow's milk. In most cases, however, this is too costly to use for such purposes, and thus commercial blends of dairy by-products (whey, lactose, buttermilk, and skim milk) are used instead. To further reduce cost, certain vegetable proteins and sugars of relatively high nutritive value are also used at variable inclusion rates. To this effect, many ingredients (e.g. wheat gluten) are processed to increase their solubility in water. Obviously, the higher the inclusion rate of high-quality dairy ingredients in a milk replacer formula, the higher its nutritive value.

In terms of nutrient specifications, a typical commercial milk replacer (dry powder form) would have about 25% crude protein, 40–50% lactose, and 10–12% lipids. Typical mixing rates range between 150 and 250 g/l, with higher rates favoring better piglet performance (Table 11.5; Azain, 1998) The physical characteristics of a high-quality milk replacer include freshness, stability in solution for up to 2–3 days, minimal fat separation (lecithin is often used as an emulsifier) and protein flocculation, high solubility, a creamy white color with a typical milk smell, and of course it should be non-hygroscopic to facilitate usage and storage.

There are two types of milk replacer products depending on the temperature of the final solution. Milk replacers that are used with cold water are almost always fortified with an organic acid (e.g. citric acid) to prevent spoilage while in solution. Milk replacers that are destined to be used with warm water do not usually contain organic acids, at least not for the purpose

Table 11.5. Effect of milk replacer mixing rate on piglet performance[a]. (Adapted from Azain, 1998.)

	150 g/l[b]	250 g/l[b]
Body weight at day 14 (kg)	7.1	8.2
Weight gain (g/day)	294	374
Feed intake (g/day)[c]	307	404

[a] Piglets were weaned at 7 days of age.
[b] Grams of powder per liter of water.
[c] All means across rows are significantly different ($P < 0.05$). There was no effect on feed efficiency.

of preserving the quality of the liquid end product. Both types are readily consumed by piglets, although a warm milk replacer is more acceptable during winter.

Management

When selecting liquid milk replacer feeders it must be kept in mind that piglets prefer to eat communally. Devices with six to eight places are better for piglets reared away from a sow, while those with only one or two places are sufficient for supplementing piglets on the sow. Feeders should be portable, durable, and easily cleaned and refilled.

Mixing milk replacer powder with cold, tepid or warm water should be done thoroughly and the manufacturer's dosages and guidelines precisely followed. Some milk replacers must never be mixed with warm water, while none should be mixed with hot water as nutrient degradation (e.g. vitamins) may occur. It is strongly recommended that a fresh solution be prepared every day, even though some mixes stay in good suspension for 2–3 days.

In the case of diarrhea, intake must be lowered and an antibiotic treatment followed. Overfeeding as well as poor hygiene conditions are the main causes of diarrhea. Veterinary supervision is necessary.

Consumption of dry feed (creep diet, starter) should be instituted as soon as possible. Piglets with high dry feed intake can be weaned earlier, with fewer post-weaning problems and certainly consume less milk replacer. Gradually reducing the milk replacer allowance forces piglets to look for dry feed as an alternative source of nutrients to satisfy their needs.

References

Azain MJ, Tomkins T, Sowinski JS, Arentson RA, and Jewell DE (1996) Effect of supplemental pig milk replacer on litter performance: seasonal variation in response. *Journal of Animal Science* 74:2195–2202.

Azain MJ (1998) Young pig nutrition, use of liquid diets examined. *Feedstuffs*, February 23:12–21.

Brooks PH (1999) The multiple benefits of liquid feed for pigs. *FeedTech* 3(5):29–31.

Brooks PH, Geary TM, Morgan DT, and Campbell A (1999) New developments in liquid feeding. *Pig Journal* 36:43–64.

Brooks PH, Moran CA, Beal JD, Demeckova V, and Campbell A (2001) Liquid feeding for the young piglet. In: *The Weaner Pig*, by Varley MA and Wiseman J (ed), 153–178. CAB International, Wallingford, UK.

Canibe N, Miquel N, Miettinen H, and Jensen BB (2001) Effect of addition of formic acid and starter cultures to liquid feed on pH, microflora composition, organic acid production and ammonia production. *15th Forum for Applied Biotechnology (Volume 66/3b)*, 431–434. Gent, Belgium.

Canibe N, Mikkelsen LL, and Jensen BB (2002) Fermented liquid feeding: an alternative feed strategy for pigs. *FeedTech* 6(4):24–28.

Demeckova V, Moran CA, Caveney C, Campbell A, Kuri V, and Brooks PH (2001) The effect of fermentation and/or sanitization of liquid diets on the feeding preferences of newly weaned pigs. In: *Digestive Physiology of Pigs: 8th Symposium of Digestive Physiology in Pigs*, by Lindberg JE and Ogle B (ed), 291–293. CAB International, Wallingford, UK.

Dunshea FR, Kerton DJ, Eason PJ, and King RH (1999) Supplemental skim milk before and after weaning improves growth performance of pigs. *Australian Journal of Agricultural Research* 50:1165–1170.

Gadd J (2003) *Pig Production Problems*. Nottingham University Press, Nottingham, UK.

Geary TM, Brooks PH, Morgan DT, Campbell A, and Russell PJ (1996) Performance of weaner pigs fed *ad libitum* with liquid feed at different dry matter concentrations. *Journal of the Science of Food and Agriculture* 72:17–24.

Geary TM, Brooks PH, Beal JD, and Campbell A (1999) Effect on weaner pig performance and diet microbiology of feeding a liquid diet acidified to pH 4 with either lactic acid or through fermentation with *Pediococcus acidilactici*. *Journal of the Science of Food and Agriculture* 79:633–640.

Jensen BB and Mikkelsen LL (1998) Feeding liquid diets to pigs. In: *Recent Advances in Animal Nutrition*, by Garnsworthy PC and Wiseman J (ed), 107–126. Nottingham University Press, Nottingham, UK.

Kim JH, Heo KN, Odle J, Han IK, and Harrell RJ (2001) Liquid diets accelerate the growth of early-weaned pigs and the effects are maintained to market weight. *Journal of Animal Science* 79:427–434.

Larsen T, Skoglund E, Sandberg AS, and Endberg RM (1999) Soaking and pelleting of pig diets alters the apparent absorption and retention of minerals. *Canadian Journal of Animal Science* 79:477–483.

Mohler J (1922) *Hogs in Kansas* (2nd edn). Kansas State Board of Agriculture, Topeka, KS.

Russell PJ, Geary TM, Brooks PH, and Campbell A (1996) Performance, water use and effluent output of weaner pigs fed *ad libitum* with either dry pellets or liquid feed and the role of microbial activity in the liquid feed. *Journal of the Science of Food and Agriculture* 72:8–16.

Scholten RHJ, van der Peet-Schwering CMC, Verstegen MWA, den Hartog LA, Schrama JW, and Vesseur PC (1999) Fermented co-products and fermented compound diets for pigs: a review. *Animal Feed Science and Technology* 82:1–19.

van Winsen RL, Urlings BAP, Lipman LJA, and Snijders JMA (2001) Effect of fermented feed on the microbial population of the gastrointestinal tract of pigs. *Applied Environmental Microbiology* 67:3071–3076.

Veum TL and Odle J (2001) Feeding neonatal pigs. In: *Swine Nutrition* (2nd edn), by Lewis AJ and Southern LL (ed), 671–690. CRC Press LLC, Boca Raton, FL.

Zijlstra RT, Whang K-Y, Easter RA, and Odle J (1996) Effect of feeding a milk replacer to early-weaned pigs on growth, body composition, and small intestinal morphology, compared with suckled littermates. *Journal of Animal Science* 74:2948–2959.

Water Nutrition

12

Introduction

Water is often called the 'forgotten nutrient', and for good reason (Brooks, 1994a). Although water is required in most physiological functions and comprises over 70% of body weight in young pigs, it has two major 'disadvantages' over other nutrients. It is relatively inexpensive and readily available, and, thus, of little commercial value. This may explain the paucity of meaningful research work on water. Yet, limited water intake or water of poor quality can seriously impair animal performance and health, especially in young pigs, in which feed consumption is strongly related to water intake. Therefore, recommendations are often based on commercial experience and field observations due to the lack of better data from the scientific community.

Water as a Nutrient

Water is the most critical component in the organism, serving a plethora of important, yet disparate, physiological functions (NRC, 1998). To begin with, water is a major structural element providing cell turgidity and body form. Water is also a solvent and transportation medium for most nutrients, metabolites, and waste products. Because of its high specific heat, water is used in thermoregulation via evaporation from the lungs. Water also takes part in most biochemical reactions (hydration, hydrolysis) within the organism. Finally, water is important in the lubrication of joints and the protection of the nervous system. In short, water plays a fundamental role in supporting life (Thacker, 2001).

The concentration of water in different tissues is dramatically variable. Lean tissue contains on average 70% water, 20% protein, and 8% fat; the remainder being minerals and carbohydrates (de Lange *et al.*, 2001). Conversely, fat tissue contains on average 15% water, 2% protein, and 75% lipids (Whittemore, 1998). It appears, therefore, that body water concentration is in direct proportion to protein and in inverse relationship with lipid concentration. As a consequence, water concentration in empty body weight (i.e. minus gastrointestinal contents) declines sharply with age as older pigs deposit progressively more fat than lean tissue (Georgievskii, 1982; Fig. 12.1). For example, a newborn piglet at 1.5 kg body weight contains less than 2% fat and over 80% water, whereas a market-age hog at 90 kg contains over 20% fat and less than 60% water (Shields *et al.*, 1983).

Although drinking water covers the majority of daily water requirements, other sources of water are available. Water is a natural component in all ingredients and therefore an integral part of all pig diets. Cereal grains contain about 12% water (air-dried basis), whereas most oilseed protein supplements contain 5–10% water. Therefore, in 1 kg of a typical pig feed there is about 100 g of available water. Wet or liquid ingredients such as wet maize and liquid whey naturally contain even more water and hence contribute more in meeting water requirements. Water is also produced during the process of metabolic oxidation of nutrients during metabolism. The oxidation of 1 kg carbohydrate, fat, or protein yields 560, 1190, or 450 g water, respectively (NRC, 1981). Therefore, 1 kg of a typical piglet feed

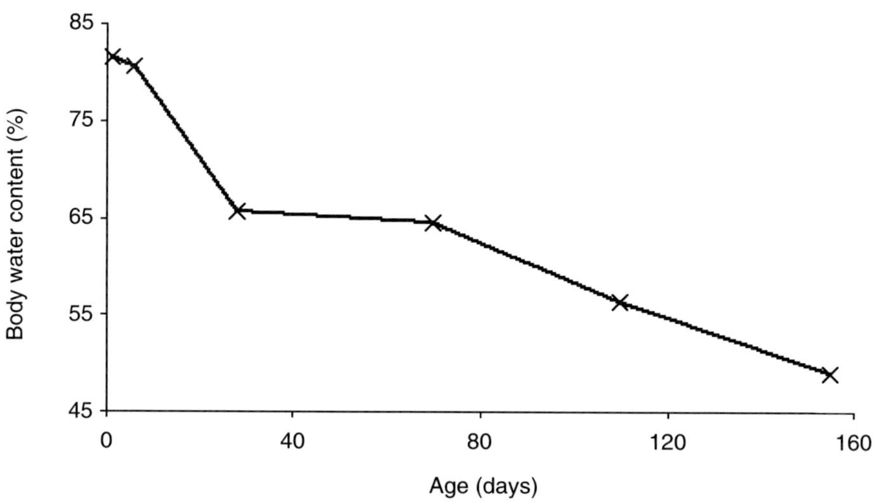

Fig. 12.1. Body water concentration in relation to age in growing pigs. (From Georgievskii, 1982.)

containing 10% moisture, 60% carbohydrate, 20% protein, 5% fat, and 5% ash should yield over 500 g water after complete catabolism for energy purposes. In reality, however, nutrient oxidation creates a net demand for water to process end products, especially with diets rich in protein and minerals (Thacker, 2001).

In pigs, water is lost from the body via: (i) respiration; (ii) defecation; (iii) evaporation; and (iv) urination. At 20 kg body weight, pigs kept at 20°C exhale about 300 ml water per day (Holmes and Mount, 1967). Increased air temperature and decreased humidity usually intensify respiration losses. Pigs also lose a considerable amount of water in manure, which is produced at a rate of about 8% of body weight and has an average water content of 70% (Brooks and Carpenter, 1993). Increased dietary fiber (Thacker, 2001) and diarrhea (Thulin and Brumm, 1991) also increase fecal water losses. Water loss from the skin is trivial because pigs have dormant sweat glands. Pigs excrete most water via urination as the kidneys maintain homeostasis by regulating the volume and composition of urine. Water excretion via urination increases when pigs are fed high-protein (Wahlstrom *et al.*, 1970) or high-mineral diets (Sinclair, 1939) and decreases when water intake is limited or lost via other routes.

Factors Affecting Requirements

Pigs must consume daily enough water to maintain constant body water concentration. Therefore, factors that increase water losses also increase water requirements. In addition, several stress factors may also increase water intake beyond physiological requirements. Water requirements and water consumption are not necessarily equivalent, because wastage contributes to increased water use. Wastage can account for up to 60% of water use under poor management conditions (Gonyou, 1996). Because it is extremely difficult to measure water requirements it is often satisfactory to assess water requirements based on consumption at moderate wastage.

Increased air temperature generally increases water intake for thermoregulation. Pigs use water to reduce body temperature under excessive heat conditions because water has a high specific heat index. For every gram of water that evaporates via respiration, 580 calories of heat are released (Thulin and Brumm, 1991). However, research has demonstrated that unless temperature exceeds 30–35°C, pigs do not increase respiration considerably to dissipate enough body heat (Holmes and Mount, 1967). Under heat stress, water intake easily increases over 50% (Brooks and Carpenter, 1993) but offering cool water reduces the amount required to regulate body temperature (Varjrabukka *et al.*, 1981). The reverse is true under low ambient temperatures.

Dietary composition may also increase requirements of water for disposal of excess nutrients. Catabolism of excess dietary protein yields ammonia which is highly toxic for the organism. Ammonia is excreted as urea in urine, but there is a limit to which urea can be concentrated in urine, after which increased dietary protein concentration increases urination and water consumption. For example, water consumption increased by 35% in 5-week-old pigs when dietary protein concentration was increased by 4 percentage units (Wahlstrom *et al.*, 1970).

In a similar pattern, proper disposal of excess ingested minerals is accomplished via increased urination (Sinclair, 1939). Growing animals can tolerate up to 8% dietary sodium chloride (i.e. common salt) given free access to fresh water (NRC, 1980), but if water is saline, restricted, or otherwise non-available, as little as 0.5% sodium chloride can be fatally toxic. Increasing dietary salt addition from 0.5% to 2.5% (a fivefold increase) increased water intake by 26% (Hagsten and Perry, 1976). Excess potassium, however, appears to have even more dramatic effects on water intake. For example, increasing dietary potassium concentration by 100% (double) resulted in about 20% increased water consumption (Brooks *et al.*, 1992). Although accidental addition of excess minerals during feed preparation is a point of concern, most incidents of 'salt poisoning' usually involve some form of water deprivation.

Pigs will also consume extra water if they feel hungry. It appears that pigs have a requirement for total volumetric intake (Brooks, 1994b), at which satiety is achieved. This was estimated at 19% of body weight (Yang *et al.*, 1981) for growing pigs. It is hypothesized that when pigs do not consume enough feed to satisfy this need, they revert to water (if available) to satisfy the demand for gut fill. The estimated total volumetric capacity for young pigs is estimated at about 13% of body weight. For example, a 8-kg pig would require a minimum of about 1 liter of gut fill per day, which may be satisfied by either feed or water. If this hypothesis holds true, it would be logical to assume that factors that increase water intake would inevitably reduce feed intake and, thus, impair growth.

Antimicrobial agents may also affect water balance, but research reports are often contradictory (McLeese *et al.*, 1992). In the absence of definitive information, it should be anticipated that antimicrobial agents that are being absorbed into the bloodstream will increase water requirements for renal clearance. Antimicrobial agents that act locally at the lumen of the gastrointestinal tract should be expected to reduce water intake by depressing diarrhea.

In studies with 35-kg pigs using tritiated water to account for spillage, it was estimated that pigs require about 120 ml/kg body weight (Yang *et al.*, 1981). But, based on practical experience and accounting for unavoidable spillage, it is often suggested that pigs consume about 3 liters of non-saline water per kilogram of ingested feed under thermoneutral conditions. Ultimately, free access to fresh water is the ideal way of meeting the water requirements in young pigs (Whittemore, 1998).

Water for Suckling Pigs

Sow's milk contains about 80% water, and therefore it is often assumed that milk-fed piglets should be able to cover their daily water requirements without supplemental water. Indeed, in many production systems, farrowing crates are not equipped with a water delivery system for piglets, and only after weaning do piglets drink water. But in such systems, it is not uncommon to observe piglets trying to reach the water devices installed for sows (Fraser *et al.*, 1993). The general consensus, however, is that: (i) supplemental water may actually benefit suckling piglets under certain circumstances; and (ii) these benefits greatly outweigh the cost of providing water for piglets in farrowing crates.

Dehydration during the first few days after birth is a common cause of death in newborn pigs, especially among light and weak piglets that fail to consume enough milk. It has been suggested that provision of drinking water may reduce pre-weaning mortality from dehydration, especially when environmental temperature is excessive. For example, water loss (mainly from evaporation) in piglets housed under common radiant heaters was about 155 g/kg body weight per day (Fraser *et al.*, 1993). Also, piglets housed at 28°C consumed four times more water than piglets housed at 20°C. Therefore, when milk intake is limited, a source of drinking water should be able to reduce dehydration and sustain life. But, if energy reserves in neonatal pigs are depleted faster than replenished via milk, supplemental water may not be sufficient to sustain life for too long.

Supplemental water may also be beneficial to suckling piglets suffering from diarrhea, which causes severe water loss from the gut. In experimental studies (Balsbaugh *et al.*, 1986; cited by Fraser *et al.*, 1993), diarrhea caused severe dehydration (measured by blood hematocrit), body weight loss, and mortality. Surviving piglets were able to withstand dehydration by adjusting intra- and extracellular fractions of body water. Thus, it is strongly recommended to provide electrolytes in addition to drinking water in pigs suffering from acute diarrhea to prevent severe dehydration.

Sow's milk is relatively high in protein (30%) and ash (25%). As fresh water is required for urinary excretion of excess nitrogen and minerals, a potential deficit could, at least theoretically, reduce milk intake and growth in suckling piglets (Lloyd *et al.*, 1978). It is interesting to note that newborn pigs are able to drink water within the first 2 hours after birth (NRC, 1998), indicating a need for water in addition to that supplied by sow's colostrum or milk.

It is also essential to provide drinking water to suckling piglets that actively consume solid feed. It has been demonstrated (Friend and Cunningham, 1966) that piglets with free access to water eat more creep feed than piglets without supplemental water (3215 versus 2166 g/pig, respectively, in the above study). The importance of drinking water in supporting vigorous intake of dry feed increases with weaning age. In production systems practicing early weaning, creep intake is rather trivial and, thus, the effect of water on feed intake is minimal (Fraser *et al.*, 1993). But, in production systems that wean pigs around 5 weeks of age, creep intake can be substantial, especially after the third week of lactation, and supplemental drinking water must always be provided.

Water for Weaned Pigs

At the time of weaning, pigs without previous experience in drinking fresh water are required to distinguish thirst from hunger and operate different devices (i.e. drinkers and feeders) to satisfy these needs via unfamiliar media (i.e. water and dry feed). This requirement for an abrupt change in drinking and feeding behavior is in sharp contrast with the way piglets used to cover their needs before weaning with sow's milk. This argument gives ground to the notion of providing fresh water and creep feed to suckling pigs, although results are often less than satisfactory.

During the first couple of days post-weaning, piglets weaned at an early age (less than 3 weeks) consume little if any dry feed. Thus, to satisfy their hunger they tend to fill up with water beyond their physiological needs (Brooks and Tsourgiannis, 2003). It is not uncommon for newly weaned pigs to drink up to 4 l water per day during the first few days post-weaning (Thacker, 2001). Pigs that fail to locate or learn how to use drinkers should be encouraged to drink from bowls filled with water to prevent dehydration. During the rest of the first week, weaned pigs reduce their intake of water as they tend to consume more feed than they can actually process.

By the end of the first week, and assuming that feed intake has reached a linearly increasing pattern, water intake parallels feed intake. During the following weeks, water intake ranges from 2 to 4 l per kg dry feed, but most often it averages around 3 l per kg feed eaten. Allowances should be made for wastage or abnormally high requirements for water during hot seasons or disease outbreaks. Average water intake during the first, second, and third week post-weaning (for piglets weaned at 3 weeks of age) is expected at about 0.5, 1.0, and 1.5 l per pig daily. Studies (Gill *et al.*, 1986) indicated that water intake may be predicted based on feed dry matter intake using the following equation:

$$\text{Water intake (l/day)} = 0.149 + [3.053 \times \text{feed intake (kg/day)}], \qquad (12.1)$$

which is very close to the 3:1 (water/feed) practical rule.

Weaned pigs housed under constant light drink more during 'day' hours (8 am to 5 pm) than during 'night' hours (Brooks, 1994a). Also, weaned pigs drink most water in association with a meal. In young pigs, 85% of drinking takes place within 10 min of a meal (Bigelow and Houpt, 1988).

It is advisable to monitor daily water intake per room using a simple water meter. Plotting water intake against time provides a visual aid in detecting irregular patterns of water intake that could be used as an indication of an imminent disease outbreak. For example, pigs start to drink more water at the onset of fever or diarrhea, before any visual symptoms become apparent. However, a distinction must be made for abnormal patterns in water intake due to elevated room temperature. To this end, monitoring daily temperature (min–max or average) along with daily water intake could prevent false alarms. Finally, water intake records from the first week post-weaning should be used with caution for monitoring health.

Water in Liquid Feeding Systems

It is often suggested that liquid feeding eliminates the need for supplemental fresh water. In theory, pigs do not require a separate source of water given that their true requirements for water are satisfied through the daily allotment of liquid feed. Yet, there are a number of unpredictable circumstances under which lack of fresh water may be detrimental to animal health and performance. Moreover, several countries require by law that all liquid-fed pigs have access to supplemental fresh water.

One of the main advantages of liquid feeding is the ability to use relatively large quantities of inexpensive agro-industrial by-products. Yet, these by-products tend to be rather variable in composition that may change from batch to batch even within the same processing plant. If these by-products are naturally high in sodium chloride or potassium (e.g. whey or molasses), a slight, yet undetected, change in production process or dry matter concentration of the by-product can lead to dramatic changes in dietary composition. Under these unpredictable circumstances pigs may receive a diet that fluctuates widely in nutrient composition including minerals that could lead to 'salt poisoning' from water deprivation. Thus, it is strongly recommended to supply at least one drinker per pen when pigs are fed with such by-products.

The assumption that liquid-fed pigs acquire enough water through their daily allotment of soup is based on the traditional 3:1 water ratio (25% dry matter) used to prepare liquid feed. But with modern delivery systems, it is possible now to effectively pump a more dense feed that has as much as 33% dry matter (2:1 ratio). Under such circumstances pigs must be provided with a supply of fresh water to compensate for any water deficit.

Finally, it is recommended to offer liquid-fed pigs a supply of fresh water when daily water requirements are expected to fluctuate widely due to environmental changes, insufficient feed intake from excessive competition, or under the stress of disease, during which period pigs tend to decrease feed intake and increase water intake.

There are, however, circumstances under which the supply of fresh water is advised to be limited or even shut off. During the first couple of days post-weaning, or when pigs are switched from dry to liquid feeding, pigs may refuse to consume sufficient quantities of liquid feed to sustain their body weight. Instead, they prefer to drink enough fresh water in an attempt to provide sufficient gut fill for satiety. It is, hence, advised to provide access to fresh water only after feed intake has reached satisfactory levels or limit it to a short period between meals. Caution should be taken to ensure that the liquid feed is properly formulated to avoid 'salt poisoning' or that feed formulation does not create palatability problems.

Aspects of Water Quality

Water is expected to be devoid of any color, taste, or aroma. Yet, water used in commercial operations comes from a plethora of sources including surface water (lakes, rivers), underground water (wells), or human/industrial water (main supply) that all affect the water's physical, chemical, and microbiological characteristics. The effects of poor water quality on pig performance and health are not well understood as they may range from minor (aversion) to lethal (poisoning). An interaction between water quality and dietary composition also exerts different effects. In short, water quality can affect pig performance and should be closely monitored.

Physical quality

Water coloration or opacity is easily detected and may be due to suspended colloidal solids such as clay or slit (harmless) or from particles originating from human, animal, or industrial waste (harmful). Flavors also indicate contamination as water is expected to be inert in this regard. On the other hand, water-soluble additives and medications administered via water may alter any of the physical characteristics of pure water in a way that could be beneficial (e.g. a flavor) or detrimental (e.g. excess chlorination) to water intake.

Microbiological quality

Water may contain a host of bacteria, viruses, protozoa, and even eggs or cysts of intestinal parasites. Bacteria pose the greatest health hazard, with salmonella, colibacili, cholera, and leptospira being the most commonly encountered in pig units. Contamination usually originates from contact with human or animal waste and from algae growth that builds up in water reservoirs. A coliform count test is usually the first step in assessing water microbiological load, but tests that identify the type of bacteria should be performed in contaminated water. A coliform count below 50 per ml water is considered acceptable for pigs (Bureau of National Affairs, 1973). Bacterial contamination is more common in surface waters (NRC, 1998).

Water sanitization at source or at delivery point (pig unit) is required if contaminated water must be used for pigs. Chlorination using a proportioner at the main incoming line (requires high pressure to avoid accidental over-chlorination) can significantly reduce microbial contamination and ensure water safety (Brooks, 1994b). Chlorination effectiveness depends on water pH (less effective over 7) and chlorination agent. Chlorine dioxide is more potent (especially against viruses) and less reactive than chlorine, but it is costly and tends to leave toxic residues (Fraser *et al.*, 1993). Excessive chlorination reduces water acceptance, but it is not clear at what level this becomes counterproductive. Nevertheless, ultraviolet sterilization may be used in place of excessive chlorination to treat heavily contaminated water, but this could be prohibitively expensive (Brooks, 1994b).

Toxins produced by blue-green algae cannot be eliminated by water treatment, but only with thorough cleaning and disinfecting of water-holding tanks and the associated piping system. Not all algae produce toxins lethal to animals but most impair water taste and reduce its acceptability. Algae grow most rapidly in open ponds and lakes and in header tanks exposed to sunlight. Water high in nitrates tends to promote heavier algae growth (Brooks, 1994b).

On a final note, water rich in iron supports rapid proliferation of iron-dependent bacteria that use inorganic ferrous iron as an energy source (Fraser *et al.*, 1993). They produce a reddish slime that plugs filters and severely reduces water flow. Moreover, decomposition of these bacteria creates foul odors that impair water taste. Iron bacteria can be controlled by shock chlorination (system stays overnight with bleach in the water followed by thorough flushing).

Chemical characteristics

The chemical characteristics of water are of most concern because they are a natural aspect of water quality. Chemical quality is affected by water source and contact with various natural geological entities that enrich it with salts. Water rich in salts is prone to cause water refusal, scouring, and loss of appetite.

Total dissolved solids

One of the most valuable tests performed to assess water quality, total dissolved solids (TDS) provides a first indication of the amount of mineral salts dissolved in water. Such salts may include carbonate and bicarbonates, sulfates, nitrates, chlorides, phosphates, and fluorides. It is generally assumed that a level of TDS below 1000 ppm is safe for pigs, whereas above 7000 ppm it becomes unfit for consumption (Fraser *et al.*, 1993;

NRC, 1998). Between these levels, the effects on animal performance and health are largely unpredictable and variable as individual salts and interactions with dietary components become more important than total salt concentration. For example, piglets offered water with up to 4390 ppm TDS experienced no adverse effects with medicated feed, but they scoured heavily and performed poorly when medication was removed from feed (McLeese *et al.*, 1992). In short, it is strongly advised to perform a detailed chemical analysis when TDS exceeds 1000 ppm.

Salinity

Salinity is usually associated with the concentration of sodium chloride (common salt), although the term salinity literally refers to total salts (similar to TDS). Regardless of its source (from water or diet), sodium chloride and all other salts require ample quantities of fresh, non-saline water for efficient excretion in urine. If only saline water is available, pigs enter into a futile cycle in which salt toxicity becomes progressively more severe as pigs become unable to excrete excess salt (Brooks and Carpenter, 1993). Water salinity should be taken into account in diet design and even complete removal of supplemental salt may be warranted. But, as most saline water sources contain more sodium than chlorine (Thacker, 2001), complete removal of dietary salt may cause chlorine deficiency that further depresses appetite.

pH

The acidity (or alkalinity) of most sources of water rarely becomes problematic as it usually falls within the acceptable level of 6.5–8.5 (Fraser *et al.*, 1993). Acidic water ($pH < 7$) may corrode metal pipes and reduce the effectiveness of water medication. In contrast, alkaline water ($pH > 7$) reduces the effectiveness of chlorination and may leave scaly deposits. Most pathogenic bacteria have an optimum growth pH of 6–7. Water acidification (e.g. citric acid) may reduce bacterial proliferation and even aid in lowering stomach pH in weaned pigs (Brooks *et al.*, 1992). But, organic acids in water tend to dislodge organic matter stuck in pipes that may result in nipple blockage.

Hardness

Hardness is the sum of calcium and magnesium expressed as calcium carbonate equivalents. Although water hardness does not affect safety, excess calcium in drinking water may reduce dietary phosphorus absorption, which can become problematic in diets marginal in phosphorus. Thus, dietary adjustment of calcium concentration is warranted in units using very hard water. In addition, hard water tends to interfere with water delivery systems as mineral deposits accumulate over time. In general, soft water contains less than 60 ppm $CaCO_3$ equivalents, whereas above 180 ppm water is classified as very hard (NRC, 1998). Water is frequently softened by ion exchange during which sodium replaces calcium and magnesium. Saline water already high in sodium should not be softened by ion exchange to prevent 'salt poisoning'. Reverse osmosis is preferable in this aspect, but cost is prohibitive (Thacker, 2001).

Sulfates

Drinking water containing above 1000 ppm sulfates may cause diarrhea in young pigs, although this may be mild and with minimal effect on performance (Fraser *et al.*, 1993; NRC, 1998). Animals can be acclimated to relatively high levels of sulfates in water, but the exact conditions under which diarrhea develops are still unclear. It is speculated that other mineral salts interfere with sulfate absorption in the gastrointestinal lumen and that sulfate intake rather than its concentration in water is more important (Fraser *et al.*, 1993). A commercial-scale study (Patience *et al.*, 1997) revealed that young pigs receiving drinking water with as much as 1634 ppm sulfate performed as well as pigs receiving similar water treated by reverse osmosis to reduce sulfate down to 15 ppm. Nevertheless, pigs receiving high sulfate water developed mild diarrhea. Weaned pigs unfamiliar with high-sulfate water are the most susceptible to develop diarrhea (Thacker, 2001). Water with over 7000 ppm sulfates is not accepted by pigs (Anderson *et al.*, 1994).

Iron, manganese, fluoride

These minerals pose no direct threat to animal health (Fraser *et al.*, 1993). But, excess iron supports proliferation of iron-dependent bacteria and will precipitate upon oxidation, causing problems in the water delivery system. Manganese can precipitate after oxidation but only at very high pH levels (> 9.5) which are seldom encountered in water supply. Excess fluoride is detrimental to tooth health but this rarely becomes an issue taking into account the relatively short life of a market pig.

Nitrates and nitrites

These nitrogenous compounds result mainly from decomposition of organic matter and from excessive application of nitrogen fertilizers. They pose limited health risk for pigs (Fraser *et al.*, 1993) as opposed to human infants or ruminants (Boyles *et al.*, 1988). Nitrate is not toxic but can be converted to nitrite (especially in the presence of iron, zinc, and lead), which is toxic and causes oxygen deprivation of the blood. Nitrates and nitrites in water also disturb utilization of vitamin A (Wood *et al.*, 1967). Water containing more than 100 ppm nitrates and 5–10 ppm nitrites is not suitable for young pigs (NRC, 1998).

Delivery Systems and Management

Drinker types

Most common types of drinkers in commercial facilities include nipples and bowls/cups. Turkey drinkers are also found in Europe, but their use is limited. There are several pros and cons regarding each drinker device. If properly installed and managed, all systems are equally effective in providing water to young pigs. Drinker design, however, has an impact on cost and water wastage. It is recommended that similar drinkers be used in farrowing crates and nursery pens to accelerate water consumption post-weaning.

Nipple drinkers (Fig. 12.2) operate by biting, moving, or pushing a valve-activating mechanism. Bite-type drinkers minimize wastage because the pig has to take the drinker in its mouth to open the valve. In general, nipples are less expensive and easier to install and maintain than bowls/cups, but they require frequent height adjustment and are prone to excessive water wastage. In contrast, bowls/cups (Fig. 12.3) are more

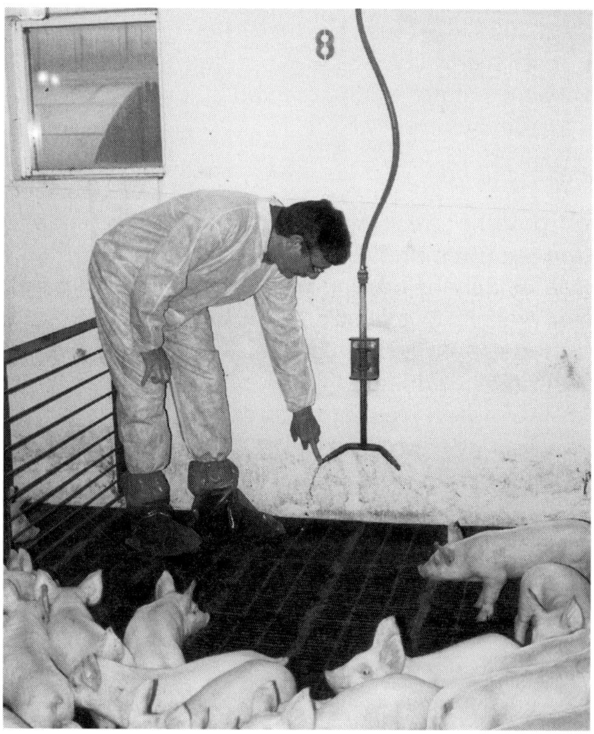

Fig. 12.2. Frequent checks of nipple drinkers are necessary to ensure piglets receive enough fresh water.

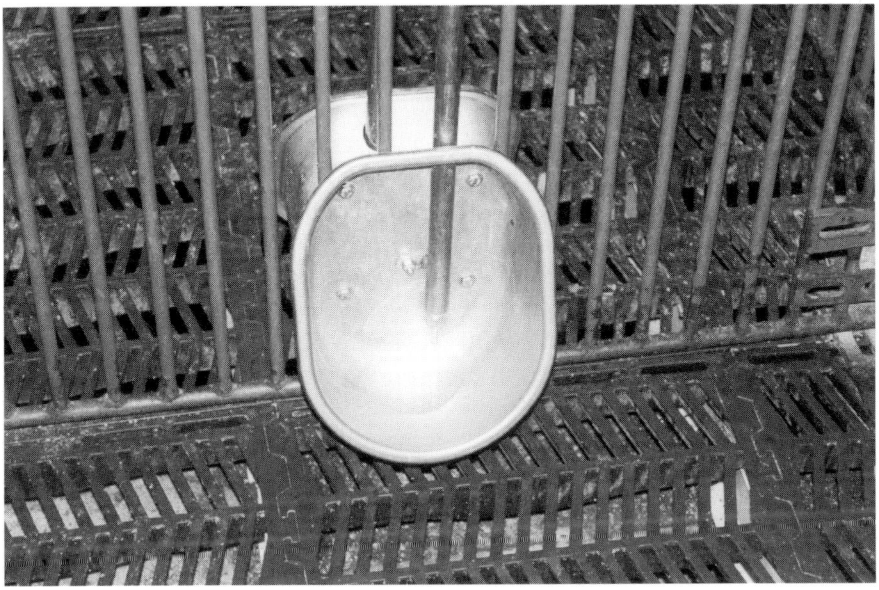

Fig. 12.3. Cup drinkers are placed near the floor to enable access for pigs of all sizes.

accessible to pigs and do not require height adjustment, but they are more expensive and are easily fouled if not properly placed and managed. Pigs clearly prefer to drink from an open-surface drinker both before and after weaning (Phillips and Fraser, 1991), but revert to nipples when faced with contaminated water (Brooks, 1994b).

Bell-shaped hanging drinkers (originally designed for turkeys) provide an open-surface water source while minimizing wastage and fouling. These drinkers also require frequent height adjustment and inspection for contamination. Turkey drinkers are more suitable for large pens. Field reports (Gadd, 1997) indicate that when properly used, these drinkers may actually improve performance in young pigs (Table 12.1). However, these observations require further verification.

Table 12.1. Turkey drinkers for weaned pigs. (Adapted from Gadd, 1997.)

	Control	Turkey drinker
Start weight (kg)	6.2	6.2
End weight (kg)	22.1	23.7
Weight gain (g/day)	388	427
Feed intake (g/day)	686	738
Feed/gain	1.77	1.73

Placement

Drinkers are frequently placed over the designated dunging area to facilitate removal of waste water, which is especially important in partially slatted facilities. But, if the distance between the feeder and drinker is excessive, feed intake may be actually impaired because water intake in young pigs is associated with meals (Bigelow and Houpt, 1988). This becomes even more relevant in large-size pens in which pigs form subgroups, as pigs become reluctant to enter another group's territory to reach a water outlet. To this end, it is recommended that drinkers be placed centrally or well dispersed in pens holding over 50 pigs. Wet/dry feeders, which provide a water source inside the feeder to enable pigs to drink during the course of a meal, may be more suitable for large-size pens, but this merits further investigation. Finally, placing cups at the dunging area or near corners further increases the probability of being fouled because cups are usually at or slightly above floor level.

The number of nipples per pen has been traditionally recommended at 10:1 (Gonyou, 1996), which is in accordance with most welfare codes. It is advisable, however, to install at least two drinkers per pen regardless of pen density to ensure uninterrupted water intake if one nipple becomes blocked. In large-size pens with 50 or more animals, one drinker per 20 animals is sufficient if water outlets are properly placed and dispersed (Thacker, 2001). Cups are able to service more pigs per drinker and, thus, it is recommended to have one cup per 20 animals (Gonyou, 1996). With cups there is no need to have a minimum of two drinkers per pen, because malfunctioning cups are easy to detect during daily inspections.

Nipple drinkers require frequent height adjustment to ensure pigs have free access to water and that wastage is minimized. It has been suggested that when a nipple is placed too low, the pig is required to drink from an angle and therefore it wastes over 60% of the water released (Gonyou, 1996). Thus, it is strongly recommended to position the tip of the nipple at pig shoulder height (horizontal nipples) or slightly (5 cm) higher (angled nipples). Nipples pointing upward are discouraged because they tend to block easier from water deposits and feed particles (Carlson and Peo, 1982). If pigs of variable size are housed in the same pen, care should be taken to ensure that even the smallest pigs have free access to water. Adjusting drinkers on a weekly basis should be enough to maintain drinkers at proper height (Fig. 12.4).

Cup drinkers may be placed at floor level, but if they have a very shallow lip, water wastage and fouling may become problematic. Thus, it is better to place cups 5–15 cm above the level of the floor (Gonyou, 1996).

Turkey drinkers must be adjusted so that pigs can easily drink without tipping the drinker to one side.

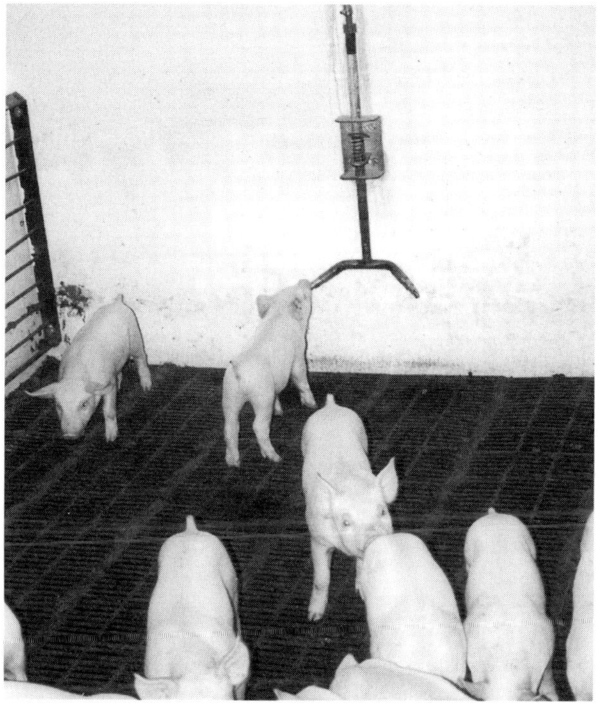

Fig. 12.4. Height of nipple drinkers should be adjusted frequently to just above shoulder level.

Water flow

Water flow rate is of paramount importance for young pigs. Insufficient flow rate reduces water intake because pigs discontinue drinking before completely quenching their thirst. It has been demonstrated (Barber *et al.*, 1989; Brooks *et al.*, 1992) that although young pigs increase drinking time as flow rate decreases, they are not prepared to devote enough drinking time to fully meet their daily water needs (Fig. 12.5). Therefore, weight gain (through reduced feed intake) is invariably reduced with insufficient water intake because of low flow rates (Fig. 12.6). Likewise, excessive flow rate not only impairs water intake because pigs cannot easily control the process of drinking, but it also increases wastage.

For young pigs, flow rate from nipples should be between 500 and 1000 ml/min. North American experts favor low flow rates (250 to 500 ml/min), especially for pigs weaned around 2 weeks of age. In contrast, most European authorities tend to favor higher flow rates (750 to 1000 ml/min), because pigs are weaned at heavier weights. Research has demonstrated (Barber *et al.*, 1989) that flow rates below 500 ml/min are likely to impair

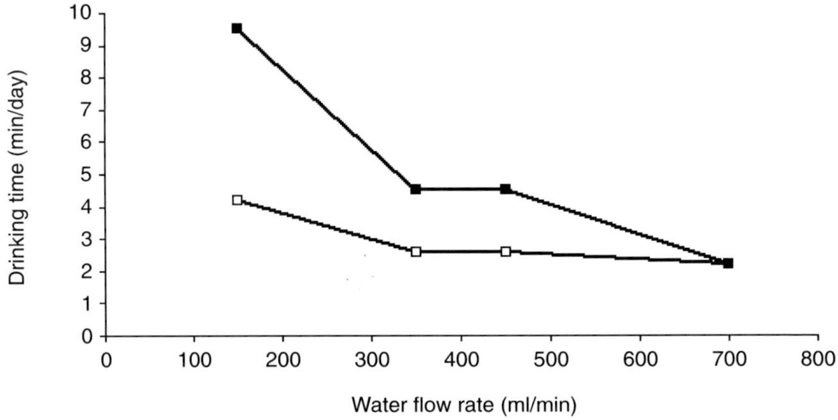

Fig. 12.5. Actual time spent drinking by piglets from drinkers at different delivery rates (□) compared with estimated time needed to consume the same amount of water as the pigs on the highest flow rate (■). Apparently, pigs did not sufficiently increase time spent drinking as water flow was reduced. (From Barber *et al.*, 1989; Brooks *et al.*, 1992.)

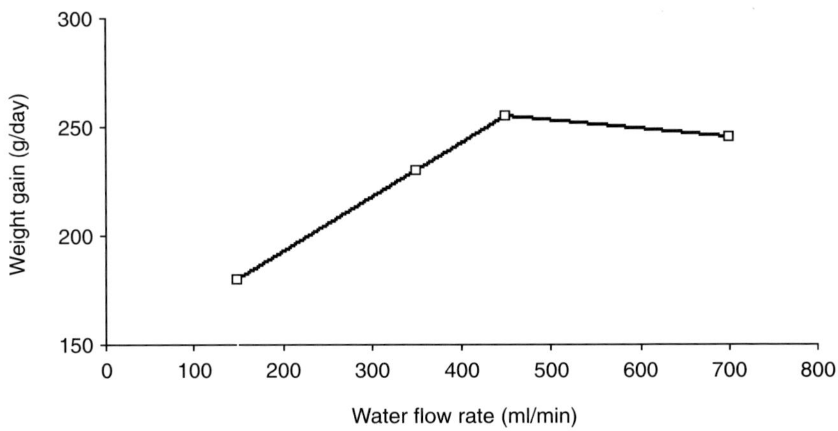

Fig. 12.6. Effect of water flow rate on growth rate in piglets. (From Barber *et al.*, 1989; Brooks *et al.*, 1992.)

growth performance (Fig. 12.6), especially when pigs have to compete for water. The flow rate from cups is rather high (1000 ml/min), because pigs must devote time to first operate drinkers and then drink.

The way flow rate is measured and adjusted can create vast differences in the actual flow rate that pigs experience. Pressure tends to fall towards the end of the pipe delivery system. For example (Brooks *et al.*, 1992), it was demonstrated that flow rate from the first to last pen down the length of a nursery room was reduced over 70% due to the loss of pressure from natural friction in the pipes (Fig. 12.7). Also, pressure is reduced with the number of drinkers in concurrent operation. Therefore, it is recommended to take multiple measurements across the length of the delivery system, preferably during feeding time when water demand is high. Taken this way, measurements in the range of 500 to 1000 ml/min should be satisfactory for nursery pigs.

Controlling wastage

Water use (wastage plus intake) in nursery facilities usually exceeds physiological requirements because: (i) young pigs with limited appetite drink water to meet satiety; (ii) pigs play with water as a measure against boredom; (iii) nursery diets are normally high in protein and minerals; and (iv) excessive activity causes accidental water release from nipples. In addition, failure to properly manage drinkers (e.g. repair, height adjustment) greatly increases wastage. Drinker type and even brand may affect wastage (Table 12.2). All these factors contribute to increased effluent volume, which is undesirable regarding legislation compliance with respect to effluent disposal, storage, and related costs.

When water wastage becomes excessive one or more of the following should be checked before the design of the water system is re-evaluated:

- Feed intake during the first week post-weaning.
- Diet design to minimize nutrient excesses (protein and minerals).
- Timely repair of leaking drinkers.
- Frequency of height adjustment and flow rate (nipples).
- Ambient temperature fluctuation throughout the day.

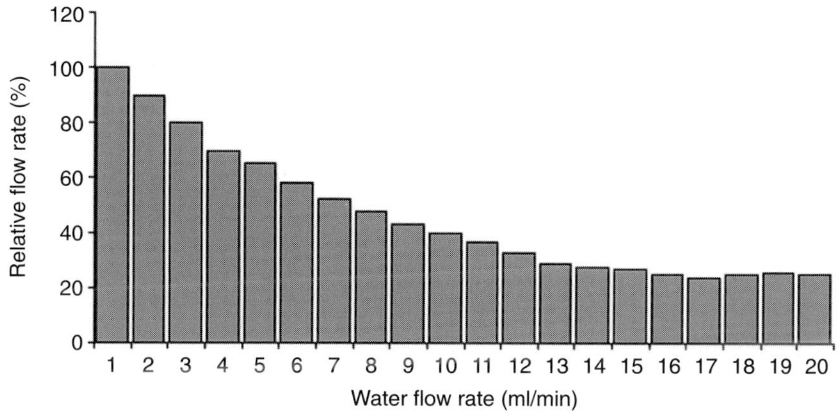

Fig. 12.7. Loss of water flow rate across the length of a nursery due to friction in the pipe system. (From Brooks *et al.*, 1992.)

Table 12.2. Water use by the best and worst tested drinker types in a university trial. (Adapted from Brooks, 1994b.)

	Best	Worst
Daily water use (l)		
5 to 10 kg (body weight)	0.9	1.6
11 to 100 kg	5.0	8.3
Total water use (l)		
5 to 10 kg	11.1	33.4
11 to 100 kg	543	907
Total water wasted (l/pig)		364

It is also suggested (Gonyou, 1996) that forcing pigs to drink while facing the drinker, as opposed to drinking at an angle, drastically reduces wastage. To this end, flanges or 'wings' can be placed on each side of a nipple drinker (Gill and Barber, 1990). Alternatively, nipples, but not cups, may be installed near corners so that pigs have to stand next to a wall while drinking.

Water-administered Compounds

It is often assumed that pigs will continue to drink water even if they stop eating feed. Therefore, water is used frequently as a medium for delivering nutrients and medications during periods of stress or disease (Fig. 12.8). Of course, wastage increases the cost of water nutrition and medication.

Electrolytes

Salts of minerals (electrolytes), often in combination with simple sugars and additives, are frequently administered to stressed pigs and especially those in danger of severe dehydration. Dehydration may result after prolonged transportation without access to fresh water or even from a prolonged stay in holding before transfer to nursery facilities. After placement in pens, several pigs may fail to consume enough or any water at all and become susceptible to dehydration. Naturally, high ambient temperatures tend to accelerate the rate of dehydration.

Commercial preparations of electrolyte solutions are available for administration via the main water supply (using a simple medicator) to all pigs, or for targeting specific pens holding stressed pigs. In the latter case, water with electrolytes is often administered from containers (e.g. bowls) but this approach requires frequent replenishing and cleaning of drinkers.

Table 12.3 presents a simple electrolyte solution that may be used for dehydrated pigs (by P.W. Blackburn; cited by Best, 1983). The main

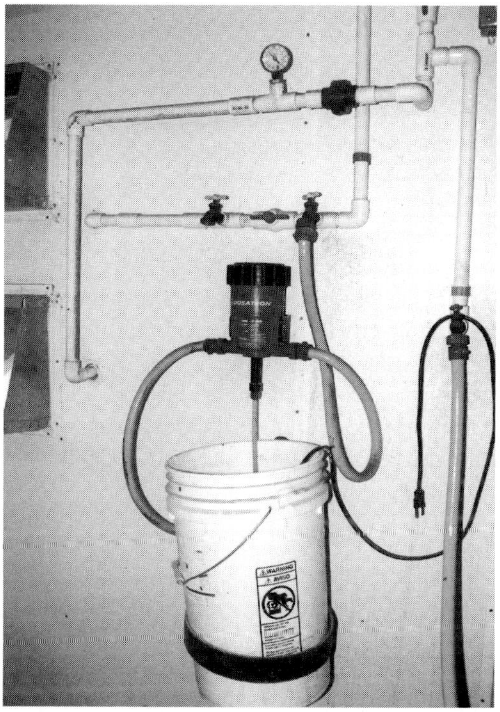

Fig. 12.8. Water medication systems are often used to administer nutritional compounds.

Table 12.3. Simple formula for home-made electrolyte solution (recommended by P.W. Blackburn). (Adapted from Best, 1983.)

	Grams per 10 liters water
Dextrose	225.0
Sodium chloride	42.5
Citric acid	2.5
Glycine	30.0
Potassium citrate	0.6
Potassium dihydrogen phosphate	2.0

components are glucose (energy), sodium, chlorine, and potassium. Sodium bicarbonate may be used for buffering purposes, whereas vitamin C (optional) is often recommended for stressed animals. A food-grade colorant (e.g. yellow or blue) is often added in commercial products along with other more complex ingredients. This solution is recommended at full strength for dehydrated pigs and double strength for pigs suffering from severe diarrhea or prolonged dehydration.

Animal plasma

It is well known that animal plasma in starter feeds markedly increases feed intake during the first couple of weeks post-weaning. Water-soluble forms of plasma-based products are commercially available for administration via drinking water. Such formulas also include an energy source (glucose or lactose) and electrolytes.

Research has demonstrated that water-soluble plasma administered via drinking water improves weight gain and survivability in early-weaned piglets, especially in lightweight pigs (Borg *et al.*, 1999). It may also reduce weight variability that is often encountered in pigs failing to establish a satisfactory feed intake pattern during the first week post-weaning. Water-soluble plasma products are used only during the first few days post-weaning, often at reducing concentrations, because of cost concerns.

Organic acids

Organic acids are often used in drinking water for newly weaned pigs. They offer the potential of sanitizing the drinking water and reducing stomach pH. Several acids such as citric acid are readily absorbed by the stomach epithelium and, thus, they may also contribute to a positive energy balance in weaned pigs. However, controlled research has failed to provide a conclusive answer whether organic acids in water truly benefit piglets, despite their widespread field use.

Citric acid is one of the most frequently used acids because it is readily available and imparts a taste in water that is strongly favored by piglets. A concentration of 0.2–0.5% (i.e. 2–5 g/l) is often satisfactory for most conditions. Other acids used frequently include lactic and formic acid. Organic acids are normally administered via the water medicator from a stock solution, but they should never be mixed with medications or other water additives.

Medications

Water medication is often practiced in large-size units because it offers several advantages over feed medication: (i) it is easy and quick to implement in an emergency disease outbreak as a new feed order does not have to be placed; (ii) handling multiple medicated feed formulas increases logistics burden, which is best avoided by modern feed manufacturers and producers; (iii) sick pigs continue to drink even if they cease to eat, and thus medication reaches them; and (iv) medication and dosage may be adjusted easily. Water medication, however, has several disadvantages: (i) it can be costly if water wastage is excessive; (ii) automatic medication proportioners require a high volume of water throughput to be effective in dispensing the right amount of medication; (iii) hand-mixing medications in portable drinkers or header tanks is labor-intensive; and (iv) some medications may impart a negative flavor in water.

Drinking water may also be used to administer vaccinations to nursery pigs (Best, 2002). Water vaccination compared to syringe injections markedly reduces manual labor and the incidence of broken needles remaining inside the animal. Water vaccines are available for a large number of diseases such as salmonella, ileitis, and erysipelas. It should be noted that water and feed antimicrobial agents should not be combined with water live vaccines because antimicrobial agents may act against live vaccines. Water chlorination also greatly diminishes the effectiveness of water vaccination and a neutralizer (e.g. skim milk or sodium thiosulfate) should be included in the vaccine preparation (according to veterinary recommendations). It is also important to ensure that all pigs drink enough treated water to ensure maximum immunization. To this end, it is recommended to administer vaccines for 4–6 h during the early morning hours when pigs are more active, especially after their first meal.

References

Anderson JS, Anderson DM, and Murphy JM (1994) The effect of water quality on nutrient availability for grower/finisher pigs. *Canadian Journal of Animal Science* 74:141–148.

Barber J, Brooks PH, and Carpenter JL (1989) The effects of water delivery rate on the voluntary food intake, water use and performance of early-weaned pigs from 3 to 6 weeks of age. In: *The Voluntary Food Intake of Pigs*, 103–104. Occasional Publication No. 13. British Society of Animal Science, Midlothian, UK.

Best P (1983) Electrolytes and the pig. *Pig International* 13(6):15–18.

Best P (2002) Vaccines in the drinking water. *Pig International* 32(10):9–12.

Bigelow JA and Houpt TR (1988) Feeding and drinking patterns in young pigs. *Physiology of Behavior* 43:99–109.

Borg BS, Campbell JM, Russell LE, Thomson DU, and Weaver EM (1999) Effects of water soluble globulin on the performance of weanling pigs. *Journal of Animal Science* 77(Supplement 1):193.

Boyles S, Fisher G, Wohlgemuth K, Lundstrom D, and Johnson L (1988) Livestock and water. *Report No. AS-954*. NDSU Extension Service, Fargo, ND.

Brooks PH, Carpenter JL, and Barber J (1992) Impact of water quality on swine welfare and productivity. In: *Advances in Pork Production*, by Foxcroft G (ed), 1–21. Banff Pork Seminar, Banff, Canada.

Brooks PH and Carpenter JL (1993) The water requirement of growing/finishing pigs. Theoretical and practical considerations. In: *Recent Developments in Pig Nutrition 2*, by Cole DJA, Haresign W, and Garnsworthy PC (ed), 179–200. Nottingham University Press, Nottingham, UK.

Brooks PH (1994a) Water – forgotten nutrient and novel delivery system. In: *Biotechnology in the Feed Industry, Proceedings of Alltech's Tenth Annual*

Symposium, by Lyons P and Jacques KA (ed), 211–234. Nottingham University Press, Nottingham, UK.

Brooks PH (1994b) Effect of water provision on pig performance: implications for breeding programmes and nutritional experiments. *IInd International Conference 'The Influence of Genetic and Non Genetic Traits on Carcass and Meat Quality'*, 101–113. Agricultural and Pedagogical University, Siedlce, Poland.

Brooks PH and Tsourgiannis CA (2003) Factors affecting the voluntary feed intake of the weaned pig. In: *Weaning the Pig – Concepts and Consequences*, by Pluske JR, Le Dividich J, and Verstegen MWA (ed), 81–116. Wageningen Academic Publishers, Wageningen, The Netherlands.

Bureau of National Affairs (1973) EPA drafts water quality criteria as required under federal order law. *Environment Reporter* 4:663–670.

Carlson RL and Peo ER Jr (1982) Nipple water position – up or down? *Nebraska Swine Report No. EC 82–219*:8–9. University of Nebraska, Lincoln, NE.

de Lange CFM, Birkett SH, and Morel PCH (2001) Protein, fat, and bone tissue growth in swine. In: *Swine Nutrition* (2nd edn), by Lewis AJ and Southern LL (ed), 65–81. CRC Press LLC, Boca Raton, FL.

Fraser D, Patience JF, Phillips PS, and McLeese JM (1993) Water for piglets and lactating sows: quantity, quality and quandaries. In: *Recent Developments in Pig Nutrition 2*, by Cole DJA, Haresign W, and Garnsworthy PC (ed), 200–224. Nottingham University Press, Nottingham, UK.

Friend DW and Cunningham HM (1966) The effect of water consumption on the growth, feed intake, and carcass composition of suckling pigs. *Canadian Journal of Animal Science* 46:203–209.

Gadd J (1997) What the textbooks don't tell you about new style weaner drinkers. *Pigs* 13(2):19.

Georgievskii VI (1982) Water metabolism and the animal's water requirements. In: *Mineral Nutrition of Animals*, by Georgievskii VI, Annenkov BN, and Samokhin VI (ed), 79–89. Butterworths, London.

Gill BP, Brooks PH, and Carpenter JL (1986) The water intake of weaned pigs from 3 to 6 weeks of age. *Animal Production* 42:470.

Gill BP and Barber J (1990) Water delivery systems for growing pigs. *Farm Building Progress* 102:19–22.

Gonyou HW (1996) Water use and drinker management. In: *Annual Research Report*, 74–80. Prairie Swine Centre Inc., Saskatchewan, Canada.

Hagsten I and Perry TW (1976) Evaluation of dietary salt levels for swine. 1. Effect on gain, water consumption and efficiency of feed conversion. *Journal of Animal Science* 42:1187–1190.

Holmes CW and Mount LE (1967) Heat loss from groups of growing pigs under various conditions of environmental temperature and air movement. *Animal Production* 7:377–384.

Lloyd LE, McDonald BE, and Crampton EW (1978) *Fundamentals of Nutrition* (2nd edn). W.H. Freeman and Co., San Franscisco, CA.

McLeese JM, Tremblay ML, Patience JF, and Christison GI (1992) Water intake patterns in the weanling pig: effect of water quality, antibiotics and probiotics. *Animal Production* 54:135–142.

NRC (1980) *Mineral Tolerance of Domestic Animals*. National Academy Press, Washington, DC.

NRC (1981) *Effect of Environment on Nutrient Requirements of Domestic Animals*. National Academy Press, Washington, DC.

NRC (1998) *Nutrient Requirements of Swine* (10th edn). National Academy Press, Washington, DC.

Patience JF, Possberg N, and Gillis D (1997) Water quality and weanling pig performance. In: *Annual Research Report*, 26–32. Prairie Swine Centre Inc., Saskatchewan, Canada.

Phillips PA and Fraser D (1991) Discovery of selected water dispensers by newborn pigs. *Canadian Journal of Animal Science* 71:233–236.

Shields RG Jr, Mahan DC, and Graham PL (1983) Changes in swine body composition from birth to 145 kg. *Journal of Animal Science* 57:43–54.

Sinclair RD (1939) The salt requirements of growing pigs. *Science of Agriculture* 20:109–119.

Thacker PA (2001) Water in swine nutrition. In: *Swine Nutrition* (2nd edn), by Lewis AJ and Southern LL (ed), 381–398. CRC Press LLC, Boca Raton, FL.

Thulin AJ and Brumm MC (1991) Water: the forgotten nutrient. In: *Swine Nutrition*, by Miller ER, Ullrey DE, and Lewis AJ (ed), 315–324. Butterworth-Heinemann, Stoneham, MA.

Vajrabukka C, Thwaites CJ, and Farrell DJ (1981) Overcoming the effects of high temperature on pig growth. In: *Recent Advances in Animal Nutrition in Australia*, by Farrell DJ and Vohra P (ed), 99–114. University of New England, Armidale, Australia

Wahlstrom RC, Taylor AR, and Seerley RW (1970) Effects of lysine in the drinking water of growing swine. *Journal of Animal Science* 30:368–373.

Whittemore CT (1998) *The Science and Practice of Pig Production* (2nd edn). Blackwell Science Ltd, Oxford, UK.

Wood RD, Chaney CH, Waddill DG, and Garrison GW (1967) Effect of adding nitrate or nitrite to drinking water on utilization of carotene by growing swine. *Journal of Animal Science* 26:259–270.

Yang TS, Howard B, and McFarlane WV (1981) Effects of food on drinking behaviour of growing pigs. *Applied Animal Ethology* 7:259–270.

Index